Juvenile Angiofibroma

Siba P. Dubey • Bernhard Schick
Editors

Juvenile Angiofibroma

Springer

Editors
Siba P. Dubey
Department of Otolaryngology-Head and Neck Surgery
Port Moresby General Hospital and School of Medicine and Health Sciences,
University of Papua New Guinea
Boroko
Port Moresby
Papua New Guinea

Bernhard Schick
Department of Otolaryngology-Head and Neck Surgery
University of Saarlands Medical Center
Homburg/Saar
Saarland
Germany

ISBN 978-3-319-45341-5 ISBN 978-3-319-45343-9 (eBook)
DOI 10.1007/978-3-319-45343-9

Library of Congress Control Number: 2016963258

Printed on acid-free paper

This Springer imprint is published by Springer Nature
The registered company is Springer International Publishing AG
The registered company address is Gewerbestrasse 11, 6330 Cham, Switzerland

In dedicating this book to our patients,
we acknowledge the major contributions
made by our predecessors.

Preface

Juvenile angiofibroma was first described by Hippocrates in the fourth century BC. Chaveau introduced the term 'juvenile nasopharyngeal fibroma'. The term 'angiofibroma' was coined in 1940 by Friedberg. Juvenile angiofibroma is a highly vascular neoplasm almost exclusively affecting adolescent males. It is distinguished by its site of origin, pattern of spread into and through the skull base spaces and abundant and intricate arterial supply. The tumor is histologically benign in appearance, but it follows a potentially malignant clinical course characterized by recurrent epistaxis and other serious morbidities. Surgical removal is difficult and the tumor frequently recurs. Juvenile angiofibroma occurs globally though its prevalence is higher, and the tumor is more extensive among patients of non-Caucasian descent.

There are 22 chapters in the book which is divided into four parts. Each chapter is contributed by an expert who volunteered to participate. The first part deals with history, surgical anatomy and tumor biology. The historical background chapter describes the evolution of all aspects of this tumor. The surgical anatomy chapter provides a description of the relevant skull base anatomy which is necessary in order to understand the extent of the tumor and the requisite surgery. The chapters on etiology, pathology and tumor biology deal with recent developments in these fields and their relevance in understanding and managing this disease. The second part deals with clinical presentation and radiological diagnosis. The staging of the tumor is important in understanding its extent and deciding on a management strategy. The third part deals with the different management options. It begins with preoperative embolization by which this tumor is made less vascular, making easier operative removal, and continues with the vital role played by the anesthetist in reducing and replacing blood loss. The subsequent chapters in the management section deal with the different surgical techniques used around the globe. They are broadly classified as endoscopic and nonendoscopic procedures and are used according to the extent of the disease and available techniques and technologies. Sometimes tumor resection may be incomplete despite all these techniques. In this situation, irradiation and chemotherapy which are beneficial are described. The last part of the book deals with the prevention and management of recurrent tumors. This section also discuses similar tumors occurring in other sites and some of the still remaining controversies about this fascinating tumor.

Editors very much appreciate contributions made by the authors of each chapter. Sincere thanks is due to Ms Dilli George, the librarian, School of Medicine and Health Sciences, University of Papua New Guinea, for her hard work in bibliography. We are very grateful to Ms Joanna Renwick, Springer UK, and her entire team and Ms Lizzy Raj, Project Manager at Spi-Global, for their superb help in all stages of the production of this book.

Port Moresby, Papua New Guinea — Siba P. Dubey, MS
Homburg/Saar, Germany — Bernhard Schick, MD

Contents

Contributors

G. Baltsavias, MD Department of Neuroradiology, Clinical Neuroscience Center, University Hospital of Zurich, Zurich, Switzerland

J. Dale Browne, MD Department of Otolaryngology, Wake Forest University, Baptist Medical Center, Winston-Salem, NC, USA

Curtis Bryant, MD, MPH Department of Radiation Oncology, University of Florida, Gainesville, Jacksonville, FL, USA

José F. Carrillo, MD Departamento de Tumores de Cabeza y Cuello, Mexico, Mexico

Head and Neck Department, Instituto Nacional de Cancerología, México, DF, Mexico

Liliana C. Carrillo, MD Subdirección de Investigación Clínica, México, Mexico

Siba P. Dubey, MS Department of Otolaryngology – Head and Neck Surgery, Port Moresby General Hospital and School of Medicine and Health Sciences, University of Papua New Guinea, Boroko, NCD, Papua New Guinea

Tiberiu Ezri, MD Department of Anesthesia, Wolfson Medical Center, Sackler Medical School, Tel Aviv University, Holon, Israel

Outcomes Research Consortium, Cleveland, OH, USA

Juan C. Fernandez-Miranda, MD Department of Neurological Surgery, University of Pittsburgh School of Medicine, Pittsburgh, PA, USA

Mitesh Gandhi, FRACR Department of Medical Imaging, Princess Alexandra Hospital and Queensland Xray, Brisbane, QLD, Australia

Paul A. Gardner, MD Department of Neurological Surgery, University of Pittsburgh School of Medicine, Pittsburgh, PA, USA

Jaana Hagström, DDS, PhD Department of Pathology, HusLab, University of Helsinki and Helsinki University Hospital, Helsinki, Finland

Alexander Izakson, MD Department of Anesthesia, Rebecca Sieff Medical Center, Galil Medical Faculty, Bar Ilan University, Safed, Israel

M. Yashar S. Kalani, MD Department of Neurosurgery, Barrow Neurological Institute, St. Joseph's Hospital and Medical Center, Phoenix, AZ, USA

Chang Lin, MD Department of Otolaryngology–Head and Neck Surgery, First Affiliated Hospital of Fujian Medical University, Fuzhou, Fujian Province, China

José Luis Llorente, MD, PhD Depto. Otorrinolaringología, Hospital Universitario Central de Asturias, Oviedo, Spain

Antti Mäkitie, MD Department of Otorhinolaryngology and Head and Neck Surgery, University of Helsinki and Helsinki University Hospital, Helsinki, Finland

Nikolay L. Martirosyan, MD Department of Neurosurgery, Barrow Neurological Institute, St. Joseph's Hospital and Medical Center, Phoenix, AZ, USA

William M. Mendenhall, MD Department of Radiation Oncology, University of Florida, Gainesville, Jacksonville, FL, USA

Charles P. Molumi, MMed Department of Otolaryngology – Head and Neck Surgery, Port Moresby General Hospital, Boroko, NCD, Papua New Guinea

Piero Nicolai, MD Department of Otorhinolaryngology – Head and Neck Surgery, Spedali Civili of Brescia, University of Brescia, Brescia, Italy

Eric R. Oliver, MD Department of Otolaryngology, Wake Forest University, Baptist Medical Center, Winston-Salem, NC, USA

Randall W. Porter, MD Department of Neurosurgery, Barrow Neurological Institute, St. Joseph's Hospital and Medical Center, Phoenix, AZ, USA

c/o Neuroscience Publications, Barrow Neurological Institute, St. Joseph's Hospital and Medical Center, Phoenix, AZ, USA

Andreas Prescher, MD Institut für Molekulare und Zelluläre Anatomie, Aachen, Germany

Margarita C. Ramirez-Ortega, PhD Departamento de Farmacología, Instituto Nacional de Cardiología Ignacio Chávez, Mexico, Mexico

S. Girish Rao, MDS, FDSRCS(Eng), FFDRCSI(Ire) Department of Oral and Maxillofacial Surgery, RV Dental College and Hospital, Bangalore, India

Suvi Renkonen, MD Department of Otorhinolaryngology and Head and Neck Surgery, University of Helsinki and Helsinki University Hospital, Helsinki, Finland

Ahmad Safadi, MD Department of Otorhinolaryngology – Head and Neck Surgery and Maxillofacial Surgery, Tel Aviv Sourasky Medical Center, Sackler School of Medicine, Tel Aviv University, Tel Aviv, Israel

Bernhard Schick, MD Department of Otolaryngology – Head and Neck Surgery, University of Saarland Medical Centre, Homburg/Saar, Germany

Alberto Schreiber, MD Department of Otorhinolaryngology – Head and Neck Surgery, Spedali Civili of Brescia, University of Brescia, Brescia, Italy

Carl H. Snyderman, MD, MBA Department of Otolaryngology, University of Pittsburgh School of Medicine, Pittsburgh, PA, USA

Department of Neurological Surgery, University of Pittsburgh School of Medicine, Pittsburgh, PA, USA

UPMC Center for Cranial Base Surgery, Pittsburgh, PA, USA

Jennifer Sommerville, FRACR Department of Medical Imaging, Princess Alexandra Hospital and Queensland Xray, Brisbane, QLD, Australia

C. Suarez, MD, PhD University of Oviedo, Oviedo, Spain

Herwig Swoboda, MD, PhD Hospital Hietzing (Lainz), Vienna, Austria

Alok Thakar, MS, FRCSEd Department of Otolaryngology – Head and Neck Surgery, All India Institute of Medical Sciences, New Delhi, India

Anton Valavanis, MD Department of Neuroradiology, Clinical Neuroscience Center, University Hospital of Zurich, Zurich, Switzerland

Eric W. Wang, MD Department of Otolaryngology, University of Pittsburgh School of Medicine, Pittsburgh, PA, USA

Jochen P. Windfuhr, MD Department of Otorhinolaryngology, Plastic Head and Neck Surgery, Kliniken Maria Hilf, Mönchengladbach, Germany

Guoxing Xu, MD Department of Ophthalmology, First Affiliated Hospital of Fujian Medical University, Fuzhou, Fujian Province, China

Yuanten Xu, MD Department of Otolaryngology–Head and Neck Surgery, First Affiliated Hospital of Fujian Medical University, Fuzhou, Fujian Province, China

Zixiang Yi, MD Department of Otolaryngology–Head and Neck Surgery, First Affiliated Hospital of Fujian Medical University, Fuzhou, Fujian Province, China

Part I
History, Anatomy and Tumor Biology

Chapter 1
Historical Background

Herwig Swoboda

Abstract Juvenile angiofibroma is a rare but characteristic disorder arising in the depth of one nasal cavity. In historic times and in less developed societies, it has been more frequent than in affluent societies. As in other rare or extinct diseases, like plague, a historical approach may assist modern research of this model disease which not only poses formidable therapeutic challenges but also promises better understanding of tissue dynamics and morphogenesis. Probably, care of juvenile angiofibroma always has been a matter of practitioners, as written Hippocratic and Salernitan records reflect wise understanding and dexterous therapy even in remote times. Pioneers of treatment of juvenile angiofibroma like Louis-François Manne (1689–1755) or Karl Otto Weber (1827–1877) provide examples not only of outstanding professional qualification but also of humane devotion.

Keywords Juvenile angiofibroma • History of medicine • Endoscopic surgery • Rhinology • Maxillofacial surgery • Cranial morphogenesis • Anthropology

Juvenile angiofibroma constitutes a rich and mysterious pathogenetic model of high anthropological interest. This benign aggressive proliferative disease of mesenchymal origin arises in the cranial base, the rigid platform of bipedalism, more precisely in the spheno-pterygoid junction which constitutes the root of the human masticatory and respiratory apparatus, a crossroad of viscerocranial structures pierced by the pterygoid canal which harbors the artery of the first branchial arch. The expansive desmoplastic and angiogenetic features of this tumor always have put major therapeutic challenges. Its exclusive occurrence in male puberty evokes relations to the sexual dimorphic human cranial morphogenesis [1]. Regional and temporal variations of incidence point to socio-environmental determinants. Its rarity in westernized countries as well as its relatively high frequency in less developed

H. Swoboda, MD, PhD
Hospital Hietzing (Lainz), Vienna, Austria
e-mail: herwig.swoboda@wienkav.at

S.P. Dubey, B. Schick (eds.), *Juvenile Angiofibroma*,
DOI 10.1007/978-3-319-45343-9_1

countries urges for joint supra-regional efforts in treatment and research – and for consultation of historical records.

In spite of its rarity in affluent countries, juvenile angiofibroma always has attracted the attention of medical practitioners and scholars. This rare but characteristic model disease bears as much explanatory power as otosclerosis, an akin disorder of cranial osteo-fibrovascular remodeling. Our age of genes and cytokines seems to glance back to ancestors like Xavier Bichat (1771–1802), the founder of histology, and Jean Cruveilhier (1791–1874) who was so interested in the dynamics of tissues, comparing fibrous lesions in the nasopharynx with similar lesions in the breast and the uterus under the heading of "transformations fibreuses" [2–4].

Clinical description mentioning nasal obstruction, hemorrhage, facial swelling, eye protrusion, and impairment of speech, deglutition, and respiration barely has changed since antiquity. The Hippocratic text *De morbis II* distinguishes five types of nasal polyps, from which the fourth type perfectly resembles juvenile angiofibroma: "something hard appears deep in the nasal cavity, near the cartilage, like flesh, but at touch sounds like stone." It recommends preliminary scalpel incision of the nose, tumor removal with cauterization of its pedicle, suture of the incision, and topical wound treatment [5].

Celsus (c25 BC–c50 AD) declared nasopharyngeal tumors as "noli me tangere." Galen (c129–c216) restricted the term polyps to the nasal cavity. Paulus of Aegina (c625–c690) compared nasopharyngeal fibrous tumors with an octopus [6, 7]. This image applies even better to angiofibroma than to classical nasal polyps. The detailed nineteenth-century studies would emphasize the fingerlike protrusions from an epicenter in the pterygopalatine fossa (v. Langenbeck) into the pharynx, the sinuses, the infratemporal fossa, the orbit, and the cranial cavity, causing dyspnea, disfiguration, proptosis, and neurologic symptoms [8].

William of Saliceto (c1210–c1280), one of the most eminent writers of the Salernitan Medical School, in lively detail described transnasal avulsion and postoperative treatment of hard nasal polyps, thus demonstrating the consummate diagnostic and therapeutic skill of the Salernitan surgeons [9].

Louis-François Manne (1689–1755) in 1717 introduced a transpalatal approach by enlarging an insufficient exposure of an "extraordinary large polyp" with pharyngeal extension with a paramedian transection of the soft palate [10].

Johann Zacharias Platner (1694–1747), in his comprehensive description of nasopharyngeal polyp resection, mentioned this preliminary longitudinal section of the soft palate, but cautioned against ensuing deglutition disorders. He described extranasal protrusion, pharyngolaryngeal obstruction, and facial deformity, advised for reclined sitting position of the patient and good illumination, curved dentated forceps (vulsella), and wrapped scalpel blades. Cancerous lesions should not be operated on, and residues of benign polyps would relapse [11].

André Levret (1703–1780) was a gynecologist-obstetrician and a pioneer of direct laryngoscopy (spatula 1743) and in 1771 reported Manne's intervention in detail in his monograph on uterovaginal and nasal pharyngeal polyps. Levret favored ligation over cauterization, excision, and avulsion and introduced own improved instruments for putting a snare around polyps, reminiscent of today's tonsillar snares. Levret described an autopsy of a young boy with enlarged face and an expansive bone thinning lesion "enveloping the crista galli." Levret proposed a classification of nasal and nasopharyngeal polyps by origin (sinuses, nasal cavity, nasopharynx) and "in essence," differentiating between curable benign, difficult to treat by "unfavorable constitution," and incurable malignant varieties [12]. Here, the concept of polyps appears as a paradigm of tumor disease, raising awareness for aggressiveness and malignancy. In Jacques Tenon's (1724–1816) 1805 lecture on nasal polyps and in the surgical encyclopedia of Johann Nepomuk Rust (1775–1840), this general view on the exemplary character of polyps (including nasopharyngeal polyps) was extensively elaborated [6, 13].

Stimulating subtle clinical evaluation, Percivall Pott (1714–1788) advised against imprudent surgical treatment of nasopharyngeal polyps, even if neither scirrhous nor cancerous. Suffering from nasal polyps and having operated on himself, Pott was clinically saddle-fast in that field. Pott pioneered carcinogen research by pointing to the association of scrotal cancer of chimney sweepers with soot and tar, paving the way for experimental chemical carcinogenesis [14]. Even earlier, in the "Annus mirabilis" (1761) of medical science (Leopold Auenbrugger, "Inventum Novum"; Giambattista Morgagni, "De causis et sedibus morborum"; Domenico Cotugno, "De acquaeductibus auris humanae internae anatomica dissertatio"), John Hill (1716–1775) in his monograph "Cautions against the immoderate use of snuff" had described five cases of nasal cancer in snuff tobacco users [15].

Research on juvenile angiofibroma benefitted from the advent of clinicopathological correlation with Jean Cruveilhier (1791–1874) who pronounced his commitment in his doctoral thesis in 1816. Since his description, the term nasopharyngeal polyp was applied to fibrous life-threatening variants of these tumors. Cruveilhier in 1823 himself had treated one 15-year-old case with ligature [3]. Beyond clinicopathological correlation, progress in surgery, general anesthesia (Wells 1845; Morton 1846), local anesthesia (Koller, Jellinek 1884: topical cocaine; Schleich 1892: infiltration anesthesia), and the laryngeal mirror with its derivative for posterior rhinoscopy (Türck, Czermak 1858) fostered mastery of the depths around the upper jaw [16, 17].

Joseph Gensoul (1797–1858) 1827 undertook maxillectomy for osteosarcoma. James Syme (1799–1870) from Scotland, in 1832, first performed maxillectomy for nasopharyngeal fibroma, but lost the patient [8]. Achille Flaubert (1813–1882) from Rouen, in 1840, successfully performed maxillectomy for juvenile angiofibroma, using bone chisel and wire saw, thus paving the way for transfacial approaches. He was the son of an eminent surgeon and the brother of Gustave Flaubert (1821–1880), the author of the novel "Madame Bovary," which he had plotted into a "health officer's" family in Rouen [8, 18].

The most threatening burden of surgery was inevitable severe hemorrhage, fraught with high incidence of mortality regardless of method and extent. Johann Friedrich Dieffenbach (1792–1847) stated about the surgery of angiofibroma: "The surgeon needs much courage for operation upon nasopharyngeal polyps, because he almost only may choose between suffocation of the patient when ligating the polyp, making him bleed to death when operating by excision or avulsion, or non-completion of surgery" [8].

German surgeon Bernhard von Langenbeck in 1859 introduced bone and soft tissue-sparing techniques, consisting in temporarily pivoting the maxilla around a medial pedicle (osteoplastic resection of the upper jaw). Langenbeck also recognized the pterygopalatine fossa as proliferative epicenter and described various venous growths arising in the sphenopalatine fossa (1860). Panas in 1858 described fibromucous polyps originating from the choanal margin [8].

Auguste Nélaton (1807–1873) in 1853 introduced a midline transpalatal approach and emphasized the almost exclusive predominance of males in the age of puberty. In 1864, he introduced electrolytic therapy for angiofibroma (galvanic cautery; Albrecht Theodor Middeldorpf 1854) [19]. This treatment modality was much acclaimed as an alternative to surgery with its inherent risk of fatal hemorrhage, especially by rhinologists. Rudolf Voltolini (1819–1879) refined this method which also was applied to induce tumor shrinkage for easier and less hazardous subsequent surgery (Paul v. Bruns 1872) [20, 21]. Nevertheless, the efficiency of electrolysis was limited, requiring very many repetitions (up to >100). Margins of surgical wounds left open for application of galvanic electrodes shrinked, rendering delayed wound closure impossible. Chronic infection of treated tumor areas in the cranial base often caused serious problems [8].

Nasal Approaches

The Hippocratic method was advised incision of nostrils not sufficiently wide for polyp removal, which probably often was the case in angiofibroma (the fourth kind of polyps in "De morbis II"). The further development modified and extended this method in many ways, namely, mobilization of cutaneous, cartilaginous, and osseous structures and tilting the pedicled nasal pyramid to the side, upward or downward, and osteoplastic reapproximation following Langenbeck's principles, first realized by him in 1859. This concept later would reappear in transnasal hypophyseal surgery (Hermann Schloffer 1906) [22]. Sublabial incisions also were used, foreshadowing midfacial degloving (Jordan 1885; Casson et al. 1974) [23].

Transoral Approaches

Manne's para-uvular midline transection of the soft palate in 1717 to gain access to a large nasopharyngeal polyp was a breakthrough comparable to the nasal incision of the ancient Greeks. Louis-Francois Manne was a skillful and courageous physician in Avignon. He contributed with determination to fight the plague in Avignon in 1720 and lost his wife in the plague [10].

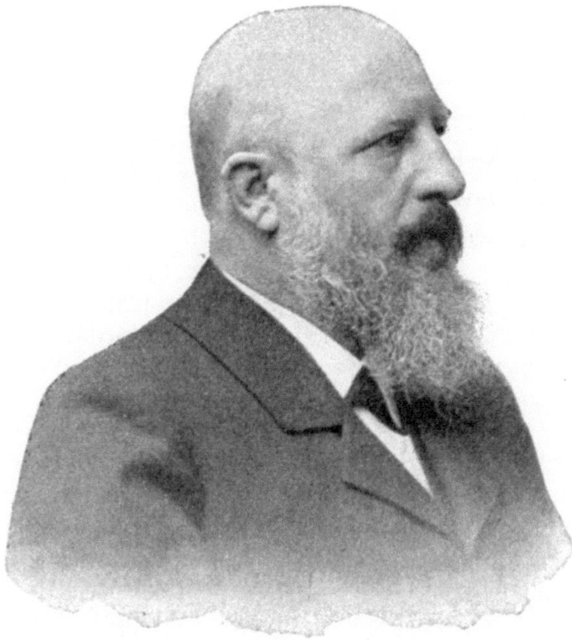

Fig. 1.1 Carl Gussenbauer 1842–1903. An authority, among many other fields, in general, laryngeal, rhino-, and neurosurgery. Refined Nélaton's transpalatal approach for juvenile angiofibroma. Alpinist and mountain guide (Source: Sport und Salon, 25 October 1902, page 9. ANNO/Österreichische Nationalbibliothek)

Numerous modifications were proposed in order to circumvent limitations of exposure and velopharyngeal insufficiency after cicatrization, namely, partial transections leaving the free margin of the soft palate (Maisonneuve 1859, "boutonnière palatine"), transverse (Dieffenbach-Böckel) or T-shaped incisions, and bone removal from the hard palate (Nélaton 1853) [19]. Transpalatal approaches were encouraged by the mainly French opinion that these fibromas originated from the pharyngobasilar fascia around the spheno-occipital synchondrosis [8].

Carl Gussenbauer (1842–1903, Fig. 1.1) shifted the transpalatal approach anteriorly into the hard palate, generously dissected the mucoperiosteum laterally after median mucoperiosteal incision, and removed the osseous plate of the hard palate with a chisel. Both tumor excision and wound closure were facilitated with this procedure [24, 25]. By this refinement of the transpalatal approach to the rhinopharynx, Gussenbauer mastered an additional field of cranial base surgery. In 1874 he reported on the first total laryngectomy, including prosthetic voice restoration. In 1895 he published transfacial subcranial ethmoid resection, and in 1902 he published osteoplastic craniotomy for brain tumor surgery (Fig. 1.1).

Transfacial Approaches

Achille Flaubert's successful maxillectomy in 1840 provided a good anterolateral exposure of a large nasopharyngeal fibroma, but at the expense of significant morbidity. Conservative variants with preservation of skeletal and soft layer support restituted the face in its normal form. Different kinds of pedicled osteocutaneous maxillary flaps were designed, following Langenbeck's principle of osteoplastic temporary upper jaw resection, a forerunner of maxillary swing and facial translocation. Besides intraoperative hemorrhage, a major drawback was facial paresis, especially of the eyelids when Langenbeck had tilted the maxilla medially. Karl Otto Weber (1827–1867) hinged the maxilla laterally, placing a paranasal incision just medial to the cheek, with lower lid and upper lip extensions as known under his and Sir William Fergusson's (1808–1877) names [8].

Many variants were designed, e.g., by Theodor Kocher (1841–1917), allowing wide unfolding of the maxillary halves [25]. Lesser variants remind of LeFort 1 osteotomy approaches [26]. Temporary removal of pedicled zygomatic arch or the complete zygoma and a suprahyoid pharyngotomy were designed to access to correspondent lateral protrusions [27].

Preliminary surgical steps other than the approach through unaffected structures included, e.g., tracheotomy with blockage of the laryngeal entrance or the trachea and arterial ligatures, either of one or both external carotid arteries or of one common carotid artery [8]. Rose's supine position with extended cervical spine was proposed for this type of maxillary surgery, but soon given up for venous congestion, following a caveat by Kocher [28].

The Twentieth Century

Intubation, anesthesia, hemosubstitution, resuscitation, neuroradiology (Arthur Schüller 1874–1957), endovascular intervention (Pierre Lasjaunias 1948–2008), endocrinology, radiotherapy, chemotherapy, genetics, and developmental anatomy (evo-devo) all contributed to further although deceptively incomplete understanding of juvenile angiofibroma. Various classification systems (Radkowski 1996) have been proposed to validate therapy. Like a golden thread, endeavors to visualize this deeply seated tumor accompany the evolution of surgical therapy of juvenile angiofibroma: from Philipp Bozzini's (1773–1809) light projector ("Lichtleiter" 1806) to rigid transnostril endoscopy (Walter Messerklinger 1920–2001; 1968), efforts to master the intricate surroundings of the pterygopalatine fossa have been relying on good direct visualization [29].

References

1. Mishra SC. Putative histogenesis of post nasal angiofibroma. Ind J Otolaryngol Head Neck Surg. 2000;52:366–70.
2. Cruveilhier J. Essai sur l'anatomie pathologique en général. Paris; 1816.
3. Cruveilher J. Traité d'anatomie pathologique générale, vol. 3. Paris; 1856, p. 609–23.
4. Roux M. Annales de la Société de Médecine d'Anvers. 1844, p. 60.
5. Gardeil J-B. Oeuvres d'Hippocrate. De morbis II. Encyclopédie des sciences médicales, 7e div. Paris; 1837, p. 143, §32.
6. Rust J N. Theoretisch-praktisches Handbuch der Chirurgie, vol. 13. Berlin Wien; 1834, p 516–51.

7. Chauveau C. Histoire des maladies du pharynx. Vol. V. Paris: J.-B. Baillière; 1906.
8. Custodis. Über die operative Behandlung der Nasenrachentumoren. Beiträge zur klinischen Chirurgie vol. 47. Tübingen; 1905, p. 37–161.
9. Saliceto, Guglielmo da. Chirurgie de Guillaume de Salicet achevée en 1275. Traduction et commentaire par Paul Pifteau. Toulouse; 1898, p. 54–7.
10. Manne L-F. Observation apologétique de chirurgie. Avignon; 1747.
11. Platner JZ. Institutiones chirurgiae. Venice; 1747, p273–76.
12. Levret A. Observations sur la cure radicale de plusieurs polypes de la matrice, de la gorge et du nez, opérée par de nouveaux moyens inventés. Paris; 1771, p. 344–433.
13. Tenon J. Mémoires et observations sur l'anatomie, la pathologie et la chirurgie. Paris; 1816.
14. Pott P. Chirurgical observations relative to the cataract, the polypus of the nose, cancer of the scrotum, different kinds of ruptures, and the mortification of the toes and feet. London; Hawes, Clarke and Collins, 1775.
15. Hill J. Cautions against the immoderate use of snuff. London; Baldwin and Jackson, 1761.
16. Pitha F, Billroth T. Handbuch der allgemeinen und speciellen Chirurgie. Erlangen; Enke, 1865.
17. Denker A. Zur operativen Behandlung der typischen Nasenrachenfibrome. Ztschr. f. Ohrenh., Wiesbaden, 1911, ixiv, 1–4.
18. Flaubert A. Observation d'ablation de l'os maxillaire supérieur en totalité, pour une affection indépendante de cet os – guérison. Arch Gen Med. 1840; 3rd series, 8:436–44.
19. Nélaton A. Sur la destruction des tumeurs par la méthode électrolytique. Académie des sciences. 1864.
20. Voltolini R. Anwendung der Galvanokaustik im Innern des Kehlkopfs und Schlundkopfs. 2. Aufl. Wien; 1872.
21. v. Bruns P. Die elektrolytische Behandlung der Nasenrachenpolypen. Berliner klin. Wochenschr. 1872:27–8.
22. Schmidt RF, Choudhry OJ, Takkellapati R, Eloy JA, Couldwell WT, Liu JK. Hermann Schloffer and the origin of transsphenoidal pituitary surgery. Neurosurg Focus. 2012;33:E5.
23. Jordan F. Extract from a clinical lecture on a new operation for nasopharyngeal or fibrous polypus. BMJ. 1885;1:888.
24. Mikulicz J. Zur Gussenbauer'schen Operationsmethode bei fibrösen Nasenrachenpolypen. Prager med Wochenschr. 1883;4:42–3.
25. Riegner O. Exstirpation eines basilaren Rachentumors nach Resektion des harten Gaumens (Methode nach Gussenbauer). Deutsche med Wochenschr. 1894:33.
26. Kocher T. Chirurgische Operationslehre. 4th ed. Jena: Gustav Fischer; 1902. p. 132–3.
27. Partsch. Lefort 1, eine neue Methode temporärer Gaumenresektion Arch f klin Chir 1898:57.
28. Rose. Operation am hängenden Kopfe. Vorschlag zur Erleichterung der Operationen am Oberkiefer. Langenbeck's Archiv vol. 18. 1874.
29. Messerklinger W. Background and evolution of endoscopic sinus surgery. Ear Nose Throat J. 1994;73:449–50.

Chapter 2
Surgical Anatomy of the Skull Base

Andreas Prescher

Abstract According to the origin and the route of spread of the juvenile angiofibroma, the relevant osseous anatomy of the central skull base and the topography of the neighbouring regions are described. Especially the posterior part of the nasal cavity, the nasopharynx, the pterygopalatine fossa and the infratemporal fossa are the main area of interest. Furthermore some embryological considerations are given, concerning the origin of the juvenile angiofibroma, which can be interpreted as a dysontogenetic tumor.

Keywords Juvenile angiofibroma • Embryology • Infratemporal fossa • Pterygopalatine fossa • Nasal cavity • Nasopharynx

Introduction

The juvenile angiofibroma (juvenile nasopharyngeal angiofibroma) is a rare, locally destructive tumor composed of fibrovascular tissue. This tumor was first described by the German surgeon and ophthalmologist Freiherr Maximilian Joseph von Chelius (1794–1846) in 1847 under the name "Fibrous Nasal Polyp". In 1940 Friedberg [1] introduced the term "angiofibroma". This tumor mostly affects young males around 14 years of age. Only in very rare cases, a female person was described, suffering from a juvenile angiofibroma [2]. The juvenile angiofibroma arises from the posterolateral roof of the nasal cavity, just above and behind the sphenopalatine foramen. Normally a strong fibrovascular stroma is present in this region where the sphenoidal process and the orbital process of the perpendicular plate of the palatine bone are fixed at the sphenoidal body. This tissue forms a thick and rigid plate at the roof of the nasopharynx. This location is in a central topographical position, so that the enlarging tumor at first fills the nasopharynx and then extends into the nasal cavity. Afterwards it can easily spread into different

A. Prescher, MD
Institut für Molekulare und Zelluläre Anatomie, Wendlingweg 2, 52074 Aachen, Germany
e-mail: aprescher@ukaachen.de

S.P. Dubey, B. Schick (eds.), *Juvenile Angiofibroma*,
DOI 10.1007/978-3-319-45343-9_2

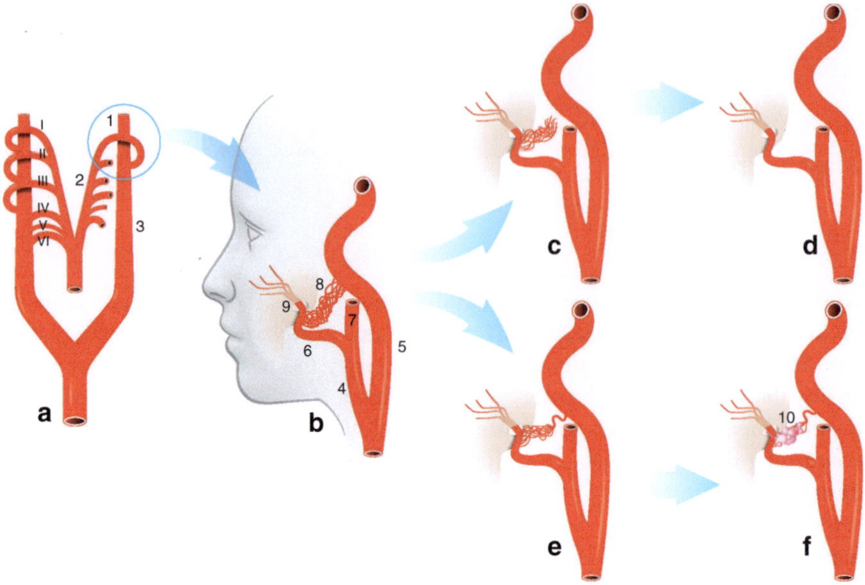

Fig. 2.1 Embryological hypothesis of juvenile angiofibroma development. *1* First pharyngeal arch artery, *2* ventral aorta, *3* dorsal aorta, *4* external carotid artery, *5* internal carotid artery, *6* maxillary artery, *7* superficial temporal artery, *8* plexus between maxillary artery and internal carotid artery resulting from disappearance of first pharyngeal arch artery, *9* sphenopalatine foramen, *10* juvenile angiofibroma developing from relics of the plexus

anatomical regions, such as the pterygopalatine fossa, the infratemporal fossa and the temporal fossa beneath the temporalis muscle. In advanced cases the paranasal sinuses, the cranial cavity, especially the cavernous sinus, and the orbit can also be involved [3].

Embryology (Fig. 2.1) According to Girgis and Fahmy [4], there are different theories concerning the origin and aetiology of juvenile angiofibroma. Many of these hypotheses are only of historical interest in our days, so that the true nature of this pathological lesion remains obscure. According to the histomorphologic investigations of Beham et al. [5], the juvenile angiofibroma can be seen as a vascular malformation. In the light of this new aspect, an embryological explanation for the juvenile angiofibroma was considered by Schick et al. [6] which should be included and repeated also in this anatomical chapter.

The clue for the embryological explanation is given in the vascularisation of the tumour tissue mainly from the maxillary artery and often also from the internal carotid artery. Therefore it must be searched for a connection of these two vessels in early development. This connection can be seen in the first pharyngeal arch artery, which occurs between the 22nd and 24th day of development. Between the 26th and 32nd day of development, this transitory artery diminishes. This process of disappearance at first forms an arterial plexus, which connects the maxillary artery with the developing internal carotid artery. Due to the developing internal carotid artery circulation, the connection is interrupted in a next step. As a result the plexus is still present at the maxillary artery and later disappears completely. Harrison [7] demonstrated vascular clefts with endothelial lining in the region of the sphenopalatine foramen and the root of the pterygoid process in a male as well as in a female foetus from the 24th week. These structures can be interpreted as remnants of the plexus from the first pharyngeal arch artery. Therefore it can be assumed that in some cases, these vestigial structures can persist and may be are responsible for the development of a juvenile angiofibroma. In this sense the juvenile angiofibroma must be classified as a further example of a dysontogenetic tumor. The development of dysontogenetic tumors is well known in pathology. For example, persisting cell clusters from the notochord may develop a chordoma, or persisting cellular elements belonging to Rathke's pouch can be responsible for a craniopharyngioma, a so-called Erdheim tumor. The embryological considerations would also easily explain that arterial "feeders" of the tumor normally arise from the maxillary artery as well as from the internal carotid artery. In advanced cases "feeders" from the vertebral artery, the ascending pharyngeal artery, the ophthalmic artery or the posterior ethmoidal artery may also be present [3, 8, 9].

According to the origin in the region of the sphenopalatine foramen and the route of growth and expansion, the anatomist has to consider the following topographic regions and structures: the nasal cavity, the nasopharynx and the central skull base. Furthermore the neighbouring pterygopalatine fossa and the infratemporal fossa are important and must also be considered. All these spaces have complicated three-dimensional architectures and contain several important nerves and vessels. Especially the vessels are of great interest, because they are feeding the tumor and should be embolised, if possible, before a surgical intervention can take place. This embolisation can be performed by interventional neuroradiology and is important, because blood loss can be minimised by such a preoperative technique [8].

Essential osseous anatomy of the central skull base (Fig. 2.2) The roof of the nasopharynx is formed in its central part by the body of the sphenoid bone and the basilar part of the occipital bone. Both structures are forming the inferior surface of the clivus (blumenbachii). In the midline we can recognise the pharyngeal tubercle, which is important for the insertion of the pharyngeal raphe and therefore marks the posterior wall of the pharynx. In the juvenile skull, the occipitosphenoid synchondrosis, which is important for the growth of the skull base, is present between the body of the sphenoid bone and the basilar part of the occipital bone. Around the age of 18 years, this normal cleft obliterates and disappears completely. The resulting osseous unit composed by the sphenoid bone and the occipital bone is also called "Os tribasilare".

Anteriorly the posterior orifice of the nasal cavity is separated by a thin osseous lamella belonging to the vomer which is an important part of the nasal septum. According to these conditions, both choanae are formed. The lateral border of choana is formed by the pterygoid process and medial by the perpendicular plate (s. verticalis) of the palatine bone. The pterygoid process of the sphenoid shows at its

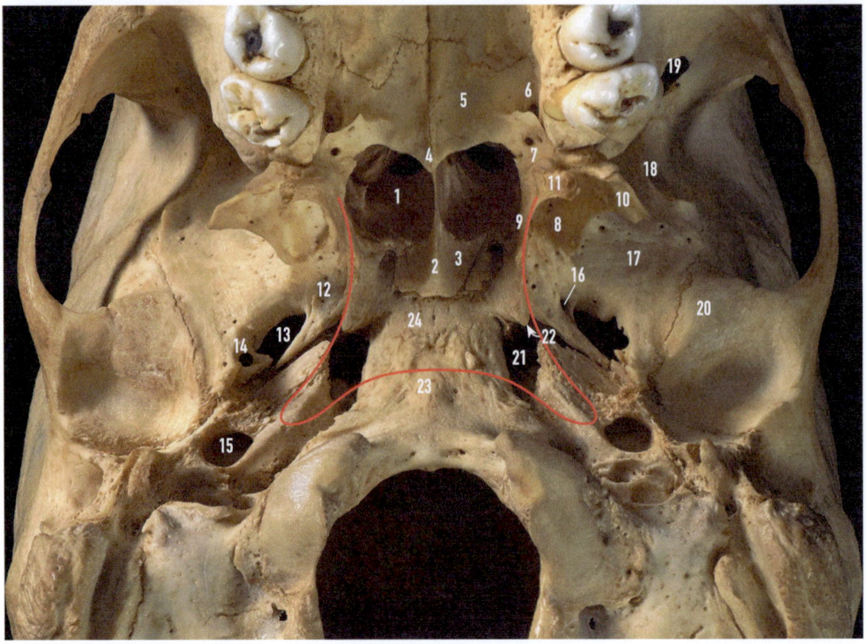

Fig. 2.2 Central skull base. *1* Choana, *2* vomer, *3* Ala of vomer , *4* posterior nasal spine, *5* horizontal plate of palatine bone, *6* greater palatine foramen, *7* lesser palatine foramen, *8* pterygoid fossa, *9* medial pterygoid plate, *10* lateral pterygoid plate, *11* pterygoid hamulus, *12* scaphoid fossa, *13* foramen ovale, *14* foramen spinosum, *15* carotid canal, *16* foramen vesalianum, *17* greater wing of sphenoid, *18* infratemporal crest, *19* inferior orbital fissure, *20* squamous part of temporal bone, *21* foramen lacerum, *22* entrance of the pterygoid canal, *23* pharyngeal tubercle, *24* inferior surface of the clivus. The *red* line marks the borders of the pharynx

posterior area a deep groove, the pterygoid fossa. This fossa is bordered by the medial and the lateral lamina of the pterygoid processes. The pterygoid fossa contains the medial pterygoid muscle, which originates from the inner surface of the lateral lamina. Cranially a small osseous crest is separated from the medial lamina and running dorsolaterally. Accordingly a small fossa is separated from the pterygoid fossa, and the former is termed as scaphoid fossa. This groove gives origin to a part of the tensor veli palatini muscle. Furthermore it is important that the medial lamella fans out into the pterygoid hamulus, which functions as fulcrum for the tendon of the tensor veli palatini muscle.

Just behind the lateral lamina of the pterygoid fossa, the foramen ovale can be seen, and through it the mandibular nerve comes out of the cranial cavity. This foramen contains not only the mandibular nerve but also a large venous plexus which connects the pterygoid plexus with the cavernous sinus inside the cranial cavity. In some cases (~40 %) somewhat anterior and medial to the foramen ovale, an emissary sphenoidal foramen (foramen vesalianum) can be seen (Fig. 2.2); it transmits a vein connecting the pterygoid venous plexus with the cavernous sinus. This venous route can be important for the spread of inflammations. Laterodorsal to the foramen ovale, the foramen spinosum is located. The middle meningeal artery passes through it into the cranial cavity as well as the recurrent meningeal nerve branch from the mandibular nerve.

In the dry skull, an irregular-shaped foramen can be seen between the clivus, the apex of the petrous bone and the greater wing of the sphenoid bone. This foramen is called the foramen lacerum due to its irregular and variable shape. This opening is completely closed by a dense, fibrous tissue, the basal fibrocartilage. This structure forms also the roof of Rosenmüller's recess. A narrow lateral extension of the foramen lacerum separates the anterior margin of the petrous bone from the greater wing of the sphenoid bone. This narrow cleft is termed as fissura sphenopetrosa. The greater and the lesser petrosal nerves are passing this fissure, whereas no essential structures are passing through the foramen lacerum.

Lateral to the pterygoid process is the roof of the infratemporal fossa, formed mainly by the inferior surface of the greater wing of the sphenoid and in a small area in front of the temporomandibular articulation by the squamous part of the temporal bone.

Nasal cavity (Fig. 2.3a, b) The lateral wall of the nasal cavity is structured by three nasal conchas, the inferior turbinate, the middle turbinate and the superior turbinate (Fig. 2.3a). In rare cases (17 %) a supreme concha can occur [10]. The inferior turbinate is a separate bone (os maxilloturbinale), whereas the other turbinates are belonging to the ethmoid. The middle turbinate must be considered as a crucial structure for endoscopic surgery, because it is a landmark for the entrance into the ethmoidal complex. Lateral to the middle turbinate, the uncinate process of the ethmoid can be identified by careful palpation (Fig. 2.3b). This thin, normally in the sagittal plane-orientated structure will be resected as a first step in ethmoid surgery (uncinectomy). Just above the uncinate process, the ethmoid bulla can be seen. This bulla ethmoidalis is a regular, large and relative constant anterior cell of the ethmoidal labyrinth. Between this bulla and the uncinate process, a distinct cleft, the hiatus semilunaris, can be easily identified. This hiatus leads into the ethmoidal infundibulum, which leads upwards into the frontal recess and medially towards the natural orifice of the maxillary sinus. The bulla ethmoidalis is also an important landmark for the identification of the anterior ethmoidal artery, which is running just above it. The exact position of this artery is dependent from the Keros type of the ethmoid. In a Keros type 1 configuration, the artery lies just below the roof of the ethmoid in a small osseous canal, the anterior ethmoidal canal. In a type 3 configuration, the artery is positioned somewhat below the ethmoidal roof, running horizontally through the ethmoid complex. The wall of the anterior ethmoidal canal may be deficient, so that the artery partly is only covered by the mucous membrane. The anterior ethmoidal artery as well as the posterior ethmoidal artery is important for surgery. If these arteries are stretched and then lacerated, they will retract into the orbit due to their elasticity. In the orbit the disrupted arteries are bleeding and a retrobulbar hematoma will result. This hematoma can cause blindness by stretching the optic nerve and is therefore a severe complication.

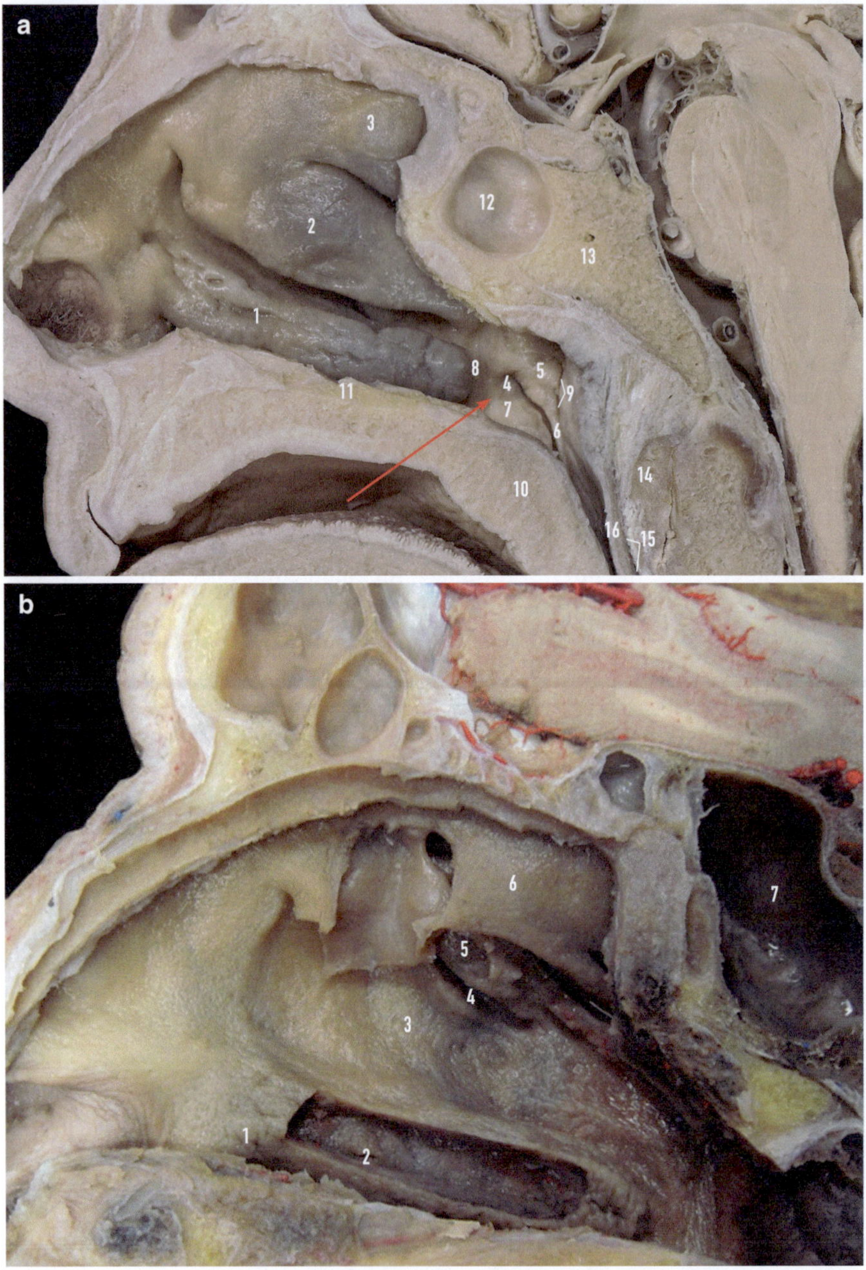

Fig. 2.3 (**a**) *1* Inferior nasal concha, *2* middle nasal concha, *3* superior nasal concha, *4* Eustachian tube opening, *5* tubal elevation, *6* salpingopharyngeal fold, *7* levator veli palatine elevation, *8* salpingopalatine elevation, *9* pharyngeal recess (Rosenmüller), *10* soft palate, 11 hard palate, *12* sphenoid sinus, *13* clivus, *14* anterior arch of atlas, *15* retropharyngeal space, *16* dorsal wall of the pharynx. The red arrow marks the route of the transpalatal approach towards the nasopharynx. (**b**) *1* Inferior nasal concha, *2* orifice of the nasolacrimal duct, *3* uncinate process, *4* hiatus semilunaris, *5* bulla ethmoidalis, *6* superior nasal concha, *7* sphenoid sinus

At the posterior end of the middle turbinate, the sphenopalatine foramen can be easily located. The osseous ethmoidal crest, which is important for the fixation of the middle turbinate, presents an essential landmark for identification of the sphenopalatine foramen and the sphenopalatine artery. According to Wareing and Padgham [11], different variations must be described, concerning the topographical relationship between the crest and the foramen. Behind the posterior ends of the nasal turbinates until the opening of the choana, the nasal cavity is termed as nasopharyngeal meatus.

The detailed anatomy of the paranasal sinuses and especially the different variations due to various grades of pneumatisation are described in the specialised literature [12–17].

Nasopharynx (Fig. 2.3a) The choanae are leading the nasopharyngeal meatus into the nasopharynx (or nasal part of the pharynx) which is bordered caudally from the oral pharynx by the soft palate. The lumen of the nasopharynx is always open, which is different from the other parts of the pharynx. Furthermore the anatomical structures of the lateral wall are important. Here we can find the somewhat triangular or slightly oval pharyngeal orifice of the Eustachian tube, which is surrounded posteriorly by the medial end of the tubal cartilage. This cartilage produces a bulging of the mucous membrane, called the tubal elevation. At its caudal end, the elevation fans out into the salpingopharyngeal fold. At the inferior border of the tubal opening, there is a soft bulging due to the levator veli palatini muscle. This moderate bulging is termed as levator veli palatine elevation. In front the tubal orifice is bordered by the salpingopalatine fold which runs into the superior surface of the soft palate. In surgery it is important not to resect the tubal cartilage under the torus tubarius, because in such cases, an abnormal opening of the Eustachian tube, the patulous tube, may result and the patient experiences autophony. Behind the tubal orifice, a slit-like lateral recess of the nasopharynx can be recognised. This lateral recess is termed as pharyngeal recess or Rosenmüller's fossa or recess. In about 35 % (autopsy) to 40 % (x-ray contrast studies), a large outpouching or diverticulum-like hollowing of the lateral recess may be present [18]. It is important that Rosenmüller's recess may have an intimate connection to the internal carotid artery (Fig. 2.4), especially if the course of the internal carotid artery is "curving", "coiling" or "kinking". Rosenmüller's recess can be seen as a gliding space which enables movement of the medial tubal cartilage [19]. Cranially Rosenmüller's recess is roofed by the thick fibrobasal cartilage, which covers the foramen lacerum. The mucous membrane of the epipharyngeal roof is up to 8 mm thick and contains lymphatic tissue which forms the pharyngeal tonsil [20]. According to Stupka [21], different structures (e.g. bursa pharyngea, Fossette pharyngienne) can be seen in the nasopharyngeal roof, which is of minor interest concerning the juvenile angiofibroma. The posterior wall of the nasopharynx is formed by the thin muscular layer of the superior pharyngeal constrictor muscle and the pharyngobasilar fascia. These structures are lying directly on the upper part of the cervical vertebral column and its prevertebral muscles. Between this posterior wall of the pharynx and the vertebral column is the retropharyngeal space. This space is only a gliding space for the pharynx and it normally contains no essential structures. In rare cases loops of the

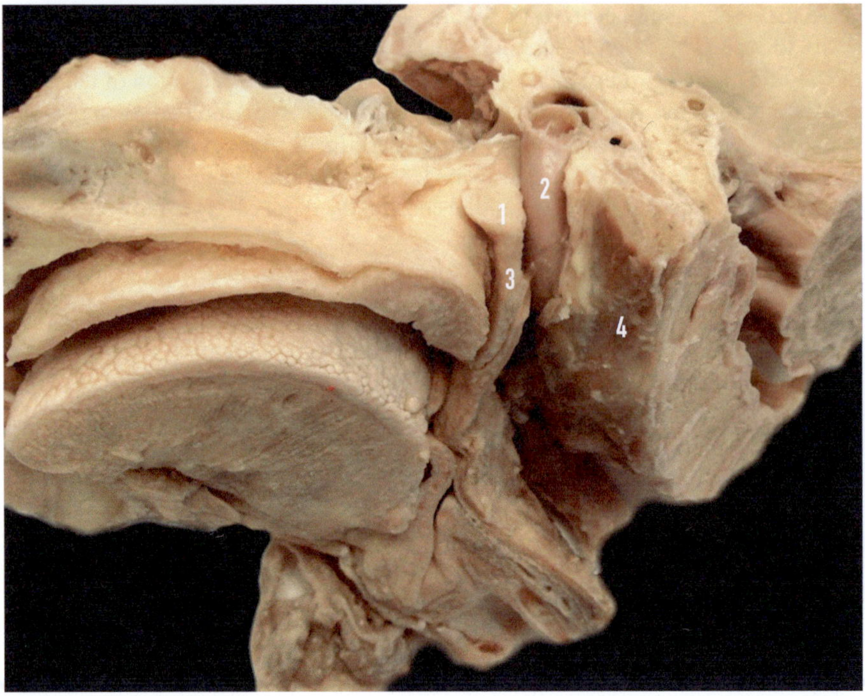

Fig. 2.4 Intimate relationship between the lateral pharyngeal recess and the internal carotid artery. *1* Tubal elevation, *2* internal carotid artery, *3* ~~Plica~~ salpingopharyngeal fold, *4* vertebral column

internal carotid artery can be dislocated in this space and therefore are running dorsolaterally or behind the pharynx [22–25] (Fig. 2.5). In such cases a slight pulsation can be seen at the patient's dorsolateral pharyngeal wall. The surgeon must be aware of these rare but important vascular anomalies.

Pterygopalatine fossa (Fig. 2.6a, b) This little but important pyramidal space lies below the orbital apex and contains important vessels and nerves. Furthermore this space contains the pterygopalatine (or sphenopalatine) ganglion, which is important for the relay of the preganglionic nerve fibres to the postganglionic fibres of the parasympathetic (secretomotor) nerves innervating the lacrimal gland and some minor glands located in the nasal, pharyngeal and palatine mucous membrane and innervates the mucous membrane of the nasopharynx behind the Eustachian tube.

The sphenopalatine foramen is the essential outlet of the pterygopalatine fossa into the three entrances, and three outlets must be described (Table 2.1). Laterally the pterygopalatine fossa communicates with the infratemporal fossa by the pterygomaxillary fissure. The medial wall shows the sphenopalatine foramen which opens in the posterior part of the nasal cavity. Furthermore there is a communication with the orbit by the inferior orbital fissure. In the posterior wall, the anterior surface of the pterygoid process (Fig. 2.6b), two orifices can be identified: the

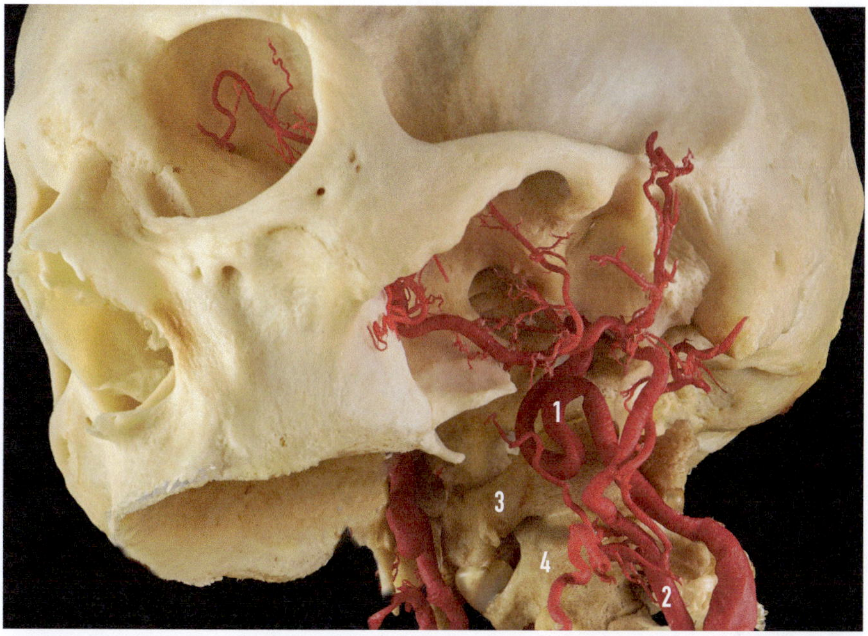

Fig. 2.5 Corrosion cast with exhaustive sling of the internal carotid artery, extending into the retropharyngeal space at the level of the nasopharynx. *1* A. internal carotid, *2* A. external carotid, *3* atlas, *4* axis

foramen rotundum and the opening of the pterygoid nerve canal. The opening of the foramen rotundum lies superolaterally to the orifice of the pterygoid canal. Caudally the pterygopalatine fossa narrows and forms the greater palatine canal, which opens with the greater palatine foramen and the lesser palatine foramina in the posterolateral region of the hard palate. The contents of these openings of the pterygopalatine fossa are also given in Table 2.1. Essential branches of the pterygopalatine ganglion are derived from the maxillary nerve, and their sensory fibres are not relayed in it. Essential branches supply orbit, nose and palate. Some orbital branches (2–3) are running through the inferior orbital fissure. The palatine nerves are forming the greater (anterior) palatine nerve and the lesser palatine nerves, which supply the hard palate as well as the soft palate. Nasal branches are separated into posterior superior lateral nasal nerves and posterior superior medial nasal nerves. The longest nerve of the medial group is termed the nasopalatine nerve (Scarpa). This nerve travels over the nasal septum towards the incisive canal and supplies the anterior region of the hard palate. At last a pharyngeal branch must be mentioned, which runs through the palatovaginal canal and distributed to the mucosa of the roof of pharynx. Sphenopalatine foramen is located at the posterior end of the middle turbinate and shows considerable topographical variations. Generally it can be assumed that the foramen lies posterior to the crista ethmoidalis, which is the osseous crest where the middle turbinate is fixed. This crest can

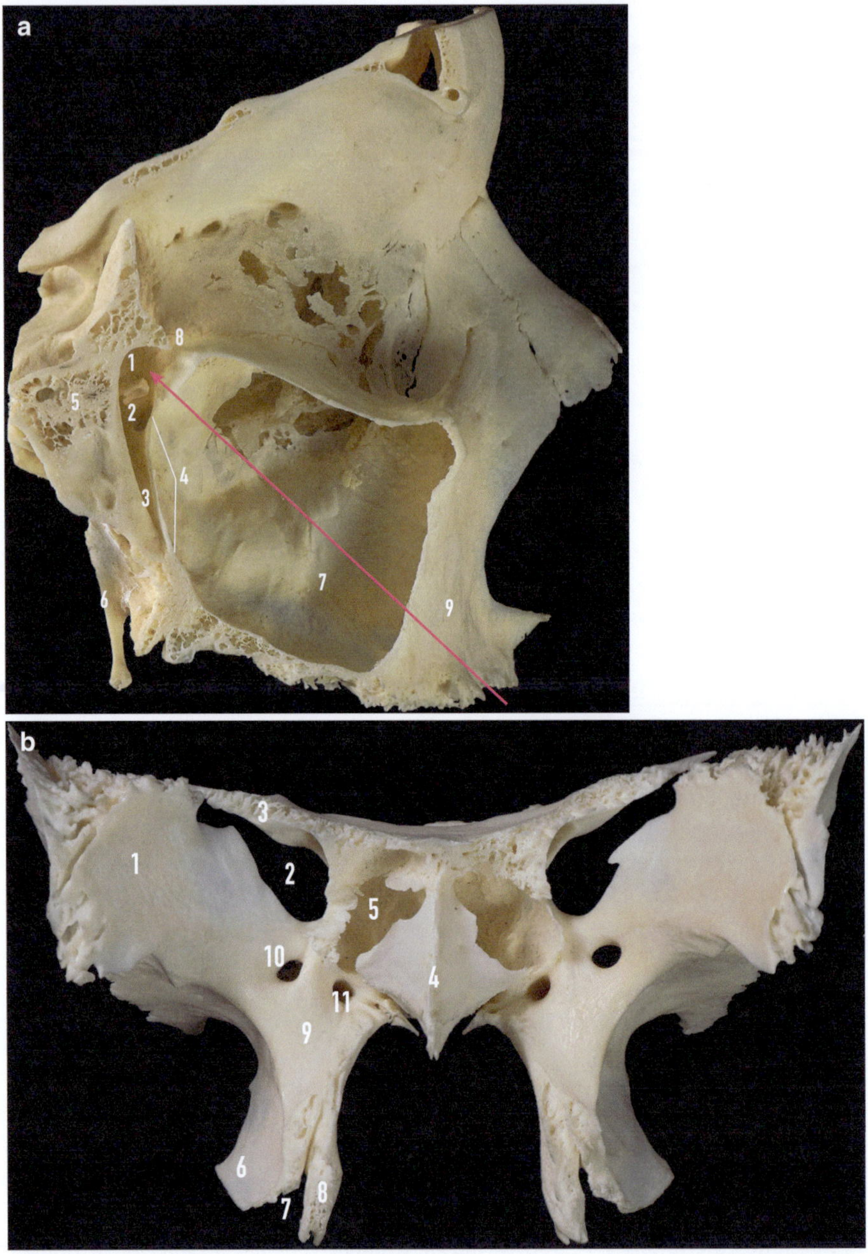

Fig. 2.6 (a) *1* Pterygopalatine fossa, *2* sphenopalatine foramen, *3* pterygopalatine canal, *4* maxillary tuberosity, *5* pterygoid process, *6* medial pterygoid plate with pterygoid hamulus, *7* maxillary sinus. The *red arrow* marks the transantral route towards the pterygopalatine fossa. (**b**) *1* Orbital surface of greater wing of sphenoid, *2* superior orbital fissure, *3* lesser wing of sphenoid, *4* rostrum of sphenoid, *5* sphenoid sinus, *6* lateral pterygoid plate, *7* pterygoid fissure, *8* medial pterygoid plate with pterygoid hamulus, *9* anterior surface of the pterygoid process forming the posterior wall of the pterygopalatine fossa, *10* foramen rotundum (canalis rotundus), *11* pterygoid canal

Table 2.1 Pterygopalatine fossa

Entry	Exit
Pterygomaxillary fissure:	Sphenopalatine foramen:
Maxillary artery	Sphenopalatine artery
	Nasopalatine and superior nasal nerves
Foramen rotundum:	Pterygopalatine canal:
Maxillary nerve	Palatine nerve
Artery and venous plexus of foramen rotundum	Descending palatine artery
Pterygoid canal:	Inferior orbital fissure:
Nerve and artery of the pterygoid canal	Infraorbital nerve and artery
	Zygomatic nerve
	Twigs from pterygopalatine ganglion

extend over the foramen, so that a superior and an inferior opening may result. The sphenopalatine artery enters the nasal cavity through this osseous foramen. It is important that according to the investigations of Simmen [26], the sphenopalatine artery is often divided into two or three branches, before entering the nasal cavity. Furthermore branches supplying the septum (Rr. septi posteriores) are running over the anterior wall of the sphenoid sinus somewhat below the apertures of these sinuses. These small branches can be responsible for bleeding, while opening the sphenoid sinus. It is important to preserve these branches, if the possibility to perform a Haddad's flap should be an option.

Infratemporal fossa This irregular space is laterally bordered by the ramus and the coronoid process of the mandible, medially by the lateral lamina of the pterygoid process and the pharynx, superiorly by the greater wing of the sphenoid bone and anteriorly by the maxillary tuberosity. The posterior border is formed by the styloid apparatus and the carotid sheath with its contents. Caudally no distinct border can be defined, so that the infratemporal fossa is in continuity with the mediastinum. The infratemporal fossa contains essential muscles, nerves and arteries. The space not occupied by these structures is filled with adipose tissue and a voluminous venous plexus, called the pterygoid plexus, which is communicating with the cavernous sinus in the cranial cavity by the basal orifices of the skull base. Therefore these orifices are important for the spread of inflammations. Furthermore this plexus is reached by the inferior ophthalmic vein and drains into the retromandibular and facial veins.

After entering the infratemporal fossa from the lateral side, the temporalis muscle inserting at the coronoid process is the first structure which can be seen. After reflecting this muscle and the coronoid process, the gross arrangement is formed by the pterygoid muscles. The lateral pterygoid muscle presents two heads, the small infratemporal one originating from the infratemporal surface and infratemporal crest of the greater wing of the sphenoid and the larger from the lateral surface of the lateral pterygoid plate. The infratemporal head inserts into the articular disc of the temporomandibular joint, whereas the pterygoidal one inserts at the pterygoid fovea located at the anterior surface of the neck of the mandible. The medial pterygoid muscle originates in the pterygoid fossa from the medial surface of the lateral pterygoid plate and with a small muscular bundle from the lateral surface of the lateral pterygoid plate as well as from the maxillary tuberosity and the pyramidal process of the palatine bone. This muscle runs downwards and inserted at the pterygoid tuberosity on the internal surface of the angle of the mandible. Between these muscular pillars, organising the infratemporal fossa, three clefts are formed: a superior cleft, a middle cleft and an inferior cleft. The superior cleft is positioned between the osseous skull base and the infratemporal head of the lateral pterygoid muscle. This cleft is traversed by the deep temporal nerves and vessels which are running into the inferior surface of the temporal muscle. The middle cleft is positioned between the two heads of the lateral pterygoid muscle, and the third cleft can be found between the pterygoidal head of the lateral pterygoid muscle and the medial pterygoid muscle. The sensory buccal nerve passes out of the middle cleft. The inferior cleft is the most important one, because it contains the inferior alveolar nerve (posterior position) and the lingual nerve (anterior position). The infratemporal fossa communicates with the orbit by means of the infraorbital fissure. The infraorbital artery passes through this osseous connection and runs into the infraorbital sulcus and then into the infraorbital canal. The infraorbital artery is not accompanied by an infraorbital vein [27].

Within the infratemporal fossa, the maxillary artery, one terminal division of the external carotid artery, is an important structure (Fig. 2.7). The maxillary artery passes horizontally forward between the neck of the mandible and the sphenomandibular ligament. In this region normally a close relationship can be seen to the auriculotemporal nerve (above) and to the maxillary vein (below) [28]. According to Krizan [29] the artery runs in 66 % of the cases between the temporalis muscle and the lateral pterygoid muscle (superficial variant), and in 34 % it is positioned between the lateral pterygoid muscle and the medial pterygoid muscle (deep variant). If the deep variant is present, the maxillary artery passes the mandibular nerve on its lateral side in 21.5 %, on its medial side in 6 %, between the inferior alveolar and the lingual nerve in 3 % and through a loop of the inferior alveolar nerve in 3.5 %. According to Urban [30] the topographic relationships of the maxillary artery are strongly depended on races. In Japanese people the artery runs only in 6.3 % medial to the lateral pterygoid muscle.

The course of the maxillary artery can be divided into three parts: the mandibular part, the pterygoidal part and the pterygopalatine part. The mandibular and the pterygoidal parts are positioned within the infratemporal fossa, whereas the pterygopalatine part belongs to the pterygopalatine fossa. All branches of the mandibular part are running into osseous canals (deep auricular artery, anterior tympanic artery, middle meningeal artery, accessory meningeal artery, inferior alveolar or dental artery). All branches of the pterygoidal part (deep temporal branches, pterygoid branches, masseteric artery, buccal artery) are supplying mainly masticatory or facial muscles. The branches of the pterygopalatine part are (posterior superior alveolar or dental artery, infraorbital artery, greater palatine artery, pharyngeal branch, artery of the pterygoid canal and sphenopalatine artery) also mainly running

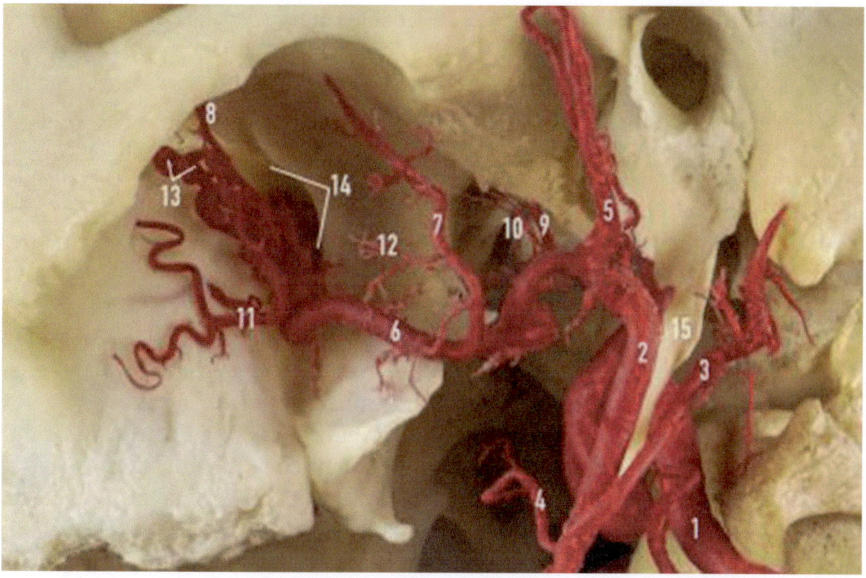

Fig. 2.7 Corrosion cast illustrating the maxillary artery and essential branches. *1* Internal carotid artery, *2* external carotid artery, *3* occipital artery, *4* ascending pharyngeal artery, *5* superficial temporal artery, *6* maxillary artery, *7* posterior deep temporal artery, *8* anterior deep temporal artery, *9* middle meningeal artery, *10* accessory meningeal artery, *11* posterior superior alveolar artery, *12* pterygoid branches, *13* ophthalmic artery, *14* pterygomaxillary fissure, *15* styloid process

into osseous canals and are important for the vascularisation of the nasal cavity, the soft and hard palate, parts of the mandibular apparatus and the orbital floor.

The maxillary artery enters the pterygopalatine fossa by the pterygomaxillary fissure (Fig. 2.7) and divides that into several branches. It can be important for surgery to have thorough knowledge of the variations occurring in this region, especially if a transantral approach (Fig. 2.6a) or a ligation of the maxillary artery according to Seiffert will be performed. An instructive table of these variations is given in literature [31].

The anterior border of the infratemporal fossa and of the pterygopalatine fossa is the tuber of the maxilla. This structure is a very thin papyraceous osseous lamella, which is also the posterior wall of the maxillary sinus (Fig. 2.6a). Juvenile angiofibroma at first presses and bends this structure easily by pressure. This typical "anterior bowing" is known in radiology as Holman-Miller sign (see Fig. 7.12). In the next step, the thin osseous lamella will be destroyed by further pressure and then the tumor enters into the maxillary sinus. The invasion of the maxillary sinus as well as of the infratemporal fossa can lead to severe deformity of the face.

If parts of the central skull base are absorbed or eroded due to enormous pressure of the expanding juvenile angiofibroma, the tumor can spread into the cranial cavity and especially into the cavernous sinus. Several cranial nerves are passing this venous chamber, positioned laterally to the sella turcica. In the lateral wall of the cavernous sinus, the oculomotor nerve, the trochlear nerve and the ophthalmic nerve are running. Within the lumen of the cavernous sinus, the abducens nerve is positioned in close relationship to the internal carotid artery. All nerves are running towards the superior orbital fissure. If the tumor expands into the cavernous sinus or reaches the apex of the orbital pyramid, intraconal as well as extraconal nerves can be destroyed, resulting in different problems of ocular motion, presenting clinically as superior orbital fissure syndrome.

Furthermore the mandibular nerve is an essential structure of the infratemporal fossa. This nerve, arising from the trigeminal nerve at the semilunar ganglion of Gasser, can be divided into a minor masticatory part and a larger, sensory part. At first the main trunk branches off the recurrent meningeal nerve (s. N. spinosus) which enters the cranial cavity through the foramen spinosum or in more rare cases through the foramen ovale. This nerve is a meningeal branch which also supplies parts of the cartilaginous Eustachian tube as well as parts of the mastoid antrum. The anterior portion of the mandibular nerve is mainly motor in function, except of the buccal nerve, which is a sensory nerve. The posterior mandibular trunk contains mainly sensory fibres, except of the inferior alveolar nerve, which carries essential motor fibres, for the mylohyoid muscle and the anterior belly of the digastric muscle.

References

1. Friedberg SA. Vascular fibromas of the nasopharynx. Arch Otolaryngol. 1940;31:313–26.
2. Svoboda DJ, Kirchner F. Ultrastructure of nasopharyngeal angiofibroma. Cancer. 1966;19:1949–62.
3. Schick B, Kahle G. Radiological findings in angiofibroma. Acta Radiol. 2000;41:585–93.
4. Girgis IH, Fahmy SA. Nasopharyngeal fibroma: its histo-pathological nature. J Laryngol Otol. 1973;87:1107–23.
5. Beham A, Beham-Schmid C, Regauer S, Auböck L, Stammberger H. Nasopharyngeal angiofibroma: true neoplasm or vascular malformation? Adv Anat Pathol. 2000;7:36–46.
6. Schick B, Plinkert P, Prescher A. Die vaskuläre Komponente: Gedanken zur Entstehung des Angiofibroms. Laryngo-Rhino-Otol. 2002;81:280–4.
7. Harrison DFN. The natural history, pathogenesis, and treatment of juvenile angiofibroma. Arch Otolaryngol Head Neck Surg. 1987;113:936–42.
8. Swoboda H, Samec P, Neuwirth-Riedl K. Zur Therapie des juvenilen Angiofibroms. Die präoperative Embolisation. HNO. 1990;38:370–4.
9. Kösling S, Bootz F. Bildgebung HNO-Heilkunde. Berlin: Springer; 2015.
10. Lang J, Sakals E. Über die Höhe der Cavitas nasi, die Länge ihres Bodens und Masse sowie Anordnung der Conchae nasales und der Apertura sinus sphenoidalis. Anat Anz. 1981;149:297–318.
11. Wareing MJ, Padgham ND. Osteologic classification of the sphenopalatine foramen. Laryngoscope. 1998;108:125–7.
12. Grünwald L. Deskriptive und topographische Anatomie der Nase und ihrer Nebenhöhlen. In: Denker A, Kahler O, editors. Handbuch der Hals-Nasen-Ohrenheilkunde Bd. 1. München: J Springer Berlin JF Bergmann; 1925.
13. Hajek M. Pathologie und Therapie der entzündlichen Erkrankungen der Nebenhöhlen der Nase. Wien: Deuticke Leipzig; 1926.

14. Lang J. Klinische Anatomie der Nase, Nasenhöhle und Nebenhöhlen. Stuttgart: Thieme; 1988.
15. Prescher A. Nasal and paranasal sinus anatomy for the endoscopic sinus surgeon. In: Stucker FJ, De Souza C, Kenyon GS, Lian TS, Draf W, Schick B, editors. Rhinology and facial plastic surgery. Berlin: Springer; 2009.
16. Prescher A. Klinische Anatomie der Nasennebenhöhlen: Systematik, Topographie und wichtige Variationen. HNO. 2009;57:1039–52.
17. Prescher A. The osseous anatomy of the skull base and related regions. In: Draf W, Carrau R, Bockmühl U, Kassam AB, Vajkoczy P, editors. Endonasal endoscopic surgery of skull base tumors: an interdisciplinary approach. Stuttgart: Thieme; 2015.
18. Khoo FY, Kanagasuntheram R, Chia KB. Variations of the lateral recesses of the nasopharynx. Arch Otolaryngol. 1967;86:456–62.
19. Bryant WS. The Eustachian tube, its anatomy, and its movements: with a description of the cartilages, muscle, fasciae and the fossa of Rosenmüller. Med Rec. 1907;71:931–4.
20. Disse J. Anatomie des Rachens. In: Heymann P, editor. Handbuch der Laryngologie und Rhinologie. Wien: Hölder; 1899. Bd. 2.
21. Stupka W. Die Mißbildungen und Anomalien der Nase und des Nasenrachenraumes. Wien: Springer; 1938.
22. Brown-Kelly A. Large pulsating vessels in the pharynx. Glas Med J. 1898;49:28–34.
23. Brown-Kelly A. Tortuosity of the internal carotid in relation to the pharynx. J Laryngol Otol. 1925;40:15–23.
24. Demme K. Ueber Gefässanomalien im Pharynx. Wien Med Wochenschr. 1901;51:2245–7.
25. Ubbens UM. Pulsating vessels in the pharynx. Pract Oto-rhin-laryngol. 1963;25:350–5.
26. Simmen DB, Raghavan U, Briner HR, Manestar M, Groscurth P, Jones NS. The anatomy of the sphenopalatine artery for the endoscopic sinus surgeon. Am J Rhinol. 2006;20:502–5.
27. Lang J. Klinische Anatomie des Kopfes. Berlin: Springer; 1981.
28. Last RJ. Anatomy: regional and applied. London: Churchill; 1966.
29. Krizan Z. Beiträge zur deskriptiven und topographischen Anatomie der A. maxillaris. Acta Anat. 1960;41:319–33.
30. Urban A. Topographie der Pars pterygopalatina der A. maxillaris aus frontaler Sicht. Würzburg: Inaug.-Diss; 1974.
31. Krmpotic-Nemanic J, Draf W, Helms J. Chirurgische Anatomie des Kopf-Hals-Bereiches. Berlin: Springer; 1985.

Chapter 3
Pathologic and Microscopic Features

Jaana Hagström, Suvi Renkonen, and Antti Mäkitie

Abstract Juvenile angiofibroma (JA) is a rare benign tumor, which almost exclusively affects adolescent males. JA is supposed to originate from the sphenopalatine foramen in the posterior wall of the nasal cavity. Although histologically benign, JA growth can be locally destructive. It grows as a polypoid mass and thus easily fills up and remodels nasal structures. Further, this phenomenon often makes its surgical treatment challenging. Histologically the tumor is composed of two elements: stroma with variable amount of cells and collagen and vascular component composed of differently sized and shaped vessels. Older lesions tend to be more collagenous and have less vascularity. The growth of the tumor is suggested to be provoked by testosterone stimulation during puberty in males. Only rare cases of transformation into malignancy have been reported.

Keywords Benign • Tumor • Nasopharynx • Vascularity • Stroma

Juvenile (nasopharyngeal) angiofibroma (JA) is a benign but potentially locally destructive tumor arising from posterolateral wall of nasal cavity without known aetiological factors or pathogenesis. The tumor is supposedly hormonally affected starting its growth during puberty in males with a peak in second decade. If females are affected, their hormonal status should be checked [1, 2].

Symptoms are neither specific nor diagnostic but usually include nasal obstruction, epistaxis, facial deformity and nasal discharge with duration from a few months to years. Despite the fact that radiological imaging with modern techniques is ably precise, the final diagnosis of JA relies on histology. Due to the tumors' rich vascularity, it has been proposed that JA could actually be a vascular malformation, but

J. Hagström, DDS, PhD (✉)
Department of Pathology, HusLab, University of Helsinki and Helsinki University Hospital, P.O. Box 21, FI-00041 Helsinki, Finland
e-mail: jaana.hagstrom@hus.fi

S. Renkonen, MD • A. Mäkitie, MD
Department of Otorhinolaryngology and Head and Neck Surgery, University of Helsinki and Helsinki University Hospital

S.P. Dubey, B. Schick (eds.), *Juvenile Angiofibroma*,
DOI 10.1007/978-3-319-45343-9_3

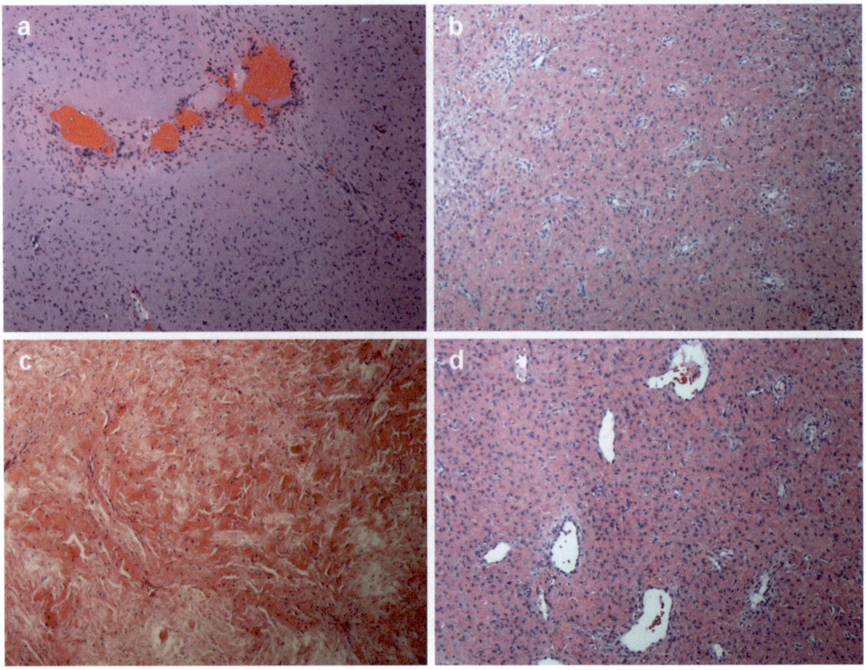

Fig. 3.1 (**a–d**) The general view of JA. Magnification 100×–200×

currently, it is still included into tumor category. JA is considered to be a biphasic tumor composed of stromal and vascular components [3–6].

In macroscopy the tumor is solid and slightly rubbery having possibly hemorrhagic content due to its vascular nature. The size is usually between 1 and 3 cm although even larger masses are encountered, and it tends to grow like a polypoid mass especially at early stage. The growth pattern will allow it to extend into sinonasal structures making its surgical resection difficult [3, 5–7].

In histology these tumors are composed of two elements: dense stroma with variable number of stromal cells and vascular component with differently sized and shaped vessels. Both components are supposed to be neoplastic by their nature. The histological diagnosis relies on morphology. Although immunohistochemistry may be helpful, there are no definitive diagnostic markers for JA (Fig. 3.1) [7, 8].

The stromal component of JA is collagen rich and contains fibroblast-like cells, usually positive for vimentin. Cell volume and shape differ from one tumor to another and some tumors appear almost acellular. Cellularity can vary from 14 to even 700 per 0.4 mm^2 (Fig. 3.2). Stromal cells may resemble epithelioid, spindle, round or stellata-like fibroblasts with sometimes mild cytological atypia (Fig. 3.3). In electron microscopy the stromal cells can be identified to be both fibroblasts, with prominent nucleoli and well-developed Golgi complexes, and myofibroblasts with plenty of rough endoplasmic reticulum. In immunohistochemistry stromal cells are found to express beta-catenin, androgen receptor, oestrogen receptor β,

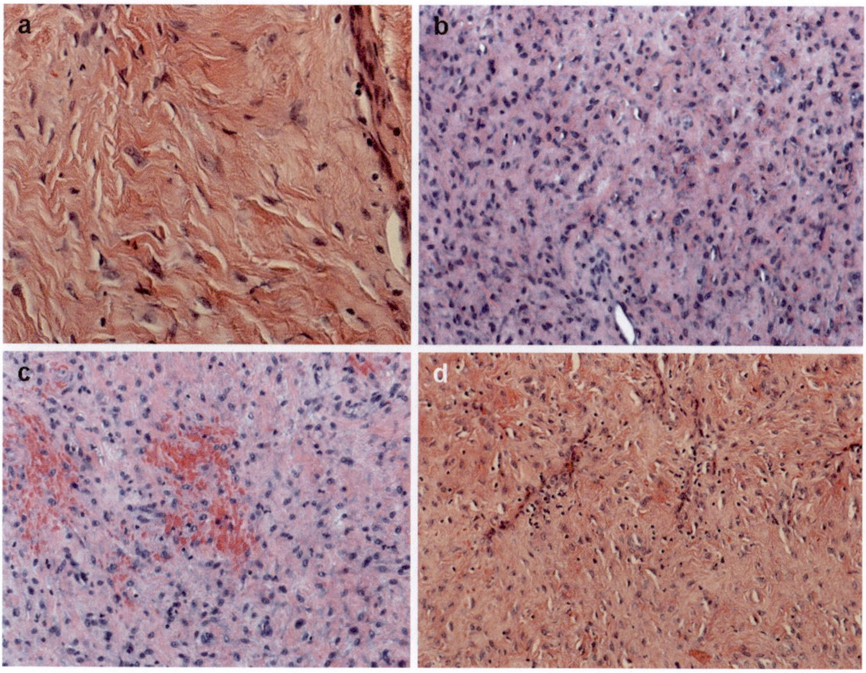

Fig. 3.2 Stroma differs in cell frequency (**a**, **b**). (**c**) Stromal hemorrhage. (**d**) Perivascular lymphocytes. Magnification 200×–400×

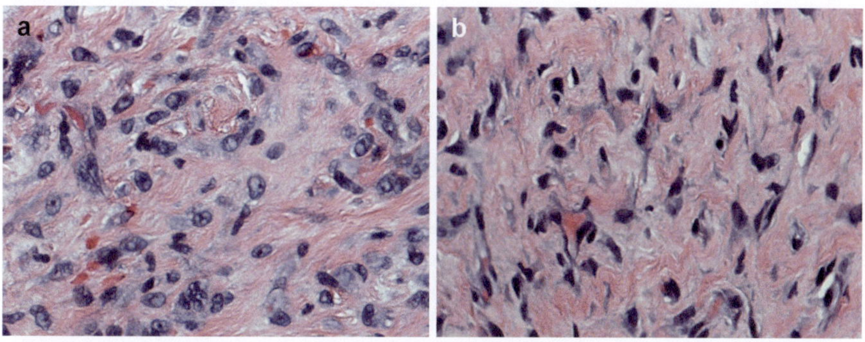

Fig. 3.3 (**a**, **b**) Differently shaped stromal cells. Magnification 600×

different MMPs, syndecan-1 and syndecan-2, C-myc and Bmi-1, although the expression intensity may vary. Sporadic tumors are supposed to have higher incidence of beta-catenin mutations. Vascular endothelial growth factor (VEGF) has been detected in stromal cells and is supposed to promote the growth of JA. The collagen fibres may express Tenascin-C with the strongest expression concentrated to the surroundings of vessels. Tenascin expression correlates to vessel density (Fig. 3.4). Stroma may contain myxoid degeneration. Myxoid features can be a

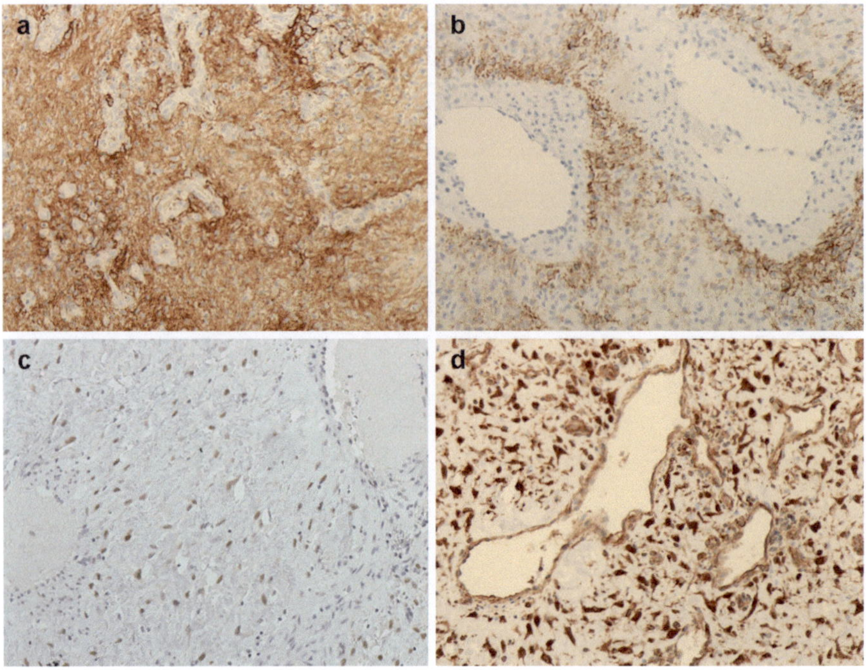

Fig. 3.4 Stromal IH expression figure. (**a**) Tenascin positivity. (**b**) Syndecan positivity. (**c**) Nuclear AR positivity. (**d**) Beta-catenin positivity

result of embolization usually performed before surgical operation to minimize perioperative bleeding. In addition to fibroblasts, stroma may contain mast cells and sometimes inflammatory cells especially in case the overlying mucosa has been ulcerated (Fig. 3.2) [4, 7–12].

Vascular structures are often thin walled and their shape, size and amount vary a lot. The shape of vascular structures may vary from stag horned to round or oval. Some vessels look immature and they are not forming normal vascular structures. These vessels look slit (stag-horned) and the luminal area is flattened (Figs. 3.5 and 3.6). In electron microscopy even these primitive capillaries have two endothelial cell layers and pericytes surrounding them. The muscular layer in vessels can be absent or patchy or surround the vessels totally. The amount of vessels varies widely from 160 to 6.200 for mm^2 and the vascularity is related to tumor recurrence rate. The vascular density within a single tumor may alternate a lot. Certain areas may be more collagenous and certain areas dense with vascular structures. Hormonal treatment may diminish the number of vessels and induce thickness of the walls [4–6, 13].

In immunohistochemistry vimentin and smooth muscle actin stain vessel-wall cells and also Syndecan-2 may be positive. In addition, MMP-9 and MMP-14 are immunopositive in vessel walls. Vascular markers CD34 and CD31 are expressed in the endothelium but stroma lacks those expressions (Fig. 3.6). It has been shown

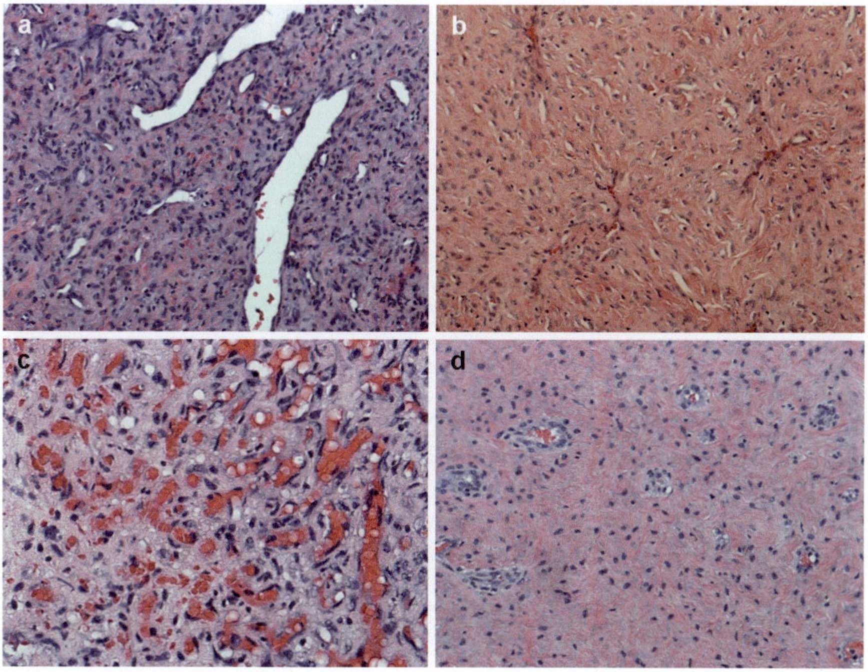

Fig. 3.5 (**a–d**) Differently shaped vessels

that vessel intensity is related to the recurrence rate, which has been reported to be from 20% even to 50%. The older lesions have less vascularity and increased amount of collagen in stroma. Furthermore, younger patients appear to have more aggressively growing tumors [6].

Some studies have suggested an association between JA and familiar adenomatous polyposis (FAP). However, also controversial studies exist with no association with FAP or evidence of inheritance in JA [14–16].

Differential diagnostic alternatives for JA include a choanal polyp, pyogenic granuloma and sinonasal haemangiopericytoma, and these should be ruled out.

Surgery is recommended as the treatment of choice for JA. Endoscopic approach is suitable for tumors limited to nasopharynx, nasal cavity and sinuses. Larger tumors with intracranial extension are challenging and carry a higher rate for complications like hemorrhage, recurrences and neurologic deficits. Small tumors may bleed more during the operation as their histology is different from that seen in older and more maturated tumors with less vasculature and more prominent fibrous component. Preoperative embolization is typically used to minimize perioperative bleeding [17–19]. However, challenges related to the surgical treatment, incomplete resection and, thus, persistent tumor growth make recurrences common. Meticulous dissection of the tumor tissue invading the sphenoid bone will obviously reduce the rate of recurrences, and even regression of residual disease has been reported [20].

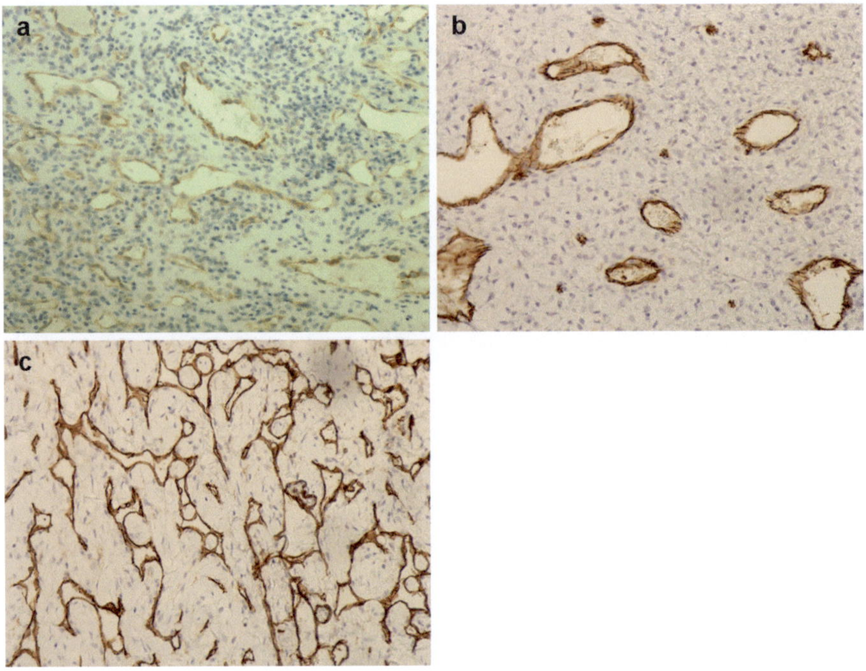

Fig. 3.6 (**a**) Syndecan-2 positivity in vessel wall. (**b**, **c**) CD 31 positivity highlights the differently shaped vessels

There are still a lot of unanswered questions concerning JA. It remains unclear if JA is a real tumor or malformation, and whether it is the stromal or the vascular component, which is the active part in it, and if this tumor truly is biphasic by its nature.

References

1. Farag MM, Ghanimah SE, Ragaie A, Saleem TH. Hormonal receptors in juvenile nasopharyngeal angiofibroma. Laryngoscope. 1987;97:208–11.
2. Neel 3rd HB, Whicker JH, Devine KD, Weiland LH. Juvenile angiofibroma. Review of 120 cases. Am J Surg. 1973;126:547–56.
3. Doyle PJ, Riding K, Kahn K. Management of nasopharyngeal angiofibroma. J Otolaryngol. 1977;6:224–32.
4. Liang J, Yi Z, Lianq P. The nature of juvenile nasopharyngeal angiofibroma. Otolaryngol Head Neck Surg. 2000;123:475–81.
5. Mistry RC, Qureshi SS, Gupta S, Gupta S. Juvenile nasopharyngeal angiofibroma: a single institution study. Indian J Cancer. 2005;42:35–9.
6. Renkonen S, Hagstrom J, Vuola J, Niemela M, Porras M, Kivivuori SM, et al. The changing surgical management of juvenile nasopharyngeal angiofibroma. Eur Arch Otorhinolaryngol. 2011;268:599–607.

7. Schuon R, Brieger J, Heinrich UR, Roth Y, Szyfter W, Mann WJ. Immunohistochemical analysis of growth mechanisms in juvenile nasopharyngeal angiofibroma. Eur Arch Otorhinolaryngol. 2007;264:389–94.
8. Renkonen S, Heikkila P, Haglund C, Makitie AA, Hagstrom J. Tenascin-C, GLUT-1, and syndecan-2 expression in juvenile nasopharyngeal angiofibroma: correlations to vessel density and tumor stage. Head Neck. 2013;35:1036–42.
9. Abraham SC, Montgomery EA, Giardiello FM, Wu TT. Frequent beta-catenin mutations in juvenile nasopharyngeal angiofibromas. Am J Pathol. 2001;158:1073–8.
10. Duerr S, Wendler O, Aigner T, Karosi S, Schick B. Metalloproteinases in juvenile angiofibroma – a collagen rich tumor. Hum Pathol. 2008;39:259–68.
11. Pauli J, Gundelach R, Vanelli-Rees A, Rees G, Campbell C, Dubey S, et al. Juvenile nasopharyngeal angiofibroma: an immunohistochemical characterisation of the stromal cell. Pathology. 2008;40:396–400.
12. Sun X, Guo L, Wang J, Wang H, Liu Z, Liu J, et al. Prognostic value of matrix metalloproteinase 9 expression in patients with juvenile nasopharyngeal angiofibroma: tissue microarray analysis. Int J Pediatr Otorhinolaryngol. 2014;78:1232–8.
13. Wang JJ, Sun XC, Hu L, Liu ZF, Yu HP, Li H, et al. Endoglin (CD105) expression on microvessel endothelial cells in juvenile nasopharyngeal angiofibroma: tissue microarray analysis and association with prognostic significance. Head Neck. 2013;35:1719–25.
14. Ferouz AS, Mohr RM, Paul P. Juvenile nasopharyngeal angiofibroma and familial adenomatous polyposis: an association? Otolaryngol Head Neck Surg. 1995;113:435–9.
15. Giardiello FM, Hamilton SR, Krush AJ, Offerhaus JA, Booker SV, Petersen GM. Nasopharyngeal angiofibroma in patients with familial adenomatous polyposis. Gastroenterology. 1993;105:1550–2.
16. Klockars T, Renkonen S, Leivo I, Hagström J, Mäkitie AA. Juvenile nasopharyngeal angiofibroma: no evidence for inheritance or association with familial adenomatous polyposis. Fam Cancer. 2010;9:401–3.
17. Sennes LU, Fortes SG, Butugan O, Saldiva P, Bernandi FC. Tissue maturation correlating to clinical manifestations in Juvenile angiofibroma. Ann Otol Rhinol Laryngol. 2005;114:705–8.
18. Browne JD, Jacob SL. Temporal approach for resection of juvenile nasopharyngeal angiofibromas. Laryngoscope. 2000;110:1287–93.
19. Bremer JW, Neel HB, DeSanto LW, Jones GC. Angiofibroma: treatment trends in 150 patients during 40 years. Laryngoscope. 1986;96:1321–9.
20. Howard DJ, Lloyd G, Lund V. Recurrence and its avoidance in juvenile angiofibroma. Laryngoscope. 2001;111:1509–11.

Chapter 4
Recent Concept of Etiology

Bernhard Schick

Abstract The etiology of the juvenile angiofibroma (JA) has been a mystery for a long time. The numerous etiologies postulated over the years could not find general acceptance being mostly able to explain only one of the specific features of the tumor. The most recent concept regarding the origin of this tumor offers for the first time an explanation that covers all specific features of this tumor and is being supported by detailed molecular studies. Herein, the etiology of JAs as a vascular malformation deriving from remnants of the first branchial arch is demonstrated.

Keywords Etiology • Malformation • Wnt-signaling • Hormones

Introduction

Juvenile angiofibroma (JA) has stimulated a huge number of physicians to speculate on the etiology of this fascinating tumor starting with Nélaton [1] who proposed in 1853 a first theory in this regard. These numerous suggested theories were however able to explain only one of the exclusive clinical features of this rare fibrovascular tumor being either: (1) a tumor originating close to the sphenopalatine foramen in the posterior nasal cavity or (2) blood supply mainly from the sphenopalatine/maxillary artery but also from the internal carotid artery even though the tumor might not be close to these vessels. Other authors presented explanation for the (3) specific tissue architecture or (4) the almost exclusive manifestation in adolescent males. However, there is the need that a theory has to be able to explain all clinical features of a specific described pathology. Recent findings postulated that the JA is a vascular malformation and molecular pathology findings were able to support this theory. Herein, this recent concept of the etiology of the JA is presented. The molecular findings are only presented in the context of this new theory and will not summarize

B. Schick, MD
ENT Department, University of Saarland Medical Centre,
Kirrberger Strasse, D-66421 Homburg/Saar, Germany
e-mail: bernhard.schick@uks.eu

S.P. Dubey, B. Schick (eds.), *Juvenile Angiofibroma*,
DOI 10.1007/978-3-319-45343-9_4

all molecular findings being reported so far. Only the main aspects being relevant for the recent concept regarding the etiology of the JAs are mentioned. For more details the listed references are excellently suited to obtain further detailed information.

Vascular Malformation: Site of Origin and Blood Supply

A fundamental process in embryology is the temporary occurrence of structures that recede during the further development. If this process is incomplete and embryological cells persist (atavism), they can be the origin for tumor, e.g., chordoma. If we consider that the JAs have embryological origin then we need to search for an embryological structure being able to explain the site of tumor origin as well as the typical tumor blood supply. The first branchial arch artery is interestingly only build up temporarily at day 22 to day 24 in human development connecting the later maxillary artery with the internal carotid artery for the time a common carotid artery has not been developed yet. For a short time period the first branchial arch artery ensures in an embryo the brain blood supply. This vessel however recedes in further development via formation of a plexus that starts first close to the internal carotid artery and finally parts of the first branchial arch artery are incorporated in the formation of the maxillary artery/sphenopalatine artery [2]. Indeed, endothelial lined vascular spaces have been found independent of the sex at week 24 close to the sphenopalatine foramen [3] presenting most probable plexus remnants of the first branchial arch artery. Thus the development of a JA based on remnants of the first branchial arch artery plexus is suited to explain its origin close to the sphenopalatine foramen since plexus remnants of the first branchial arch artery are mainly found here if the regression is incomplete (Fig. 4.1a). In addition to the normal blood supply by the internal maxillary/sphenopalatine artery, there may be direct communication between the plexus and internal carotid artery (Fig. 4.1b).

As an additional hint, it is worthwhile to consider the assumption that the JAs are a vascular malformation bringing an interesting light regarding the atypically located JAs. Vascular processes in the embryological development might be able to explain also these locations as it would be possible to define an incomplete vascular regression at the site of the detected atypical JAs.

Vascular Malformation: Tissue Architecture

A characteristic feature in JA is the histological finding of irregularly configured vessels with only endothelial lining as well as and vessels with an incomplete vascular wall (pericytes located only in parts of the vessel wall) embedded in a fibrous stroma, being infiltrated by additional inflammatory cells. The vascular architecture has been studied in detail by immunohistological end electronmicroscopic analayses suggesting that JAs are vascular malformations [4]. Meanwhile, laminin α2 has been detected

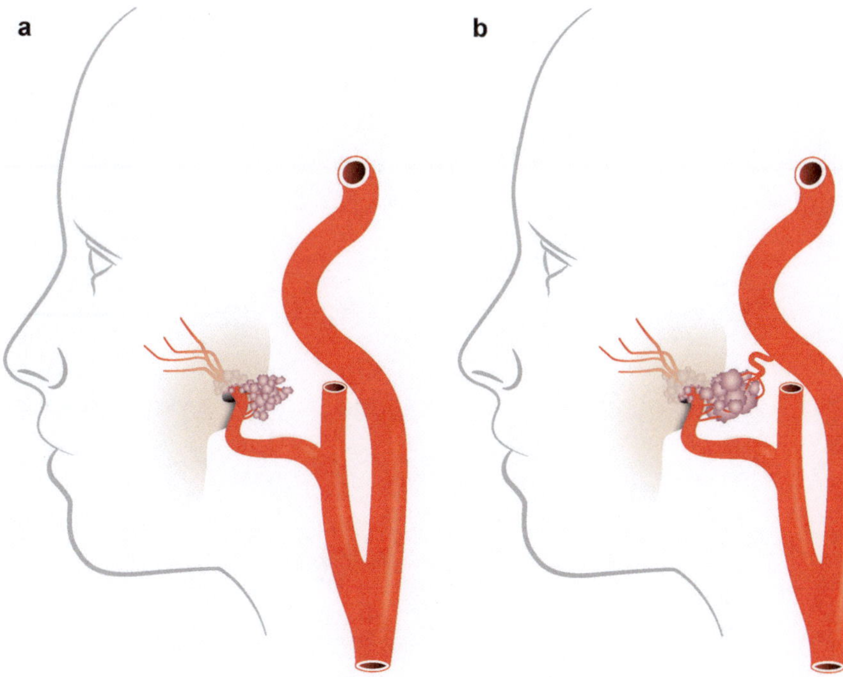

Fig. 4.1 Plexus remnants of the first branchial arch artery near the sphenopalatine foramen are the origin of the illustrated juvenile angiofibroma (**a**). Due to the still persistent communications of plexus remnants of the first branchial arch artery to the internal carotid artery, blood supply deriving from the internal carotid artery as well as from the maxillary/sphenopalatine artery is drawn into the JA example (**b**)

in the perivascular layer of JA tumor vessels, a marker that is typically found in embryological brain vessels. In addition, TSHZ1 (teashirt zinc finger homebox) has been recognized in JAs being described to be expressed in the first and second branchial arch artery [5]. Analysis of collagen Iα1 and collagen Iα2 expression profile as well as collagen VI expression in JAs fit to the assumption of embryological vessels [5]. These findings support strongly the theory of JAs as being a vascular malformation arising from remnants of the first branchial arch artery.

Vascular Malformation: Cellular and Molecular Embryological Keystones

The epithelial to mesenchymal as well as the mesenchymal to epithelial transition are important cellular changes in the embryological development. The theory of remnants of first branchial arch artery to be the origin of JAs does not need to claim the endothelial cells as being the origin of the tumor. Also perivascular/mesenchymal cells can be the possible cell of origin of the tumor as

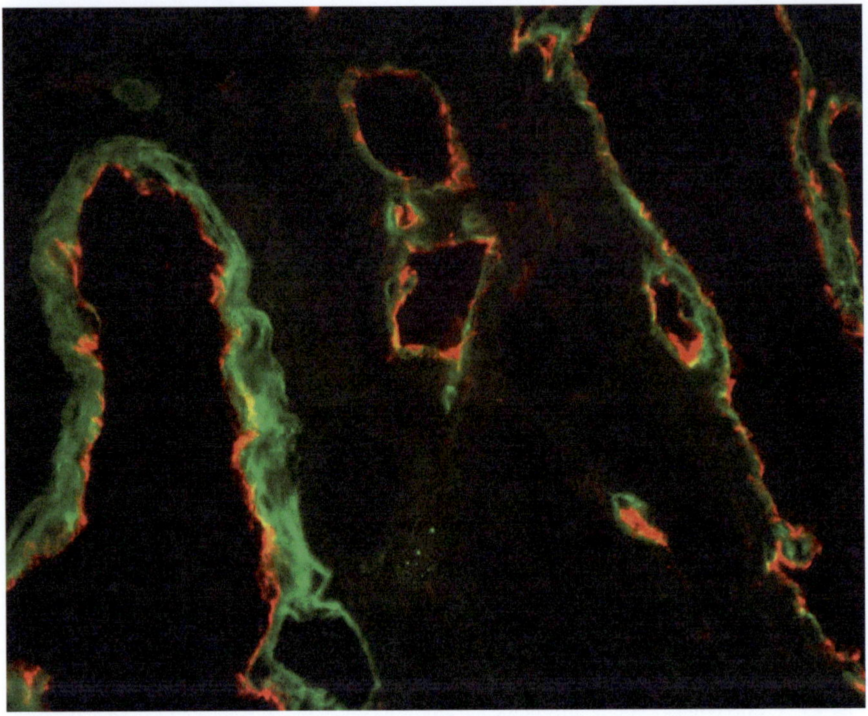

Fig. 4.2 Immunofluorescence staining of JA vessels by CD31 for endothelial cells (*red*) and laminin α2 (*green*) indicate embryological vessels as well as the irregular vascular architecture in a JA

mesenchymal-endothelial transition has been observed in cell lines derived from JAs (Fig. 4.2) [6].

As an important finding, aberrant Wnt-signaling has been detected as a common event in JAs [7]. After description of frequent β-catenin mutations, additional mutations and amplifications of the β-catenin gene (CTNNB1) have been noted with an additional Axin 2 splice variant in JAs [8]. The Wnt-signaling pathway is important not only in tumor biology. This pathway is of great importance especially in embryological development.

Vascular Malformation: Hormone Sensitivity

For a long time immunohistological stainings of hormone receptors were in the focus to understand the exclusive manifestation of JAs despite of normal hormone blood levels and inconspicuous clinical examinations of the affected adolescents. Since aromatase changes are being able to explain testosterone transformation into estrogens, this has been described in JAs as the possibility of not only the testosterone to influence but also the estrogen to have an effect on JAs. Highly interesting was the discovery/isolation of mRNA of the androgen receptor and estrogen receptor α, follicle-stimulating hormone receptor, and luteinizing hormone receptor in JAs. Since the hormones LH and FSH are not only important in adolescence but there is already a hormone peak of both of them early in childhood, this might be an explanation for the early JA manifestations, before adolescence [9].

Summary

Despite the fact that the tumorous cell of origin has not clearly been proven, there is convincing evidence to judge JAs are vascular malformations deriving from remnants of the first branchial arch artery. The origin of the tumor from tissue remnants of the first branchial arch artery gives for the first time the chance to explain its typical tumor features: tumor origin, blood supply, and tumor histology. Molecular proofs were able to define numerous embryological vascular markers in JAs. An aberrant Wnt-signaling pathway is an important finding in JAs. Even though more research work is needed to understand exactly the tumor biology, the most recent findings regarding hormone receptors enable us to understand the almost exclusive tumor manifestation in male adolescents. Additionally, the recent findings regarding the etiology JAs provide the option to understand atypical locations and tumor manifestation at an unusual age.

References

1. Nélaton M. Polype fibreux de la base du crane. Considérations générales. Gaz Hop. 1853;26:22.
2. Schick B, Plinkert PK, Prescher A. Aetiology of angiofibromas: refelction on their specific vascular component. Laryngorhinootologie. 2002;81:280–4.
3. Harrison DFN. The natural history, pathgenesis, and treatment of juvenile angiofibroma. Arch Otolaryngol Head Neck Surg. 1987;113:936–42.
4. Beham A, Regauer S, Beham-Schmid C, Kainz J, Stammberger H. Nasopharyngeal angiofibroma: true neoplasm or vascular malformation? Adv Anat Pathol. 2000;7:36–46.
5. Schick B, Wemmert S, Willnecker V, Dlugaiczyk J, Nicolai P, Siwiec H, Thiel CT, Rauch A, Wendler O. Genome-wide copy number profiling using a 100 K SNP array reveals novel disease-related genes BORIS and TSHZ1 in juvenile angiofibroma. Int J Oncol. 2011;39: 1143–51.
6. Kulas P, Willnecker V, Dlugaiczyk J, Laschke MW, Schick B. Mesenchymal-endothelial transition in juvenile angiofibromas? Acta Otolaryngol. 2015;135:955–61.
7. Abraham SC, Montgomery EA, Giardiello FM, Wu TT. Frequent beta-catenin mutations in juvenile nasopharyngeal angiofibromas. Am J Pathol. 2001;158:1073–8.
8. Wemmert S, Villnecker V, Kulas P, Weber S, Lerner C, Berndt S, Wendler O, Schick B. Identification of CTNNB1 mutations, CTNNB1 amplifications, and an Axin 2 splice variant in juvenile angiofibromas. Tumour Biol. 2016;37:5539–49.
9. Schick B, Dlugaiczyk J, Wendler O. Expression of sex hormone receptors in juvenile angiofibromas and antiproliverative effects of receptor modulators. Head Neck. 2014;36:1596–603.

Part II
Clinical and Radiological Diagnosis

Chapter 5
Clinical Presentation

Siba P. Dubey and Charles P. Molumi

Abstract Juvenile angiofibroma (JA) is a benign tumor. It occurs mostly in prepubescent or pubescent males. From its point of origin, the tumor grows simultaneously in multiple directions and in multiple projections. The topographical understanding of these extensions is important for complete removal of the tumor at operation. The patient initially presents with unilateral nasal obstruction and recurrent unprovoked nosebleed as soon as the tumor occupies the nasopharynx. The tumor grows bigger. Consequently, the nasal obstruction becomes bilateral, epistaxis becomes more frequent, and rhinolalia and obstructive sleep apnea becomes apparent. At this stage the patient used to develop conductive hearing loss due to obstruction of the Eustachian tube by the tumor.

The tumor increases in size, pushes the soft palate down, and produces bulge in it. With further increase in size, the tumor extends caudally and enters into the oropharynx. At this stage, the patient used to have additional complaint in the form of offensive odor, muffled voice, snoring, and even bleeding from the oropharyngeal part of the tumor. The patient used to swallow this blood as it is difficult to regurgitate in presence of the tumor. The patient also develops difficulty in breathing in lying on supine position. The tumor extends anteriorly into the nasal cavity, and the patient additionally develops mucoid or mucopurulent nasal discharge, facial asymmetry, and even obstruction to lacrimal drainage.

Superior extension leads the tumor to sphenoid sinus and then to pituitary fossa and optic chiasma. As a consequence the patient complains of reduced vision and even blindness. The incidence of lateral extension of JA into pterygopalatine fossa is quite high. The tumor spreads further laterally to infratemporal and temporal fossae, orbit, and cheek. The patient develops swelling of the cheek and temple and proptosis. The tumor enters the cranial cavity through the superior orbital fissure or through the middle or anterior cranial fossa floor. Intracranial tumor leads to headache, cranial nerve palsy, and visual aberrations. In rare situation the tumor can enter the parapharyngeal space and produce medial bulge of the lateral wall of the oropharynx.

S.P. Dubey, MS (✉) • C.P. Molumi, MMed
Department of Otolaryngology – Head and Neck Surgery, Port Moresby General Hospital, Boroko, NCD, Papua New Guinea
e-mail: dr_sp_dubey@yahoo.com; pmolumi@gmail.com

S.P. Dubey, B. Schick (eds.), *Juvenile Angiofibroma*,
DOI 10.1007/978-3-319-45343-9_5

Keywords Juvenile angiofibroma • Extension • Clinical features • Intracranial extension

Introduction

Juvenile angiofibroma (JA) is a fibrovascular tumor presenting almost exclusively in adolescent males. Histologically, JAs are benign. However these tumors are highly aggressive and associated with significant morbidity. The exact pathogenesis and site of origin have been debated for a long time and all aspects are still not understood. What is clearer in JAs are their routes of extensions. With the help of superior imaging modalities, we are now able to trace the routes of extensions and correlate them with the clinical features. The embryological explanation about the origin of the tumor is discussed in Chap. 2. The tumor grows in all directions through multiple projections, and these projections have distinct rates of development [1]. Some tumors show preference to grow laterally, while others toward a posterior, medial, anterior, or superior direction [1]. The explanation why this happens is still unknown.

Incomplete understanding of the invasion pattern of JA is one explanation for significant postoperative recurrence [2]. The possible pathways of extensions and location of JA are described in Fig. 5.1. This chapter describes the clinical presentation of the patients according to the locations of the tumor.

Tumor in Nasopharynx

A tumor growing medially enlarges the sphenopalatine foramen and enters nasopharynx. The early clinical features of JA are those due to the tumor in the nasopharynx. They are unprovoked epistaxis, unilateral nasal obstruction, and hearing loss. The tumor is visualized by passing an endoscope through the nose (Fig. 5.2).

Epistaxis is more pronounced in the younger age group. There is reduced tendency of tumor bleeding after the age of 20. The reason for it is explained in Chap. 3. At our institution, 14.0 % patients was in the first, 77.9 % in the second, and 8.1 % in the third decade of life; the youngest patient was 6 years and oldest 32 years old. The largest number of patients was at 13 years in our series. The duration and volume of blood loss during epistaxis apparently reduce as the volume of the tumor increases; the explanation of it is given in Chap. 3. Younger patients with smaller tumors used to bleed severely and the hemoglobin level may go as low as 6 gm%, and blood transfusion at this stage to raise the hemoglobin level may lead to continued bleeding. It is extremely unlikely that severe bleeding leads to preoperative mortality in JA patients.

Unilateral nasal obstruction is the commonest presenting symptom in owver 80 % of cases [3]. When the entire nasopharynx is occupied by the tumor, the contralateral nasal airway is also obstructed. The patient presents with bilateral nasal obstruction, epistaxis from nasal cavities, rhinolalia clausa, and obstructive sleep apnea.

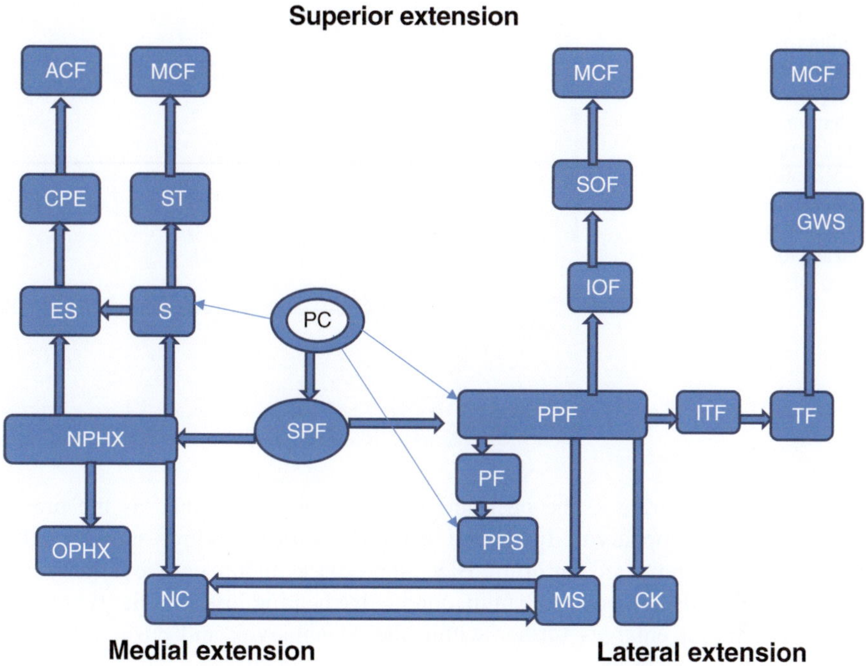

Fig. 5.1 Schematic diagram showing possible pathways of extension and location of JA taking the sphenopalatine foramen as the reference point. *Key to abbreviations: ACF* anterior cranial fossa, *CK* cheek, *CPE* cribriform plate of ethmoid bone, *ES* ethmoid sinus, *GWS* greater wing of sphenoid, *IOF* inferior orbital fissure, *ITF* infratemporal fossa, *MCF* middle cranial fossa, *MS* maxillary sinus, *NC* nasal cavity, *NPHX* nasopharynx, *OPHX* oropharynx, *PC* pterygoid canal, *PF* pterygoid fossa, *PPF* pterygopalatine fossa, *PPS* parapharyngeal space, *S* sphenoid sinus, *SOF* superior orbital fissure, *SPF* sphenopalatine foramen, *ST* sella turcica, *TF* temporal fossa

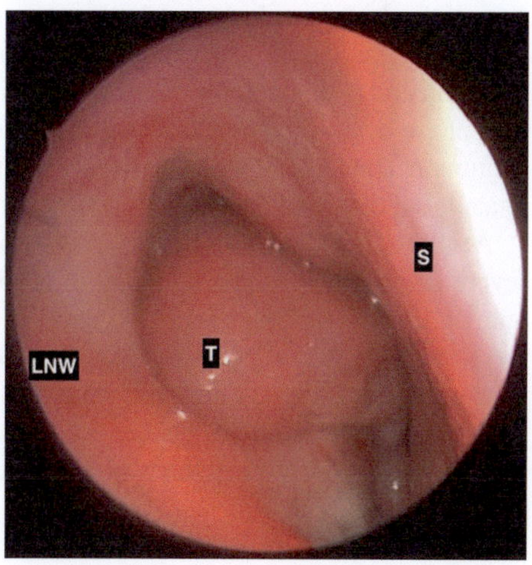

Fig. 5.2 Endoscopic picture of juvenile angiofibroma (*T*) between the nasal septum (*S*) and lateral nasal wall (*LNW*)

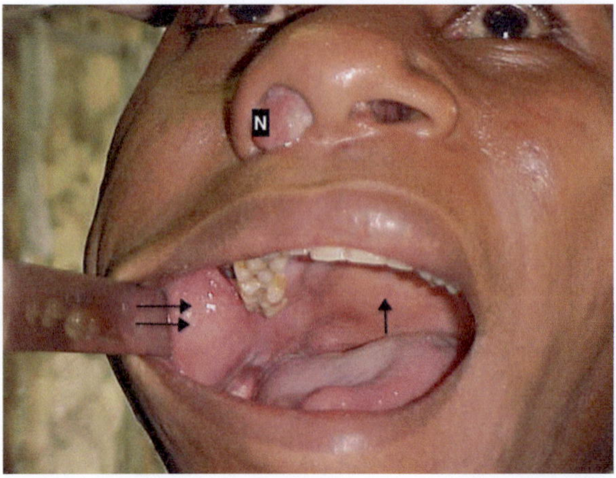

Fig. 5.3 JA expansion within nasopharynx causing the bulging of the soft palate (*arrow*), extension of the tumor to the external nose (*N*), and cheek mucosal swelling (*double arrow*) due to extension of tumor over the anterolateral wall of the maxillary sinus

Hearing loss is due to the obstruction of the Eustachian tube as the tumor expands in the nasopharynx. Ipsilateral serous otitis media follows subsequently. Otoscopy shows retracted ear drum. Bleeding into the middle ear from the tumor happens and leads to hemotympanum, conductive hearing loss, and flat tympanogram. The tumor enlarges further within the nasopharynx and pushes the soft palate caudally and produces clinically apparent bulging of the palate (Fig. 5.3).

Tumor in Oropharynx

With further increase in size, the JA extends down behind and below the level of the soft palate to the oropharynx. The patient presents with halitosis and muffled voice. The tumor is visible when the patient opens his mouth. The patient uses the oral passage for both breathing and feeding. Consequently, the patient eats small volume of food to prevent obstructive apnea while feeding. The caudal-most part of the tumor ulcerates by the food on the tongue as the latter moves up during the pharyngeal phase of swallowing. It may lead to bleeding from the oropharyngeal part of the tumor. The patient ends up swallowing the blood because it is difficult to regurgitate it out due to the tumor in the way.

At this stage both nasal and oral passages are obstructed and the patient has severe obstructive sleep apnea and loud snoring. The patient keeps the head over many pillows with hyperextended neck to maximize the space in the oral passage for breathing. When the tumor expand further to the level of the posterior one third of the tongue, breathing becomes more difficult. The patient becomes drowsy and sweaty and peripheral cyanosis occurs. At this rare stage, an urgent tracheostomy is required to relieve airway obstruction [4]. The authors encountered three such cases (Fig. 5.4).

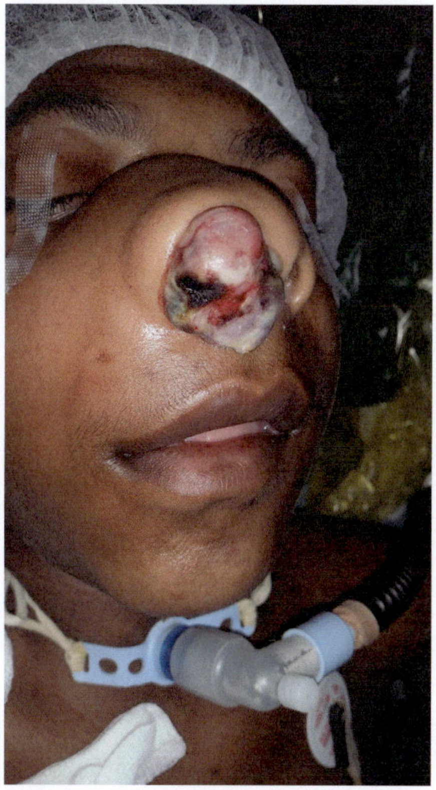

Fig. 5.4 A patient with nasal and oral airway obstruction by JA who required tracheostomy to relieve the airway obstruction

Tumor in Nasal Cavity

The tumor extends anteriorly to fill up the free space in the nasal cavity. With further growth, the JA exerts pressure on the walls of the nasal cavity. It widens the lateral wall and dorsum of the nose with consequent facial asymmetry (Fig. 5.4). Pressure on the lateral wall leads to the flattening of the turbinates. Ipsilateral epiphora results due to obstruction of the nasolacrimal duct [5]. In rare situation, the thin lacrimal bone is eroded by the pressure of large intranasal tumor causing persistent epiphora due to obstruction to the lacrimal sac. The pressure of the tumor pushes the nasal septum medially causing nasal septal deviation and obstructing the contralateral nasal passage. The patient develops mucoid or mucopurulent nasal discharge due to obstruction to sinonasal drainage. The patient also develops hyposmia due to lack of airflow through the nasal passages. Tumor grows further and protrudes out of the anterior naris. The part of the tumor outside the nose is easily traumatized and ulcerated and covered with crusts.

Tumor in Ethmoid Sinus

The tumor in the nasopharynx directly involves the posterior ethmoid sinus. The ethmoid sinus is also invaded by direct extension from the anterior face of the sphenoid sinus [6]. Patients with huge tumor in the nasal cavity can present with total ethmoidal opacification from the tumor. In very rare occasions, the tumor in the ethmoid sinus expands to erode the cribriform plate of the ethmoid bone to enter into the anterior cranial fossa [7, 8]. The symptoms are nonspecific and have features of sinusitis which is overshadowed by more severe symptoms of tumor within the nose, nasopharynx, and other extensions.

Tumor in Sphenoid Sinus

Superiorly, the expanding tumor erodes the anterior face and floor of the sphenoid sinus and fills the sinus cavity [6]. Alternatively, the tumor may arise from the intra-sphenoid part of the pterygoid canal and destroys its medial aspect to enter into the sphenoid sinus [2]. The tumor eventually occupies and expands first in the ipsilateral sinus followed by the contralateral one. Further expansion within the sphenoid leads to "ballooning" of the sinus, erosion of its roof, and displacement of the pituitary gland, and tumor extends into the sella turcica [9]. Pressure on the optic chiasma causes visual field defects (bitemporal hemianopia) and later ipsilateral and contralateral reduced vision or even blindness (Fig. 7.19). The ophthalmological features are described in details in Chap. 6.

Tumor in Pterygopalatine Fossa

From the origin the tumor extends laterally and enters into the pterygopalatine fossa. In males, the craniofacial growth occurs up to the age of 18 years especially between 12 and 14 years [1]. Consequently, the bony walls of the pterygoid fossa are not rigid before puberty and are easily expandable [1]. Hence JA extension in the pterygopalatine fossa creates a passive separation of the articulated bones and allows the tumor to expand in different directions [1]. Invasion of pterygopalatine fossa occurred between 81.81 % and 93.5 % of cases in different series [1, 2]. Subsequently, the tumor extends to infratemporal and temporal fossa, cheek, maxillary sinus, and orbital and cranial cavities. It is the main route by which tumor extends to middle cranial fossa [1].

Tumor in Infratemporal and Temporal Fossa

From the pterygopalatine fossa, JA expands laterally into the infratemporal fossa through the pterygomaxillary fissure. The JA expands to fill up the space of the infratemporal fossa presenting clinically as fullness under the zygoma. JA expands further under the zygoma and extends into the temporal fossa which is seen as dumbbell-shaped swelling in both infratemporal and temporal region and a "relative depression" over the zygomatic bone (Fig. 5.4).

Tumor in Maxillary Sinus and Cheek

As JA expands in the pterygopalatine fossa, it exerts pressure on posterior wall of the maxillary sinus. Figure 7.12 shows anterior bowing of the posterior maxillary wall. The maxillary sinus can be invaded through its posterior wall by the tumor in the pterygopalatine fossa; alternatively, tumor from the nasal cavity may enter the maxillary sinus through its medial wall or vice versa after filling the maxillary sinus [1]. Maxillary sinus invasion by JA may produce features of sinusitis. Rarely, the tumor within the maxillary sinus erodes its anterolateral wall. In most cases the tumor spreads over the posterolateral to the anterolateral wall of the maxillary sinus, and the patients present with cheek bulge intraorally and externally (Figs. 5.3 and 5.4).

Tumor in Orbit and Ophthalmological Features

The tumor in the pterygopalatine fossa moves superiorly to enter the posterior end of the inferior orbital fissure and then to the orbit. In this location, JA pushes the orbital contents outward and the patient develops proptosis. The pressure on the orbital content is from below upward. Hence the proptosis is more marked in the superior orbit as evident by more stretching of the upper eyelid in comparison to the lower one (vide Figs. 6.2 and 6.3 in chap. 6). The details of the ophthalmological features of JA are described in Chap. 6.

Tumor in Parapharyngeal Space

The tumor grows into the pharyngeal recess posterior to the medial pterygoid plate, resulting in invasion of the pterygoid fossa and parapharyngeal space [1]. It may also be possible that parapharyngeal extension occurs when the tumor

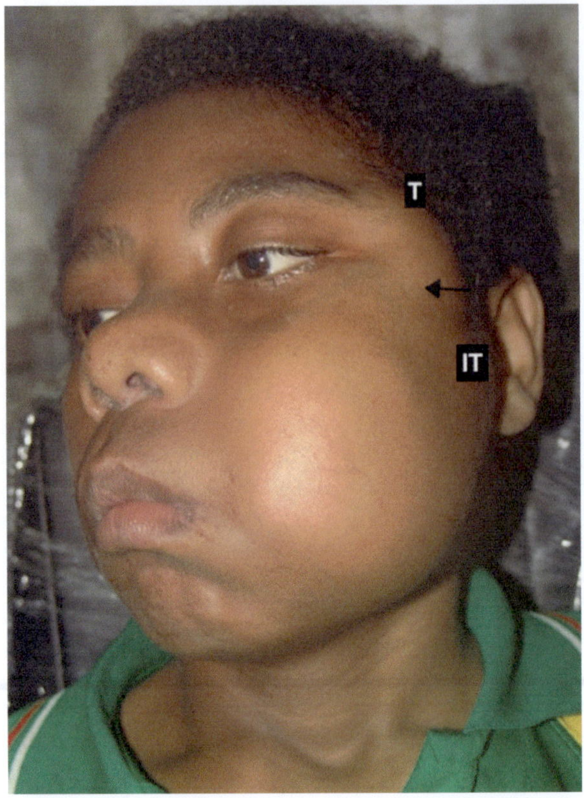

Fig. 5.5 Left JA extension to the orbital apex and lateral extension to the infratemporal and temporal fossa and cheek presenting with cheek swelling, proptosis, dumbbell-shaped swelling in both infratemporal (*IT*) and temporal (*T*) region, and "relative" depression (*arrow*) over the zygoma

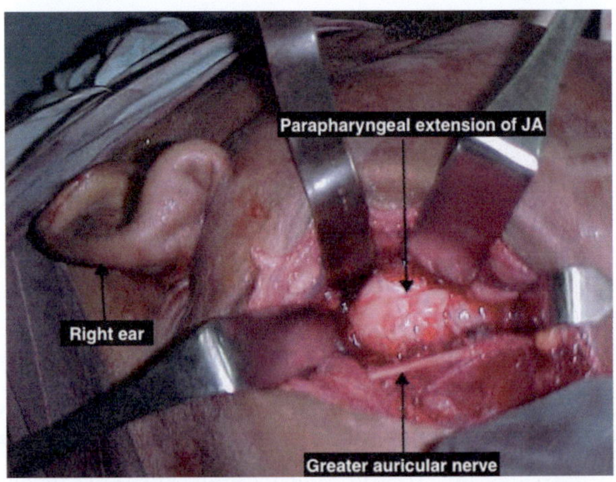

Fig. 5.6 Parapharyngeal extension of JA removed by the lateral cervical approach

arises from the posterior end of the pterygoid canal. The patient presents with swelling below and behind the angle of the mandible and the lateral pharyngeal wall is medialized [10]. An upper lateral cervical approach was needed to remove the parapharyngeal extension in one of our patients (Fig. 5.6).

Intracranial Tumor

In a recent series, intracranial spread at the time of presentation was seen in almost 30 % of patients [11]. Firstly, from the orbit the tumor enters into the middle cranial fossa via superior orbital fissure [1] (Fig. 7.20). In our institution, most intracranial extensions occurred by this route. Secondly, tumor also enters the intracranial cavity by erosion of the bony greater wing of the sphenoid bone forming the floor of the middle cranial fossa between the foramina of rotundum, ovale, and lacerum [12]. Facial pain associated with divisions of trigeminal nerve is noticed in this type of extension [6]. Direct extension superiorly from the sphenoid sinus through the sella turcica to the middle cranial fossa can occur [1, 6]. Very rarely the tumor can enter anterior cranial fossa through the cribriform plate of ethmoid [7, 8]. Aggressive JA may invade the cavernous sinus and threaten III, IV, V1, V2, and VI cranial nerves, the internal carotid artery, the hypophysis, and the optic chiasma [12]. Intracranial tumors give rise to headache, proptosis, diplopia, cranial nerve palsy, ophthalmoplegia, optic atrophy, reduced vision or blindness, papilledema, and facial numbness [7, 8, 11].

Angiofibroma in Adult and Elderly

There are few reports of angiofibroma presenting in the adults and elderly above the age of 30 years and beyond [13–18]. They usually present with blood-stained nasal discharge instead of epistaxis [14, 16, 18, 19]. The reason for this is explained in Chap. 3. Unilateral nasal discharge or blood-stained mucous discharge in adult indicates a malignant process, and hence, the diagnosis of angiofibroma is ignored and usually diagnosed after a biopsy [13, 16, 18, 19] or from the postoperative specimen [14, 15, 17]. Many of the origin and extensions of angiofibroma in adult and elderly are not typical like JA in prepubescent or pubescent males [15, 17]. Immunohistochemical analysis helps to confirm the diagnosis [15, 17].

References

1. Sennes LU, Butugan O, Sanchez TG, et al. Juvenile angiofibroma: the routes of invasion. Rhinology. 2003;41:235–40.
2. Liu Z, Wang D, Sun X, Wang J, Hu L, Han L, Dai P. The site of origin and expansive routes of juvenile nasopharyngeal angiofibroma (JNA). Int J Pediatr Otorhinolaryngol. 2011;75:1088–92.
3. Bremer JW, Neel HB, De Santo W, Jones GC, Rochester MN. Angiofibroma: treatment trends in 150 patients during 40 years. Laryngoscope. 1989;96:1321–9.
4. Singh HP, Kumar S, Vashistha M, Aggarwal SP. Stridor: an unusual presentation of juvenile angiofibroma. BMJ Case Rep. 2014;7:1–4.
5. Llorente JL, Lopez F, Suarez V, Costales M, Suarez C. Evolution in the treatment of juvenile nasopharyngeal angiofibroma. Acta Otorrinolaringol Esp. 2011;62:279–86.

6. Spector JC. Management of juvenile angiofibromata. Laryngoscope. 1988;98:1016–26.
7. Jafek BW, Krekorian EA, Kirsch WM, Wood RP. Juvenile nasopharyngeal angiofibroma: management of intracranial extension. Head Neck Surg. 1979;2:119–28.
8. Gill G, Rice DH, Ritter FN, Kindt G, Russo HR. Intracranial and extracranial nasopharyngeal angiofibroma. Arch Otolaryngol. 1976;102:371–3.
9. Dubey SP, Molumi CP, Apaio ML. Total maxillary swing approach to the skull base for advanced intracranial and extracranial nasopharyngeal angiofibroma. J Craniofac Surg. 2011;22:1671–6.
10. Johnson JE, Yang PJ, Koopmann Jr CF, Heffner DK. Parapharyngeal angiofibroma. Am J Neuroradiol. 1987;8:1152–3.
11. Mattei TA, Nogueira GF, Ramina R. Juvenile nasopharyngeal angiofibroma with intracranial extension. Otolaryngol Head Neck Surg. 2011;145:498–505.
12. Bales C, Kotapka M, Loevner LA, Al-Rawi M, Weinstein G, Hurst R, Weber RS. Craniofacial resection of advanced juvenile nasopharyngeal angiofibroma. Arch Otolaryngol Head Neck Surg. 2002;128:1071–8.
13. Pradillo JA, Rodriguez HA, Arrayo JF. Nasopharyngeal angiofibroma in the elderly: report of a case. Laryngoscope. 1975;85:1063–5.
14. Sukumaran P, Pillai B. Nasopharyngeal angiofibroma in the fifth decade. Indian J Otolaryngol. 1977;29:17–8.
15. Zhang H, Wang J, Liu Z, Wang D. Management of nasopharyngeal angiofibroma in a 72 years old male through a sublabial and buccolabial incision approach: a case report and literature review. Oncol Lett. 2015;10:1267–70.
16. Szyfter W, Popoko M, Leszczynska M, Gawecki W. Exclusively endoscopic approach for juvenile angiofibroma in adult-a case report. Videosurg Other Non Invasive Tech. 2010;5: 107–9.
17. Sarafoleanu C, Enache R, Sabaru I. Unusual case of nasopharyngeal angiofibroma in adult male patient. Rom J Rhinol. 2011;1:218–20.
18. Panigrahi R. Angiofibroma in an elderly-a case report. Indian J Res Rep Med Sci. 2012;2:31–2.
19. Lukomski M, Danilewicz, Pajor A. Juvenile angiofibroma in adults. Otolaryngol Pol. 2008; 63:20–6.

Chapter 6
Juvenile Angiofibroma and Eye

Guoxing Xu and Yuanten Xu

Abstract Juvenile angiofibroma is a rare vascular hamartoma that often occurs in adolescent boys. The continuous growth of tumor can cause bone resorption and destruction of the medial orbital wall, optic canal, chiasmatic–sellar region, clivus, etc. In addition, juvenile angiofibroma may also invade the eye through the inferior orbital fissure. According to the abovementioned reasons, there are a series of eye symptoms and signs among which exophthalmos and ocular dysmotility are common. Optic nerve and chiasma compression result in visual acuity impairment, metamorphopsia, visual field defects, and even blindness. The compressed cavernous sinus could lead to tortuous retinal veins, retinal edema, and palpebral edema. Pressure over oculomotor, trochlear, and abducens nerve could induce paralysis of the corresponding extraocular muscles and presenting as strabismus.

Keywords Juvenile angiofibroma • Orbit • Optic nerve • Visual acuity • Visual field defect

Effects of Juvenile Angiofibroma Compressing Orbit and Visual Pathway

Compressing the Orbit

Seven skull bones join together to form the orbit and between each of which exists a bony interval. The medial wall of the orbit is the ethmoid sinus; behind the medial wall is the sphenoid sinus. Above and in front of the orbit is the frontal sinus, and below the orbit is the maxillary sinus. The main route of orbital invasion by juvenile angiofibroma mass is the inferior orbital fissure, or it can compress the intraocular contents through bone walls of the paranasal sinuses. Pressure from the growing tumor could erode the bone of the medial and inferior orbital wall and compressing

G. Xu, MD (✉) • Y. Xu, MD
Department of Ophthalmology and Otolaryngology–Head & Neck Surgery,
First Affiliated Hospital of Fujian Medical University, Fuzhou,
Fujian Province, China, 350005
e-mail: fjmuxgx@163.com

S.P. Dubey, B. Schick (eds.), *Juvenile Angiofibroma*,
DOI 10.1007/978-3-319-45343-9_6

the bulbus oculi through the ethmoid and the maxillary sinus wall. This may cause exophthalmos and ocular dislocation. The tumor spreads to the pterygopalatine fossa, inferior orbital fissure, and superior orbital fissure and then into the orbital and cranial fossa and compresses the eye, optic nerve, and chiasma [1].

Compressing Optic Nerve and Optic Chiasma

Juvenile angiofibroma may grow into the cranium causing compression on the optic nerve and elevated intracranial pressure. Large juvenile angiofibromas involve the optic nerve and chiasm. When the optic nerve is compressed and displaced, visual impairment is detected. On condition that optic nerve was not obviously involved, visual acuity, the b-wave amplitude in electroretinography (ERG), and P-wave latency in visual evoked potential (VEP) could be normal. When proptosis was accompanied by visual acuity impairment, the b-wave amplitude in ERG decreased and P-wave latency in VEP elongated. The tumor mass originates from the sphenopalatine foramen or near the medial wall of the pterygoid canal. In such a situation, optic nerve and optic chiasma are affected by a rapidly growing juvenile angiofibroma Alternatively, juvenile angiofibroma could destroy the sella turcica and its surrounding bones through the sphenoid sinus and compress optic nerve, optic chiasm, the cavernous sinus, and internal carotid artery. Optic nerve edema, disk edema, and a pale optic disk are detected via fundus examination. At this stage, the visual symptoms are visual acuity impairment, metamorphopsia, and visual field defects.

Foster–Kennedy syndrome (FKS) is usually caused by a frontal lobe glioma or an olfactory groove meningioma. Juvenile angiofibroma is a rare cause of FKS. FKS presents as one atrophic and one papilledematous optic nerve head of bilateral asymmetric optic atrophy. The mechanism of direct optic nerve compression in one eye and increased intracranial pressure is not the only way to develop FKS. Both compression and increased intracranial pressure cause disk swelling by interrupting of axoplasmic transport. And ophthalmic examination would reveal no light perception in one eye and mildly decreased visual acuity in another one. In order to avoid FKS, surgical resection is the most common primary treatment for the early case [2].

Compressing the Cavernous Sinus

The cavernous sinus receives blood via the superior and inferior ophthalmic veins through the superior orbital fissure and from superficial cortical veins and is connected to the basilar plexus of veins posteriorly. The internal carotid artery and cranial nerves III, IV, V (branches V1 and V2), and VI all pass through this blood-filled space. Tumor mass near the sphenopalatine foramen and the lateral plate of pterygoid process may destroy sella turcica and the adjacent bone and compress the cavernous sinus and internal carotid artery through sphenoid sinus, thus obstructing the backflow from central retinal vein [3]. Since the central retinal vein is one of the important sources of drainage

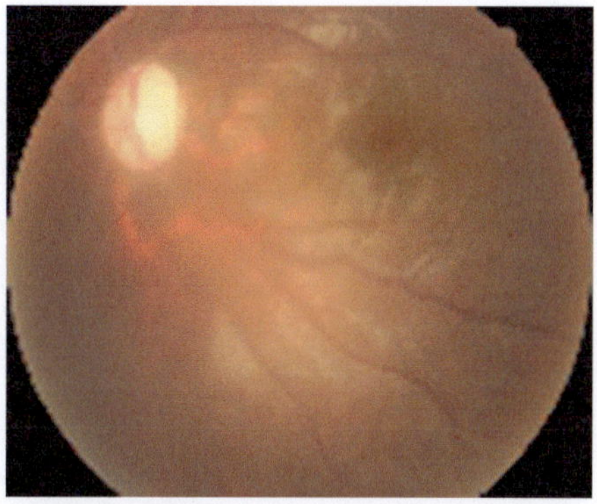

Fig. 6.1 When the optic nerve, cavernous sinus, and internal carotid artery are compressed by juvenile angiofibroma, white, edematous retina and retinal artery occlusion are noted via fundus examination

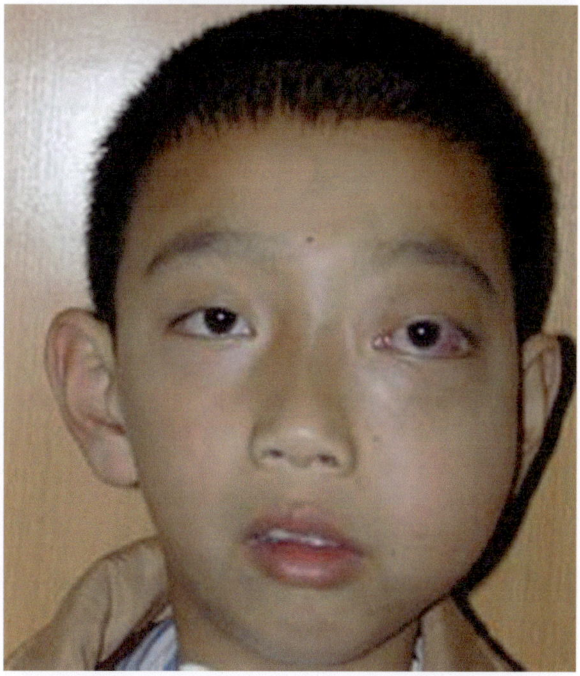

Fig. 6.2 Photograph showing proptosis due to intraorbital extension of JA; extension to the cheek is also visible

from the retina, such occlusion can lead to severe damage to the retina, namely, ischemia and edema. The patients may encounter visual acuity impairment and distorted vision, and the fundus examination shows tortuous retinal veins and retinal and macular edema (Fig. 6.1). In addition, angular vein joins the superior ophthalmic vein, and the latter passes below the Zinn's ring, along the lateral wall of the superior orbital fissure, and finally enters the cavernous sinus. For this reason, backflow obstruction in the cavernous sinus or its distal stump could result in varicosity of the palpebral and superior ophthalmic vein, and patient develops swelling of the eyelids and even ptosis (Figs. 6.2 and 6.3). Salcone and Pepin [4] reported a case of patient with juvenile angiofibroma whose early manifestation was left esotropia, followed by severe visual loss. Extensive involvement

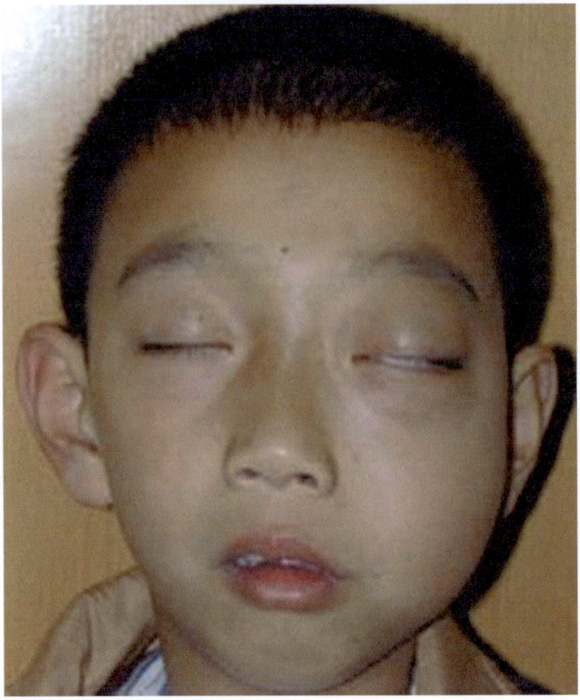

Fig. 6.3 Photograph showing swelling of the eyelids due to the obstruction of the palpebral and superior ophthalmic veins secondary to obstruction of the cavernous sinus

of the cavernous sinus leads to paresis of the sixth and the fourth cranial nerve, resulting in the dysfunction of the superior oblique and lateral rectus muscles, with the manifestation of esotropia. It is proved that decompensation of a preexisting phoria or monofixation syndrome is the most common cause of acute esotropia [5].

Juvenile Angiofibroma and Retrobulbar Neuritis

At early stage, no abnormalities are noted in the fundus of patients with retrobulbar neuritis. Later visual acuity impairment, visual field defects, absent light perception, and moderately dilated pupil are detected in the patients. The direct pupillary light reflex becomes sluggish or disappears, while the indirect pupillary light reflex still presents. Nasosinusitis is the main cause of retrobulbar neuritis. Inflammation in the nasal cavity and paranasal sinus spreads to the optic nerve directly or via blood and lymph indirectly. The bony wall between the ethmoid sinus, sphenoid sinus, and the optic nerve is as thin as paper. For this reason, it is easy for inflammation to involve the optic nerve. Zhang and Sun [6] have reported a case of juvenile angiofibroma which was mistaken as retrobulbar neuritis at the beginning. A patient who complained of no light perception in the left eye for 1 week, with left nasal cavity full of tumor mass, was admitted in the Department of Ophthalmology.

There is no improvement after 1 week of conservative treatment. During the tumor resection, ENT surgeons found that the posterior ethmoidal cells and the sphenoid sinus had fused together, while the internal mucosa was edematous and congested. Pathological examination showed the tumor mass to be juvenile angiofibroma.

Ocular Complications Following Preoperative Embolization

In most cases, juvenile angiofibroma receives blood supply from external carotid artery and sometimes from internal carotid artery. In cases of advanced disease, internal carotid artery contributes to the vascular supply [7]. Because juvenile angiofibroma is a highly vascular benign tumor, intraoperative tumor bleeding is one of the major concerns during operation. Hence, most authors consider it to be necessary to have preoperative embolization; in order to minimize intraoperative bleeding, this procedure should be performed within 24–48 h prior to surgery [8, 9]. However, McCombe et al. [10] assume that embolization may be the cause of recurrences because embolized tumor shrinks, and its removal from remote areas becomes complicated. Besides, embolization procedure may have some severe thromboembolic complications such as central retinal artery occlusion (CRAO). CRAO is an ocular emergency that causes abrupt and generally irreversible visual loss unless retinal circulation is reestablished before irreversible ischemic damage occurs. As it is well known, retina receives its blood supply from two sources. The choriocapillaris of the choroid nurtures the outer retina, whereas the central retinal artery (CRA) and its end branches feed the inner retinal layers. Therefore, the occlusion of the CRA deprives the entire inner retina of its blood supply unless a cilioretinal artery is present (in 15–30 % of eyes). Fundus examination of a patient with juvenile angiofibroma who lost his vision in the left eye following embolization showed (i) prominent segmentation of the blood column in the narrowed arterioles and venules, (ii) the retina appears white as a result of cloudy swelling caused by intracellular edema, and (iii) as the central fovea is devoid of these layers, the orange reflex from the intact choroidal vessels beneath the foveola stands out in contrast to the surrounding opaque retina, giving rise to the "cherry-red spot" appearance. The pupillary response to direct illumination was poor with a dense relative afferent pupillary defect (RAPD). Visual acuity impairment, visual field defects, and even no light perception are found in patients with CRAO [11, 12].

Postoperative Complications After Tumor Excision

If the retina, macula, and optic nerve are only mildly affected by juvenile angiofibroma, tumor excision and the following optic nerve decompression may return the eye to the normal position and restore visual acuity. However, the relationship between the orbit and the origin of juvenile angiofibroma is intricate; therefore, surgery may bring some complications [1, 13, 14].

Ocular Complications Related to Pterygopalatine Ganglion Injury

Tear comes from basal and reflex secretion, with the latter secreted by lacrimal gland. It serves to clean and lubricate the eyes in response to an irritation of the eyes. The parasympathetic and sympathetic nerve root joins in the vidian canal to form a single nerve (the vidian nerve) before entering the pterygopalatine ganglion. The lacrimal secretion is coordinated by the efferent pathway from the vidian nerve and pterygopalatine ganglion to the lacrimal glands. Pterygopalatine fossa is a small pyramidal space that houses the pterygopalatine ganglion. Studies indicate that, in most cases, angiofibroma takes origin in the pterygopalatine fossa at the opening of the vidian canal. Juvenile angiofibroma extends along the pterygoid canal and invades the cancellous bone of the pterygoid base and greater wing of the sphenoid [15]. The most common site involved by juvenile angiofibroma was pterygopalatine fossa (100 %); it was followed by nasal cavity (94.7 %), then sphenoid sinus (84.2 %), and nasopharynx (73.7 %) [16]. Lin C et al. [17] found that in 15 out of 35 patients with juvenile angiofibroma, the tumor was near the sphenopalatine foramen, and others mainly originated from the posterior of lateral nasal wall. Yi et al. [18, 19] also suggested that juvenile angiofibroma mainly originated from the sphenopalatine foramen. The vidian nerve carries fibers for lacrimation. However, the pterygopalatine ganglion and vidian nerve may be removed or damaged during the surgical process, resulting in postoperative lacrimal hyposecretion [20]. Lacrimal dysfunction should be considered an expected consequence of surgery [20, 21]. After bilateral vidian neurectomy, bilateral sensory neurons of the trigeminal nerve and sympathetic nerve could be damaged, the exact mechanisms of which remained unknown. Lin et al. [22] speculated that a strong aberrant electric current might flow through the vidian nerve to the trigeminal ganglion and then damage the sensory fibers and possibly the sympathetic fibers in the ophthalmic nerve, finally resulting in the decrease of lacrimation and corneal epithelial defect, with the manifestation of neurotrophic keratopathy.

Pyocele of the Lacrimal Sac After Operation

When the surgery for juvenile angiofibroma involves the maxillary sinus, the resection of the medial wall of the maxillary sinus is indicated. Management of the nasolacrimal duct may be a challenge. Classically simple section of the duct is sufficient but in some cases, the section is done very close to the sac. The anatomy may be highly distorted, sequel of the previous surgery for juvenile angiofibroma. As a result, the patient can experience intermittent or persistent epiphora, which usually did not draw patient's attention until infection occurred. A mucocele of the lacrimal sac results from a combination of a complete occlusion of the nasolacrimal duct and the presence of mucoid secretions within the sac. In case of an acute bacterial infection, a skin fistula can occur. Open surgery for juvenile angiofibroma with a complete removal of the sinus mucosa leads to the formation of crusts and fibrosis in the operated cavities. This can contribute to a stenosis of the remnant part of the "lacrimal duct." Clinical manifestations of the patient are intermittent, persistent tearing and even acute dacryocystitis [23].

Rare Eye Complications due to Juvenile Angiofibroma

According to a case report, a patient had concomitant combined juvenile angiofibroma and hamartoma of the retinal pigment epithelium and retina in the ipsilateral eye. Combined hamartoma of the retina and retinal pigment epithelium is a rare disorder that causes a benign, unilateral lesion comprised of a slightly elevated pigmented mass without signs of inflammation. These lesions are characteristically composed of elements of retinal pigment epithelium, retina, and vascular origin. Presenting symptoms include painless visual loss, strabismus, floaters, occasional ocular pain, and leukocoria, and it may be mistaken for a malignant tumor, such as retinoblastoma or choroidal melanoma. The diagnosis of juvenile angiofibroma was based on histopathology of the excised tumor, and the diagnosis of the combined hamartoma was based on the typical ophthalmoscopic and fluorescein angiographic appearance of the fundus lesion. It has been suggested that juvenile angiofibroma may arise from abnormalities of differentiation at the nonchromaffin paraganglionic cells of the terminal end of the maxillary artery or as a desmoplastic response of the nasopharyngeal periosteum to an ectopic focus of vascular tissue. Recently, it has been shown that activated transforming growth factor b1, a cytokine involved with vascular proliferation and stromal cell proliferation, is localized to the fibroblasts and endothelial cells within juvenile angiofibroma tumors. It may be possible that factors, such as transforming growth factor b1, which lead to the elaboration of the angiofibroma, also lead to the development of the combined hamartoma [24].

Giant Juvenile Angiofibroma Invading the Skull Base

Giant juvenile angiofibroma not only invades the orbit but also has a tendency of intracranial extension, extensively involving the sella turcica and clivus. If the tumor extends to middle cranial fossa and anterior cranial fossa, it would affect the optic tract, pituitary gland, cavernous sinus, and internal carotid artery. According to our experience, the dura mater is intact in most cases [14]. The dura mater is a tough fibrous membrane, the excellent elasticity of which makes it tolerate the stress induced by tumor. Giant juvenile angiofibroma could be removed via the infratemporal fossa, middle fossa, or anterior fossa approach, even a combined intracranial–extracranial procedure [25, 26].

Conclusion

An early diagnosis to avoid orbital invasion by juvenile angiofibroma, an adequate approach to deal with it, total tumor resection to achieve optic nerve decompression, and efforts by a team of ENT specialists and ophthalmologists is most likely to yield optimal results. In all cases, preoperative angiography and, if possible, endovascular embolization of tumor feeders are essential, even if the tumor is supplied both from external and internal carotid arteries. In addition, it is important to be aware of the surgical complications of juvenile angiofibroma. Protecting lacrimal passage during surgery should be taken into consideration. Dissecting an intact and displaced pterygopalatine ganglion and vidian nerve from the tumor to preserve their function, while not compromising excision of the tumor, still remains a surgical challenge. In conclusion, learning the mechanism of ocular complications by juvenile angiofibroma would be of great benefit in treating the tumor.

References

1. Xu Y, Lin G, Lin C, Fang Z, Li Z, Zhou A, et al. Treatment and prognosis of nasopharyngeal angiofibroma involving the eye and optic nerve. J Laryngol Otol. 2012;126:1108–13.
2. Aga A. Juvenile nasopharyngeal angiofibroma presenting as Foster Kennedy Syndrome. Ethiop Med J. 2001;39:251–60.
3. Guoxing Xu, editor. Fundamentals of ophthalmology. New Wun Ching Developmental Publishing Co., Ltd., Taipe; 2008. p. 10–30.
4. Salcone EM, Pepin SM. Intermittent esotropia as the initial presentation of juvenile nasopharyngeal angiofibroma. J AAPOS. 2004;8:201–3.
5. Lyons CJ, Tiffin PA, Oystreck D. Acute acquired comitant esotropia: a prospective study. Eye. 1999;13(Pt 5):617–20.
6. Zhongfang Z, Zhongyi S. Nasopharyngeal angiofibroma misdiagnosed as optic neuritis in 1 case after the ball. J Clin Otorhinolaryngol. 1999;13:502.
7. Nicolai P, Villaret AB, Farina D, Nadeau S, Yakirevitch A, Berlucchi M, et al. Endoscopic surgery for juvenile angiofibroma: a critical review of indications after 46 cases. Am J Rhinol Allergy. 2010;24:e67–72.
8. Midilli R, Karci B, Akyildiz S. Juvenile nasopharyngeal angiofibroma: analysis of 42 cases and important aspects of endoscopic approach. Int J Pediatr Otorhinolaryngol. 2009;73:401–8.
9. Bleier BS, Kennedy DW, Palmer JN, Chiu AG, Bloom JD, O'Malley Jr BW. Current management of juvenile nasopharyngeal angiofibroma: a tertiary center experience 1999–2007. Am J Rhinol Allergy. 2009;23:328–30.
10. McCombe A, Lund VJ, Howard DJ. Recurrence in juvenile angiofibroma. Rhinology. 1990;28:97–102.
11. Onerci M, Gumus K, Cil B, Eldem B. A rare complication of embolization in juvenile nasopharyngeal angiofibroma. Int J Pediatr Otorhinolaryngol. 2005;69:423–8.
12. Finis D, Gumbel H. Central retinal artery occlusion after embolization in juvenile nasopharyngeal angiofibroma. Klin Monbl Augenheilkd. 2009;226:579–80.
13. Patrocinio JA, Patrocinio LG, Martins LP, da Cunha AR. Vision recovery following nasopharyngeal angiofibroma excision. Auris Nasus Larynx. 2002;29:309–11.

14. Li KK, Lucarelli MJ, Bilyk JR, Joseph MP. Optic nerve decompression for compressive neuropathy secondary to neoplasia. Arch Otolaryngol Head Neck Surg. 1997;123:425–9.
15. Lloyd G, Howard D, Phelps P, Cheesman A. Juvenile angiofibroma: the lessons of 20 years of modern imaging. J Laryngol Otol. 1999;113:127–34.
16. Cruz AA, Atique JM, Melo-Filho FV, Elias Jr J. Orbital involvement in juvenile nasopharyngeal angiofibroma: prevalence and treatment. Ophthalmic Plast Reconstr Surg. 2004;20:296–300.
17. Chang Lin, Zhi-chun Li, Jin-mei Cheng, Gongbiao Lin, Ai-dong Zhou, Yi Zixiang. Nasopharyngeal angiofibroma of pathological features and clinical treatment. Chin J Otolaryngol Head Neck Surg. 2008;43:763–6.
18. Yi ZX, Li ZC, Cheng JM, Zhang R, Lin C, Zhou AD, et al. Huge nasopharyngeal angiofibroma with intracranial extension: change in the dura mater and choice of surgical management. J Laryngol Otol. 2007;121:1108–12.
19. Yi Z, Li ZC, Lin C, Ye S. Huge lobulated juvenile angiofibroma: sites of extension and selection of procedures for management. J Otolaryngol. 2003;32:211–6.
20. Rong Z, Zixiang Y, Chang L, Guoxing X, Sheng Z, Yuanteng X, et al. Lacrimal hyposecretion: a surgical complication of juvenile nasopharyngeal angiofibroma. Am J Otolaryngol. 2008;29:367–71.
21. Hillel AT, Metzinger RC, Nemechek AJ, Nuss DW. Loss of reflex tearing: an expected consequence of juvenile nasopharyngeal angiofibroma. Otolaryngol Head Neck Surg. 2005;133:605–10.
22. Lin PY, Cheng CY, Wu CC, Yen MY, Wang SJ, Liao KK, et al. Bilateral neurotrophic keratopathy complicating Vidian neurectomy. Am Ophthalmol. 2001;132:106–8.
23. Eloy P, Bachy V, Grulois V, Bertrand B. Pyocele of the lachrymal sac: a late and unusual complication after surgery for a juvenile nasopharyngeal angiofibroma. Clin Ophthalmol. 2008;2:211–5.
24. Fonseca RA, Dantas MA, Kaga T, Spaide RF. Combined hamartoma of the retina and retinal pigment epithelium associated with juvenile nasopharyngeal angiofibroma. Am J Ophthalmol. 2001;132:131–2.
25. Hardillo JA, Vander Velden LA, Knegt PP. Denker operation is an effective surgical approach in managing juvenile nasopharyngeal angiofibroma. Ann Otol Rhinol Laryngol. 2004;113:946–50.
26. Donald PJ, Enepikedes D, Boggan J. Giant juvenile nasopharyngeal angiofibroma: management by skull-base surgery. Arch Otolaryngol Head Neck Surg. 2004;130:882–6.

Chapter 7
Radiological Diagnosis

Mitesh Gandhi and Jennifer Sommerville

Abstract The clinical presentation of juvenile angiofibroma (JA) combined with the pathognomonic imaging features of the tumor are usually sufficient to make the diagnosis. The characteristic features of JA on cross-sectional imaging together with specialised MR and CT techniques currently used are delineated in this chapter. The growth patterns of the tumor (which vary from patient to patient) are described, being of some importance in surgical planning and preoperative counselling. The role of angiography in preoperative imaging is briefly mentioned. Potential mimics of JA on imaging are rare and usually not difficult to differentiate from JA. The use of imaging following surgical resection to detect residual disease is discussed. The rare entity of extranasopharyngeal angiofibroma is also described.

Keyword Juvenile angiofibroma • Imaging • CT • MRI • Angiography

Introduction

Juvenile angiofibroma (JA) is a unique tumor for many reasons. As it is a rare tumor, there are no prospective studies looking at a statistically large cohort of JAs. All studies of this condition are based on retrospective studies of varying number of patients. The opportunity to challenge or interrogate this tumor with various novel imaging techniques including diffusion-perfusion MRI, spectroscopy, molecular imaging with PET and high-resolution ultrasound using robust well-designed prospective studies has not yet been utilised due to the infrequent occurrence of this condition and the absence of designated JA centres where relatively large populations can be studied.

The imaging and management of this neoplasm currently relies on the triumvirate modalities of CT, MRI and interventional angiography. Plain film radiology is rarely utilised as a first-line investigation but may be performed in the setting of a primary care centre or in areas where cross-sectional imaging is not available.

M. Gandhi, FRACR (✉) • J. Sommerville, FRACR
Department of Medical Imaging, Princess Alexandra Hospital and Queensland Xray, Brisbane, QLD, Australia
e-mail: miteshalka@gmail.com; jensommerville@me.com

S.P. Dubey, B. Schick (eds.), *Juvenile Angiofibroma*,
DOI 10.1007/978-3-319-45343-9_7

The initial diagnosis of a JA relies on the clinical presentation (adolescent and exclusively male, presenting with a blocked nose with epistaxis), flexible nasendoscopy (FNE) findings of a vascular submucosal nasopharyngeal mass and imaging. Direct endoscopic visualisation of the tumor does not usually give a true indication of the size and extent of the lesion and may just see "the tip of the iceberg". Cross-sectional imaging in particular is therefore essential in assessing the true anatomical extent of the tumor. Biopsy is difficult given the vascular nature of the lesion [1, 2] and generally is not recommended or required for diagnosis in the presence of pathognomonic imaging.

Historically, the cumulative results of cross-sectional imaging studies have derived theories on the origin of the tumor and descriptions of its patterns of growth. In turn, staging systems have been described, and the predominantly surgical management of this condition has evolved. Preoperative angiographic embolisation has been utilised to control blood loss at surgery.

Imaging continues to play a role in post surgical surveillance to detect recurrences (in reality residual tumor which has grown) that may lead to further surgical treatment but may also be used to monitor the effects of radiotherapy when utilised in conjunction with surgery to treat intracranial extension.

Brief History

The angiofibroma is said to have been first described by Hippocrates in 4 BC when he removed a hard nasal polyp through a midline nose-splitting incision [3]. Liston in 1841 performed the first documented resection of a JA like "fibrovascular" lesion at University College Hospital, London [4], and in 1847 Chelius described the JA as a "fibrous polyp" occurring in adolescent males [5]. Legouest in 1865 associated JAs with young males. In 1873 Gosselin hypothesised that the tumors regressed as they were not seen after sexual maturity [6]. In 1906 Chaveau coined the term "juvenile nasal fibroma" [7], whereas Friedberg coined the term "juvenile nasal angiofibroma" in 1940 [8].

The discovery of the X-ray in 1895 by Wilhelm Conrad Roentgen marked the beginning of the imaging "journey" of this condition. In 1927 Egas Moniz performed the first cerebral angiogram. The technique of angiography entered a new and safer phase with the advent of transfemoral catheterisation introduced by Sven-Ivar Seldinger in 1953. This was followed by the technique of interventional embolisation in the 1960s. The next major modality breakthrough was in 1972 with the introduction of computed tomography by Godfrey Hounsfield. In 1973 Paul Lauterbur published the first MR image.

This time line parallels the appearance in the literature of the imaging manifestations of JA with the plain film descriptions of nasopharyngeal tumors appearing in the 1920s leading up to CT descriptions in the late 1970s and MR descriptions appearing in the 1980s.

Classic Imaging Descriptions of Primary Presentations

Modalities Used

Plain Films

Plain films are no longer used in the initial workup of a suspected nasopharyngeal lesion and therefore will not be reviewed in detail. The characteristic plain-film changes are well described [1, 9] but are rarely seen in practice. The findings are:

1. A soft tissue mass in the nasopharynx, sphenoid sinus or nose with displacement of nasal septum, maxillary or ethmoid or frontal sinuses
2. Anterior bowing of posterior maxillary wall, a sign of a slowly growing mass, known as the Holman-Miller sign
3. Erosion of the orbital margins
4. Erosion of the zygomatic arch
5. Erosion of bony margins of the nasopharynx

The JA is a slow-growing neoplasm which produces pressure changes on adjacent bone which can consist of bowing as in the Holman-Miller sign or erosion of bone. There may be reactive sclerosis around the expanding lesion as a healing response to the lesion.

Cross-Sectional Imaging

Both CT and MRI are now used as complementary tools in the preoperative assessment of a JA [2]. CT may be used in isolation in hospitals where MRI is not readily accessible or in the situation in which the patient cannot have an MRI (due to claustrophobia or because of the presence of ferromagnetic implant/foreign body in the patient).

The breakthrough in the understanding of the origin, nature and growth patterns of JA developed with the advent of computed tomography (CT) in the 1970s [10–13]. Initially with the "single slice" scanners, coronal and axial projections were obtained with the patient's head being placed in a hyperextended position for the coronal imaging. Intravenous iodinated contrast was and is used to depict the intensely enhancing tumor and to differentiate it from the surrounding soft tissues.

These techniques have evolved with the advent of spiral CT technology with rapid scans now being acquired as a volume of tissue acquisition with subsequent computer post-processing producing images in all three dimensions and generating 3D-rendered images. The scan may take only a few seconds using a volume of 100 mLs of water-soluble iodinated contrast. With this technology, CT angiography is now available and may be used to show the arterial supply to the lesion.

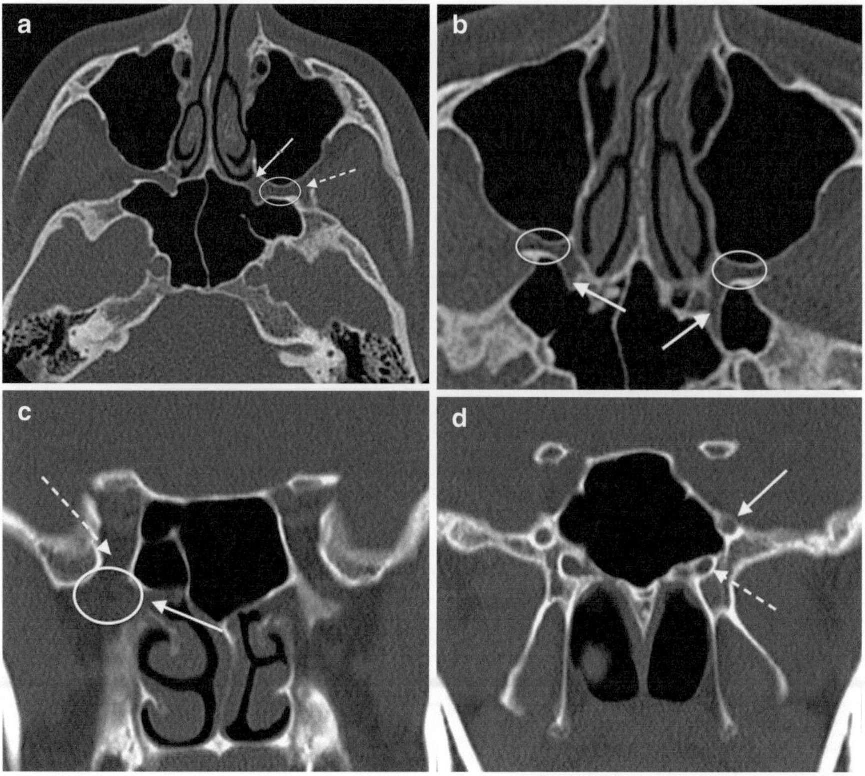

Fig. 7.1 CT demonstrates the skull-base foramina in the anterior skull base exquisitely in proximity to the site of origin of the JA, (**a**) demonstrates the pterygopalatine fossa (*oval* area) with the adjacent sphenopalatine foramen (*arrow*) and pterygomaxillary fissure (*broken arrow*) and (**b**) shows pterygopalatine fossa (*oval* area) and the vidian or pterygoid canal (*arrow*). (**c**) Coronal CT demonstrates the sphenopalatine foramen (*arrow*) and the inferior orbital fissure (*broken arrow*) in relation to the pterygopalatine fossa (*oval* area) and (**d**) shows the foramen rotundum (*arrow*) and the vidian canal (*broken arrow*), which is more inferior and medial on the coronal CT

CT is helpful in delineating bony anatomy and in particular demonstrating bony foramina and fissures (Fig. 7.1). It is also increasingly used both for surgical planning and to allow image-guided surgery with or without the placement of fiducials on the head. The data obtained is loaded on a computer in theatre and allows precise anatomical localisation during surgery using trackable instruments.

MRI is helpful in differentiating tumor from obstructed secretions in air passages and in accurately delineating the three dimensional relationship of the tumor to blood vessels, nerves, dura and marrow [14]. The standard "workhorse" sequences used in imaging of the skull base are a T1-weighted sequence, a T2 fat-saturated (fs) sequence and a post-gadolinium sequence. The T1- and T2-weighted sequences are acquired in the axial and coronal planes with the post-gadolinium images often acquired as a 3D sequence and presented in three orthogonal planes.

High field strength magnets have now come into clinical use particularly 3 Tesla (T) field strength magnets (as opposed to the older 1.5 T magnets). The higher field

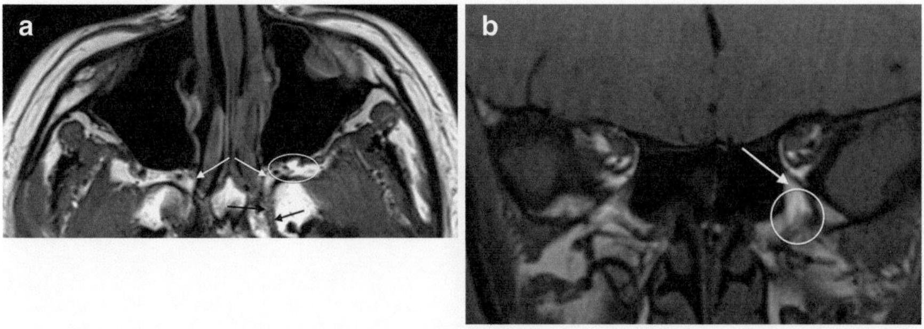

Fig. 7.2 T1-weighted ("fat-weighted") sequences showing the normal juxtaforaminal fat pads of the anterior skull base. (**a**) Axial image demonstrates the pterygopalatine fossa (*oval* area) with the adjacent sphenopalatine foramen (*white arrows*) and vidian canal (*black arrows*). (**b**) Coronal image demonstrates the inferior orbital fissure (*white arrow*) opening into the pterygopalatine fossa (*oval* area)

strength magnets allow high-resolution images to be obtained in less time and allow complex techniques such as time resolved angiography to be performed relatively quickly. Where available, most skull-base MRI scanning is performed on 3 T magnets.

The T1- or "fat-weighted" sequence most effectively depicts the relationship of the tumor to fatty marrow in the skull base and demonstrates the infiltration of normal juxtaforaminal fat pads in the region of the pterygopalatine fossa and superior and inferior orbital fissures (Fig. 7.2).

The T2- or "fluid-weighted" sequence in particular differentiates obstructed airspace secretions from actual tumor (Fig. 7.3).

The post-gadolinium sequences delineate the margins of the enhancing tumor with respect to the dura, cranial nerves and cavernous sinuses (Fig. 7.4). The contrast sequence can now be performed as a "time-resolved" angiogram with rapid repeated imaging through a volume of tissue just prior to and then following an intravenous bolus of paramagnetic contrast. This can exquisitely demonstrate the arterial supply to the tumor, the rapidity of enhancement of the lesion and the venous drainage (Fig. 7.5). This in itself may be helpful prior to embolisation and surgery.

More complex MRI techniques such as diffusion-perfusion imaging and MR spectroscopy may have a role in the future but are not used currently.

CT and MRI Features of JA

On CT the JA presents with the following features:

1. A soft tissue mass that is lobulated, nonencapsulated and heterogenous in density. The lesion is always located around the sphenopalatine foramen in the pterygopalatine fossa and probably originates close to or from the pterygoid canal according to several authors [2, 14] (Fig. 7.6).

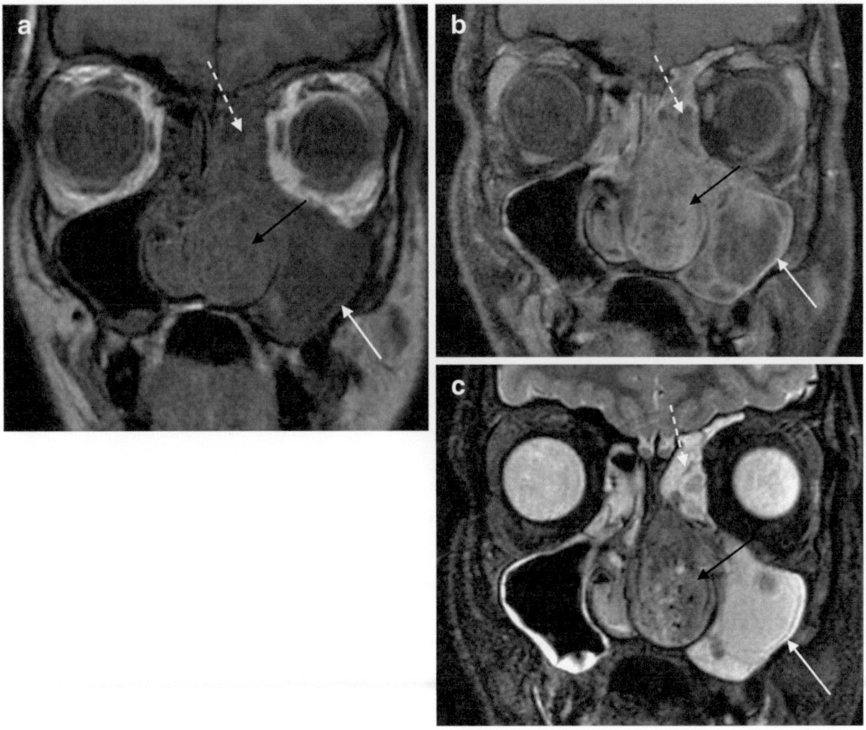

Fig. 7.3 The "workhorse" sequences of skull-base MRI, T1 (**a**) post-intravenous gadolinium, T1 with fat saturation (**b**) and T2 with fat saturation (**c**). Of the three sequences, the T2 fat-saturated sequence clearly differentiates the hypercellular "grey" tumor (*black arrow*) from the inflamed T2-bright mucosal lining of the sinuses (*white arrow*) and from the high T2 signal of the obstructed secretions (*broken arrow*). The inflamed mucosa in addition enhances on the T1 post-gadolinium sequence as much as the tumor. The obstructed secretions do not enhance. On T1-weighted sequences the only clue to the tumor is that it is slightly hyperintense compared to the other two

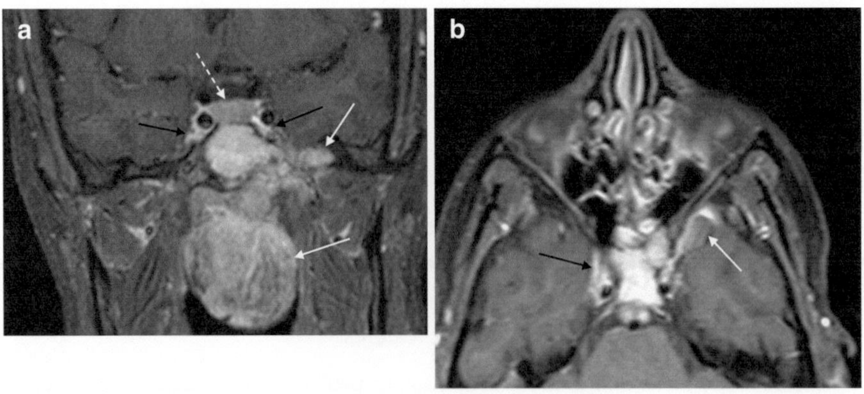

Fig. 7.4 The post-gadolinium fat-saturated (fs) sequence, in coronal (**a**) and axial (**b**), delineates the homogeneous enhancement of the cavernous sinus (*black arrow*), the slightly lower signal but enhancing pituitary gland (*broken arrow*) and the extradural as well as oropharyngeal JA (*white arrows*)

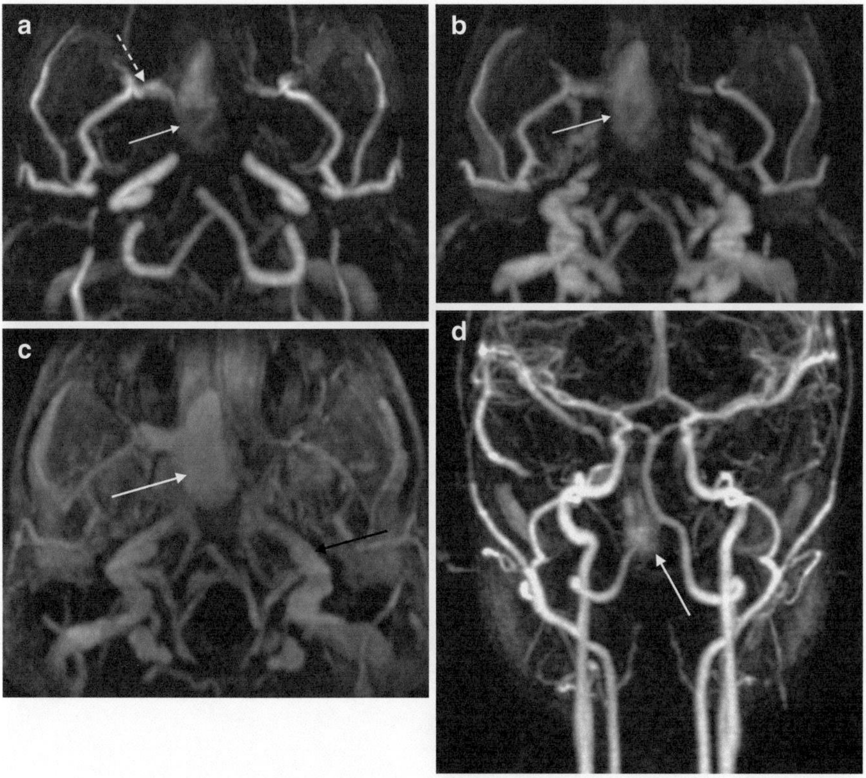

Fig. 7.5 "Time-resolved" MR angiography with intravenous gadolinium. Scans are performed rapidly through the volume of interest following a bolus of intravenous gadolinium. The enhancement pattern and the main arterial feeding vessels can be determined. The three images below (**a–c**) are at the same anatomical level and show the hypertrophic right internal maxillary artery (*broken arrow*) supplying the JA (*white arrow*) with early enhancement. Note the venous phase of the study with opacification of the internal jugular veins (*black arrow*). Note that the acquisition is in the coronal plane (**d**) but can be reconstructed in any plane

2. There is intense enhancement after iodinated contrast administration.
3. The lesion characteristically erodes or expands the skull base fissures and foramina, especially the pterygopalatine fossa and its exit/entry foramina. In particular, the sphenopalatine foramen, the pterygoid or vidian canal, the inferior orbital fissure and the pterygomaxillary fissure (Figs. 7.7, 7.8, 7.9, 7.10, and 7.11).
4. The lesion invariably erodes the posterior wall of the sphenopalatine foramen and then by extension the base of the medial pterygoid plate.
5. If the lesion extends into the pterygomaxillary fissure, it may, through pressure and slow enlargement, produce forward bowing of the posterior maxillary wall – the CT equivalent of the plain-film Holman-Miller sign (Fig. 7.12).
6. Posterior extension may mean erosion of the sphenoid and extension into the marrow cavity or cancellous bone (Fig. 7.13).

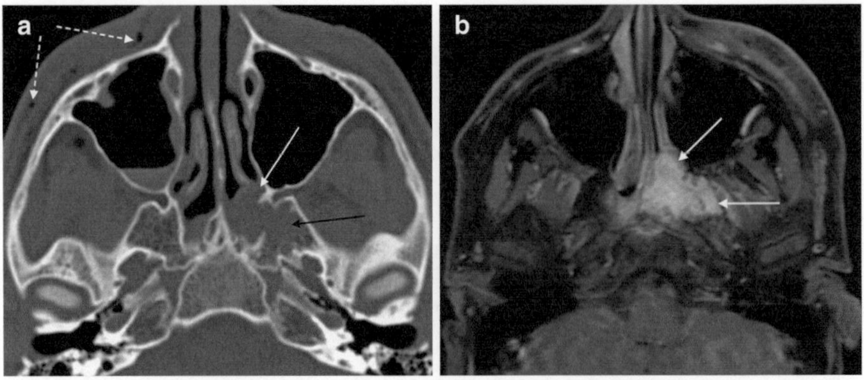

Fig. 7.6 A 19-year-old male in casualty after punch injury to the right cheek (**a**). Surgical emphysema (*broken arrows*) in the soft tissues of the right cheek, following a fracture to the maxillary sinus. The lesion (*white arrow*) in the right postnasal space adjacent to the sphenopalatine foramen erodes the pterygoid process and extends into the marrow cavity posterolaterally (*black arrow*). This was missed until the patient presented again with a nosebleed (**b**). The MRI shows the enhancing JA (*white arrow*) with a predominantly posterolateral vector of growth

Fig. 7.7 Axial CT showing erosion and widening of the right sphenopalatine foramen (*broken arrow*) with JA in the pterygopalatine fossa (*white arrow*)

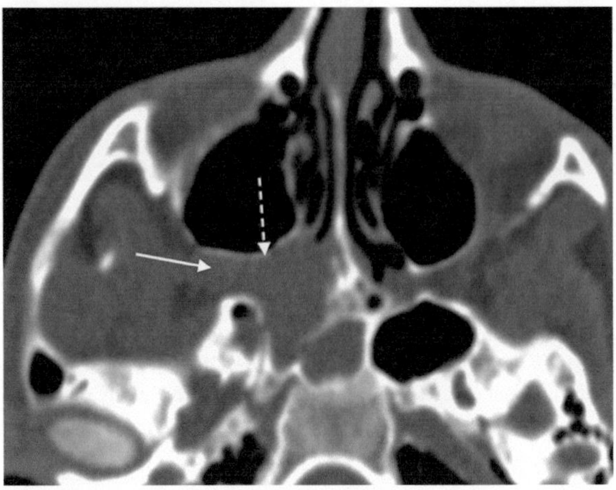

Fig. 7.8 Coronal CT showing a JA with erosion of the vidian canal on the left (*white arrow*), as compared to the normal canal on the right (*broken arrow*)

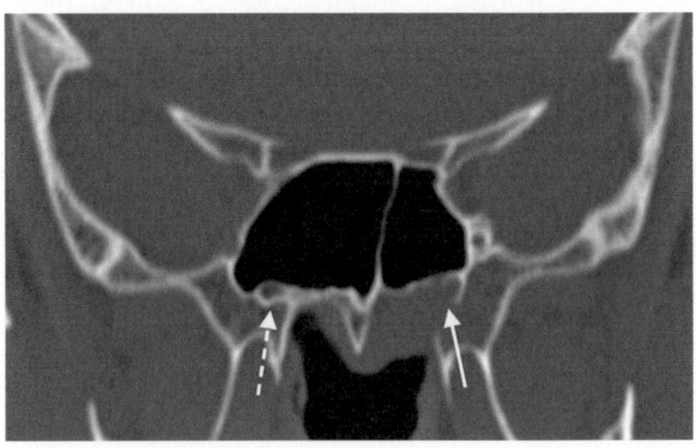

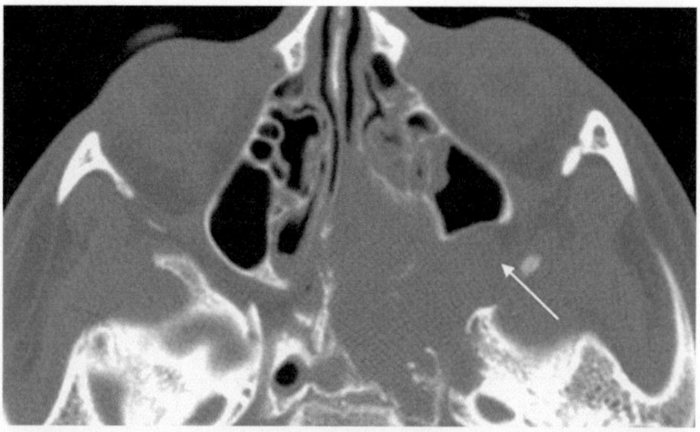

Fig. 7.9 JA causing widening of the left pterygomaxillary fissure with extension into the infratemporal fossa (*white arrow*)

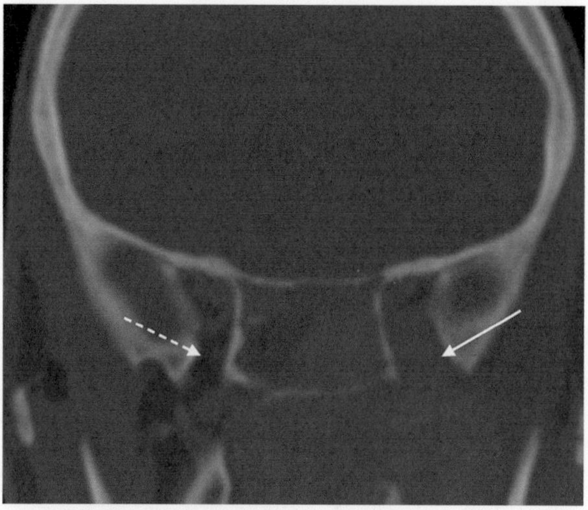

Fig. 7.10 Coronal CT demonstrating widening of the left inferior orbital fissure (IOF) (*white arrow*) as compared to the normal IOF on the right (*broken arrow*)

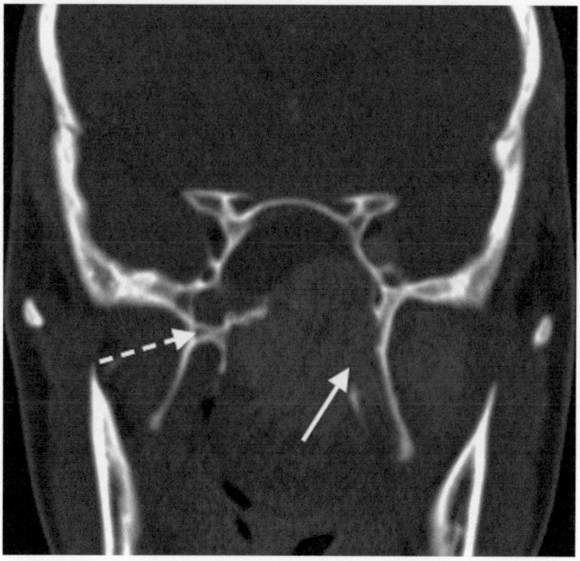

Fig. 7.11 JA eroding the base of the pterygoid on the left (*white arrow*). The normal pterygoid plate is demonstrated on the right (*broken arrow*)

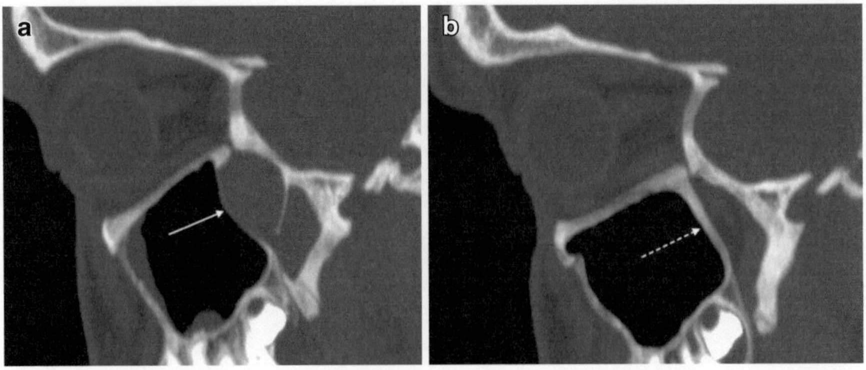

Fig. 7.12 Sagittal CT (**a**) showing a JA producing bowing of the posterior wall of the left maxillary antrum (*arrow*), the CT equivalent of the plain-film Holman-Miller sign, and (**b**) demonstrates the normal contour of the posterior wall of the right maxillary antrum in the same patient

Fig. 7.13 JA with posterior extension to infiltrate the sphenoid sinus (*white arrows*)

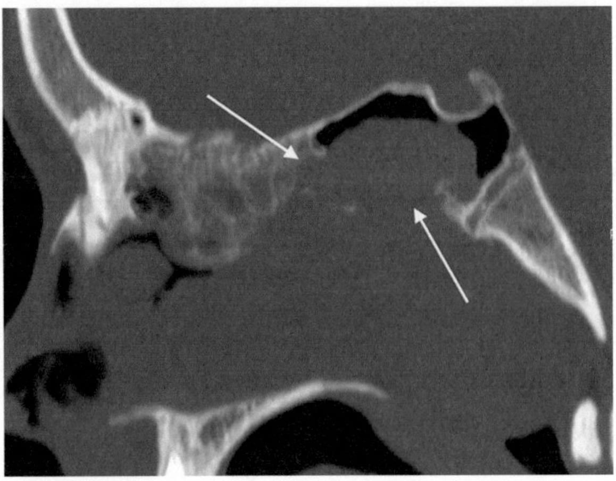

7. Calcification within the tumor has not been described.
8. The tumor is unilateral but may extend to the contralateral side. Bilateral synchronous tumors have been rarely described [15].

On MRI:

1. The lesions are isointense to hyperintense on T1- and T2-weighted scans.
2. There may be multiple flow voids within the lesion related to neovascularity (Fig. 7.14).
3. They enhance intensely following intravenous gadolinium.
4. There is early arterial enhancement and rapid homogenous enhancement on time-resolved MR angiography.

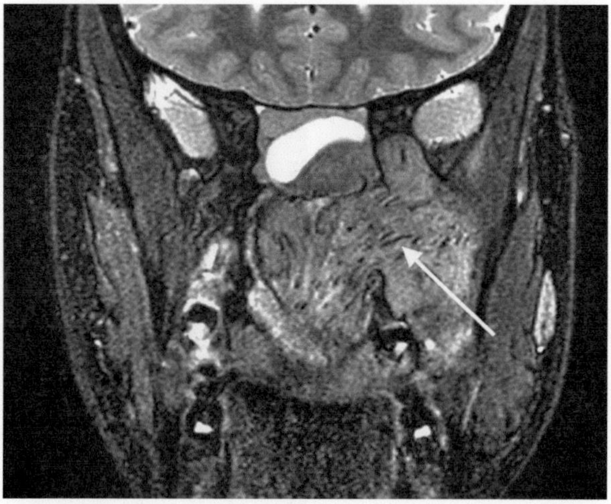

Fig. 7.14 Flow voids (the *dark* linear and punctate areas in the tumor) (*arrow*) which are related to small high flow vessels supplying the JA

Cystic changes within the tumor on both CT and MRI are said to be a sign of tumor regression usually following chemoradiation [16]. Spontaneous regression has been rarely documented in the literature in both an untreated tumor [17] and treated residual disease [18]. Distant metastatic disease has not been described [19].

Growth Patterns of JA on CT and MRI

JAs show growth patterns independent of the age of the patient or the size and staging of the tumor, and a large tumor may only show one direction of growth. The reason for a preferential growth pattern is not known. Unlike many other expansile tumors, it does not always follow the pathway of least resistance, as seen in its propensity to cross the sphenopalatine foramen into the low-volume pterygopalatine fossa [20]. This pattern of growth is of importance in surgical planning and preoperative patient counselling and is well described in the literature [21, 22].

Anterolateral Spread

Anterolateral spread through the pterygopalatine fossa is the commonest growth direction of a JA (Fig. 7.15). As it fills the pterygopalatine fossa, it can bow the posterior wall of the maxillary antrum anteriorly. It may extend through the pterygomaxillary fissure into the infratemporal fossa and parapharyngeal space (Fig. 7.16). From there, a lesion may extend to the cheek or the temporal fossa.

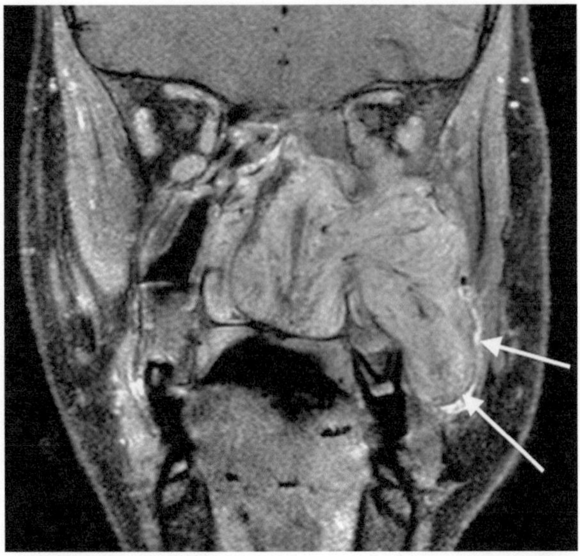

Fig. 7.15 JA with a predominantly anterolateral vector of growth extending through the pterygomaxillary fissure into the infratemporal fossa and into the deep cheek (*white arrows*)

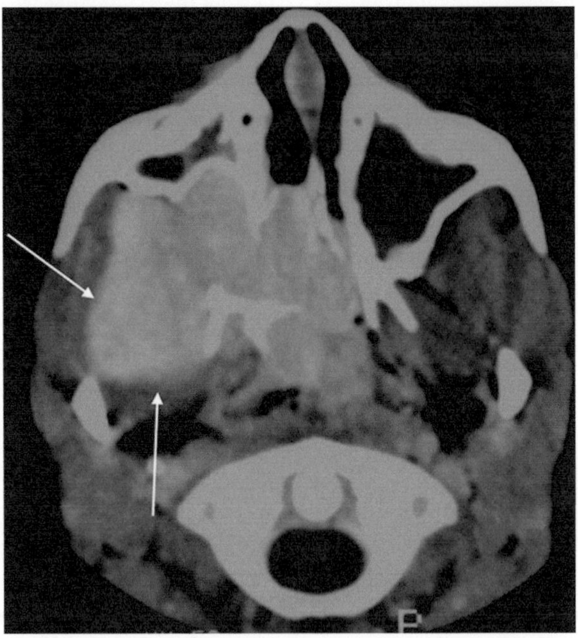

Fig. 7.16 Axial CT post-contrast demonstrates a large JA with anterolateral spread to the infratemporal fossa and parapharyngeal space (*arrows*)

Medial Spread

Medial spread occurs from the sphenopalatine foramen into the nasopharynx and to the contralateral side (Fig. 7.17). The JA is generally an asymmetrical disease process.

Anterior Spread

Anterior spread occurs directly through the posterior wall of the maxillary antrum or medially into the nasal cavity and from there can anteriorly involve the ethmoid, frontal and maxillary sinuses (Fig. 7.18).

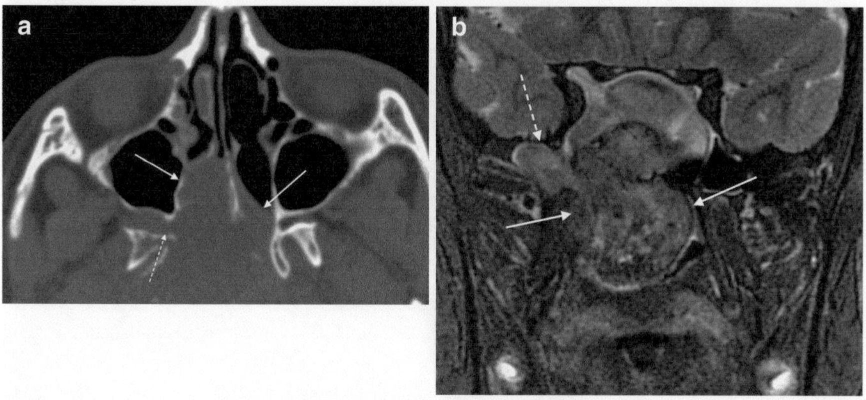

Fig. 7.17 Axial CT (**a**) and coronal T2-weighted MRI (**b**) showing JA with a predominantly medial vector of growth crossing the midline to fill both sides of the postnasal space (*white arrows*). Note the likely origin of the tumor adjacent to the right sphenopalatine foramen with a tongue extending into the pterygopalatine fossa (*broken arrow*)

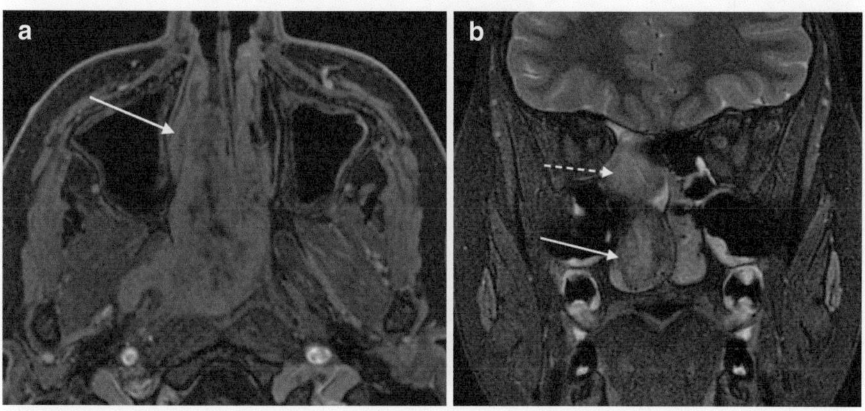

Fig. 7.18 Axial T1fs post-contrast (**a**) and coronal T2fs (**b**) images demonstrate a JA with a predominantly anterior pattern of growth as tumor is extending anteriorly into the nasal fossa (*white arrow*) and is filling the ethmoid sinus on the right (*broken arrow*)

Superior Spread

Superior spread into the inferior orbital fissure will lead to involvement of the orbital apex. From here the tumor can extend intraorbitally in the extraconal space (Fig. 7.19). If the lesion involves the superior orbital fissure, there may be posterior extension into the cavernous sinuses and along the extradural space of the middle cranial fossa (Fig. 7.20). There may be encasement of the cavernous internal carotid arteries. Rarely there is dural infiltration. Intra-axial spread is not described.

Fig. 7.19 Axial CT post-contrast of a large JA, with involvement of the orbital apex bilaterally (*arrows*), in a patient who presented with blindness in both eyes. There is associated proptosis of the globes and distortion of the optics nerve (*broken arrow*)

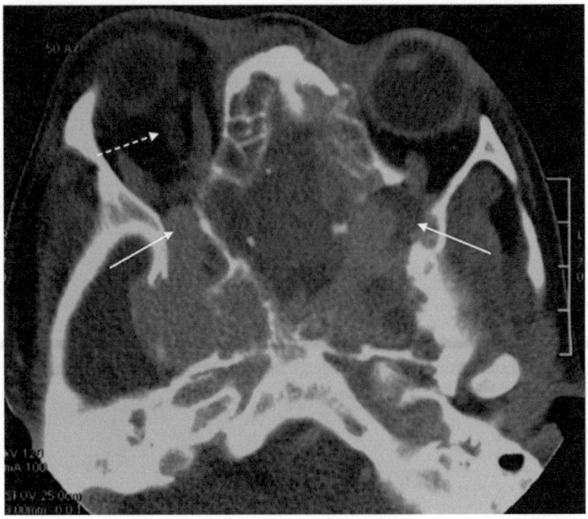

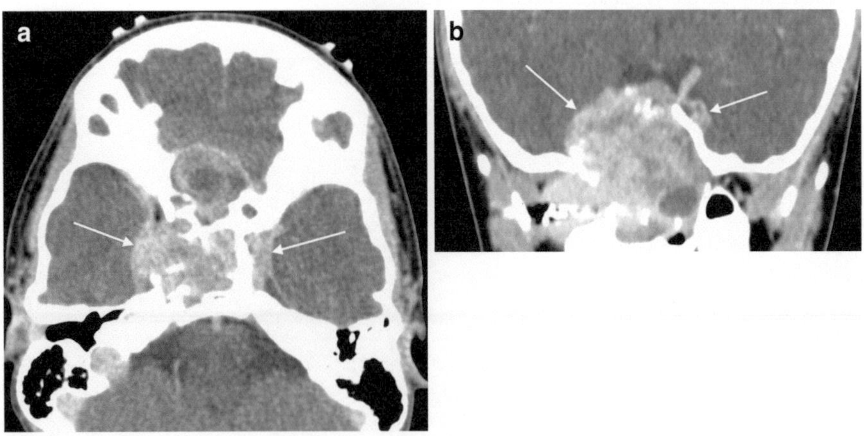

Fig. 7.20 Axial (**a**) and coronal (**b**) CT post-contrast demonstrating a JA with a predominantly superior and posterior direction of growth with infiltration of the cavernous sinuses (*arrows*)

Posterior Spread

Posterior spread occurs via three routes:

(a) Direct pressure erosion of the pterygoid plates.
(b) Deep infiltration of the marrow of the sphenoid bone with extension into the sphenoid sinus and potentially intracranial extension via the margins of the sphenoid sinuses. This type of spread is associated with highest rate of recurrence following surgery [2] (Fig. 7.20).
(c) Posterolateral spread between the pterygoid plates to the parapharyngeal space.

Dural Infiltration

This is a potential but rare consequence of intracranial extension as JAs more often displace rather than infiltrate dura [23]. Imaging is poor at differentiating between extradural disease and transdural disease. Features that may lead one to suspect dural transgression are the absence of a cleavage plane between the tumor and dura, encasement of the internal carotid artery and feeding vessels from the brain parenchyma extending into the tumor [24]. However in our experience and the experience of most authors, the JA is always extradural.

Staging on Imaging

There are multiple staging systems for the preoperative assessment of juvenile angiofibromas. These are described in Chap. 8. These stagings are based on imaging and assess the extension of tumor and intracranial extension. Some classification systems also include the amount of residual vascularity within the lesion following embolisation.

Important imaging criteria that affect staging include:

1. Involvement of the orbit or infratemporal fossa
2. Extradural but intracranial extension
3. Intradural extension
4. Involvement of the cavernous sinus, pituitary or optic chiasm

The Role of Diagnostic Angiography in JA Imaging

Diagnostic angiography as opposed to embolisation does not currently have a role in the imaging workup of JA but has been used extensively in the past before the advent of cross-sectional imaging to make the diagnosis in conjunction with the plain-film findings [1]. The role and techniques of embolisation are described in

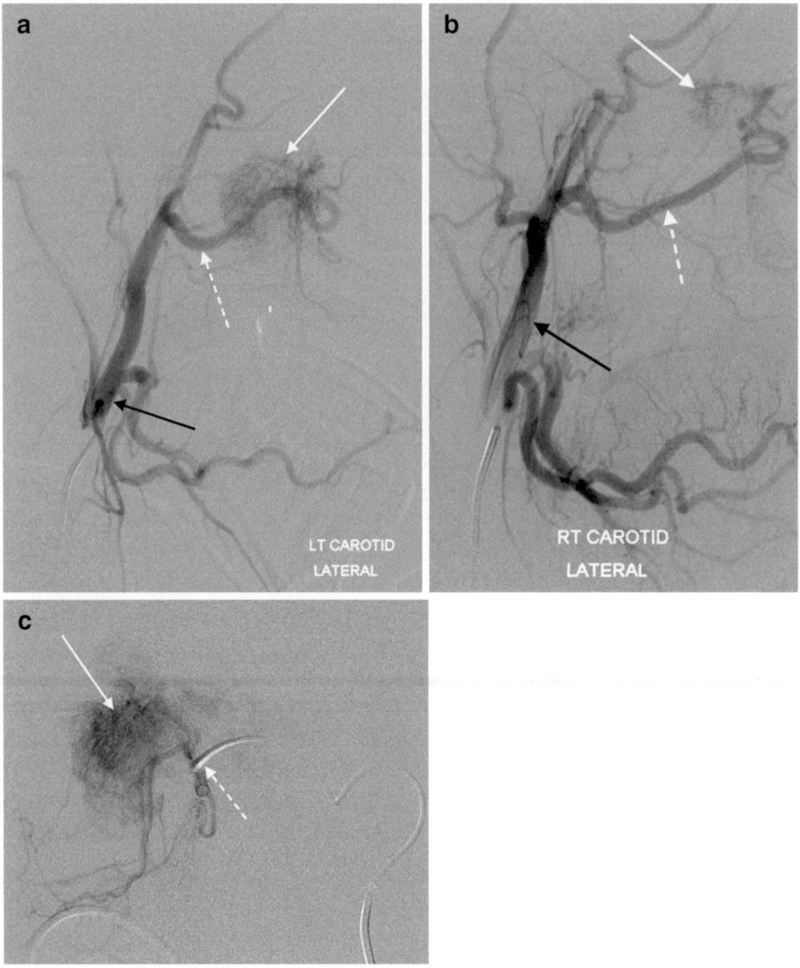

Fig. 7.21 Digital subtraction angiogram (DSA). (**a**) Selective catheterization of the left external carotid artery (ECA) (*black arrow*) showing intense early enhancement of left-sided JA (*white arrow*) supplied by the internal maxillary artery (*broken arrow*). (**b**) Selective catheterization of the contralateral right ECA (*black arrow*) showing a supply to the JA (*white arrow*) from the contralateral internal maxillary artery (*broken arrow*). (**c**) Super selective catheterization of the terminal left internal maxillary artery (*broken arrow*) prior to embolization of the JA (*white arrow*)

Chap. 9. Preoperative angiographic embolization has been used to control blood loss and thereby enhance visualization at surgery.

Angiography is performed usually via a femoral artery puncture using a Seldinger technique. To delineate the full extent of arterial supply to the tumor, one may need to selectively catheterise each internal and external carotid artery and each vertebral artery (Fig. 7.21). As the tumor grows, it may gain supply from a combination of both ipsilateral and contralateral arteries. Bilateral vascular supply has been quoted as occurring in 36 % of patients when multiple studies are combined [25].

The tumor is commonly supplied, however, by the terminal branches of the ipsilateral internal maxillary artery, a terminal branch of the external carotid artery and branches of the ascending pharyngeal artery. As the tumor gets larger, it usually gets supply also from internal carotid artery branches. There is intense early enhancement of the tumor with dense staining during the capillary phase of the angiogram [1]. This is said to be a characteristic feature of this tumor.

Other Modalities

Other imaging modalities such as ultrasound and technetium-labelled red cell scanning with single-photon emission computed tomography (SPECT) [26] have been sporadically described in the literature and are not currently used in the diagnosis of this lesion. Ultrasound may show a heterogenous vascular mass [27] when the tumor is large enough to extend into the infratemporal or temporal fossa or the deep face outside the confines of the bone.

Differential Diagnosis

The JA is a rare tumor with unique demographics, anatomical site of occurrence and growth patterns. It is therefore difficult to confuse it with other entities.

Vascular lesions of the nasal vault which expand into the nasopharynx or nasopharyngeal lesions which expand anteriorly without involvement of the sphenoid, medial pterygoid plates or pterygopalatine fossa are highly unlikely to be JAs. In this situation, hemangiomas (Fig. 7.22) (particularly in their proliferative phase), the angiomatous polyp (Fig. 7.23) [28] or vascular malformations should be considered. Rhabdomyosarcomas and lymphoproliferative disease may be included in the differential. Besides their atypical anatomical location and growth pattern, these entities may show atypical angiographic features such as lack of early arterial enhancement (in the case of the hemangioma or polyp) on time-resolved MR angiography and a predominant supply from the ethmoidal arteries.

Imaging Surveillance

Recurrent JAs are almost certainly residual JAs that have grown. The disease "recurs" in up to 40 % of patients in some series with potentially less-experienced surgeons [2]. The likelihood of recurrent or residual disease is increased when the tumor is difficult to totally remove surgically. This may happen when there is deep medullary infiltration of the sphenoid bone [29] (the posterior growth pattern) or there is intracranial extension (posterior and superior growth patterns). Some

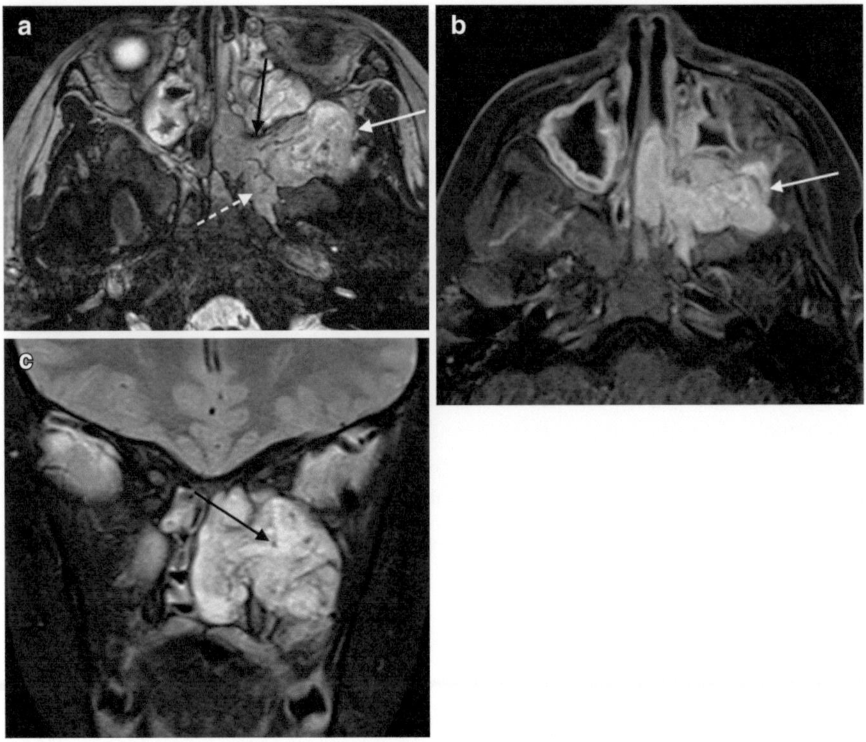

Fig. 7.22 JA mimics. A 6-year-old girl presented with a nosebleed. Imaging eventually culminating in an MRI showed a mass in the left nasal fossa extending across a widened sphenopalatine foramen (*black arrow*) into the pterygopalatine fossa and through the pterygomaxillary fissure (*white arrow*) into the infratemporal fossa (**a**, **b**). There was also involvement of the vidian canal (*broken arrow*). The lesion has the signal characteristics of a JA on MRI. Note the flow voids within the lesion on c (*black arrow*). The patient even had a chromosomal analysis to confirm that she had female chromosomes. However, formal surgical biopsy revealed a proliferative hemangioma, which was subsequently treated successfully with propranolol

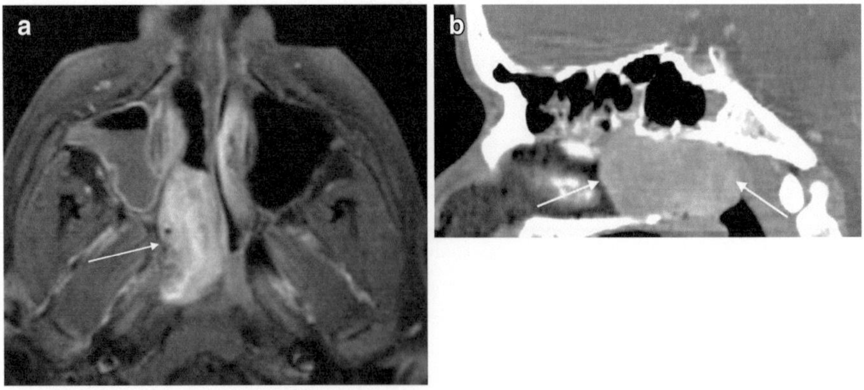

Fig. 7.23 JA mimics. A 13-year-old boy with nasal obstruction and a nosebleed. MRI (**a**) and CT (**b**) demonstrate a vascular-enhancing lesion in the right nasal cavity and nasopharynx (*white arrows*). Note that the lesion does not involve the sphenopalatine foramen or the pterygopalatine fossa. This was an "angiomatoid" polyp on histology

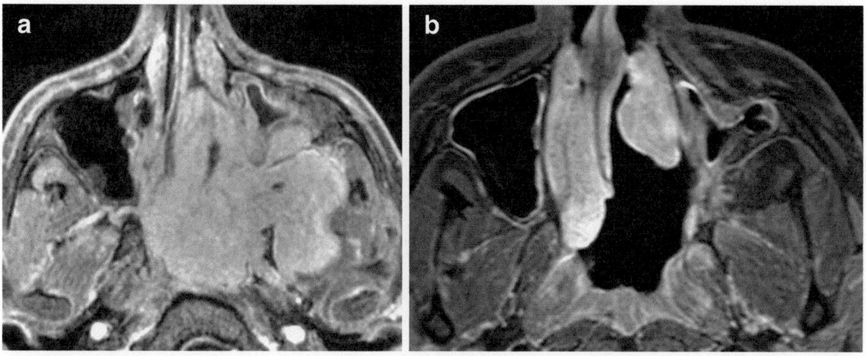

Fig. 7.24 Postsurgical surveillance. A 19-year-old patient with a laterally growing JA (**a**) excised endoscopically. The 6-month follow-up study (**b**) shows a surgical cavity in the left nasal fossa and postnasal space with no residual lesion evident

authors have suggested that preoperative embolisation increases the risk of recurrence as there may be incomplete tumor resection [2, 30]. Most recurrences occur within the first 12 months following surgery [31, 32].

Early follow up of surgically treated patients has been described at 1–4 days using CT following treatment [33]. This allows the surgical bed to be assessed before significant post-operative oedema occurs to confuse the imaging. An enhancing lesion in the surgical bed is taken to be residual disease that may require further surgical measures. However, tumor that has deeply infiltrated the bone may not be identified. Also tumor that has been subjected to embolization prior to surgery may not enhance at this early stage. Based on small numbers, the specificity of early post-operative CT in detecting residual disease in this study was 83 %, with a sensitivity of 75 %.

There is a school of thought that early post-operative imaging is not necessary particularly if there is a small residual, which may require long-term observation. In addition the choice of modality should be MRI in the long-term follow-up to avoid the radiation dose from repeated CT studies to a young patient.

Longer term follow up consists of a combination of clinical examination, FNE and cross-sectional imaging. A clinical recurrence is deemed when the patient's symptoms recur. FNE identifies mucosal recurrences and MRI/CT will identify extramucosal and extranasal recurrences (Figs. 7.24, 7.25, and 7.26). The recurrence of tumor and its prevention is dealt with in Chap. 20.

Chagnaud and his colleagues [34] devised an algorithm for the longer-term follow-up of postsurgical JAs consisting of a follow-up CT or MRI at 3 months:

(a) If the patient is negative for recurrence clinically, on FNE and on CT/MRI, then he is only followed clinically.
(b) If the patient is positive for recurrence on follow up at 3 months, then further treatment is initiated.
(c) If the patient is clinically and FNE negative at a 3-month follow-up but has an enhancing extranasal lesion, then further imaging is performed at 6 months. Non-enhancing and enhancing masses that are not tumor may occur in the post-surgical patient due to fibrosis and/or mucosal thickening.

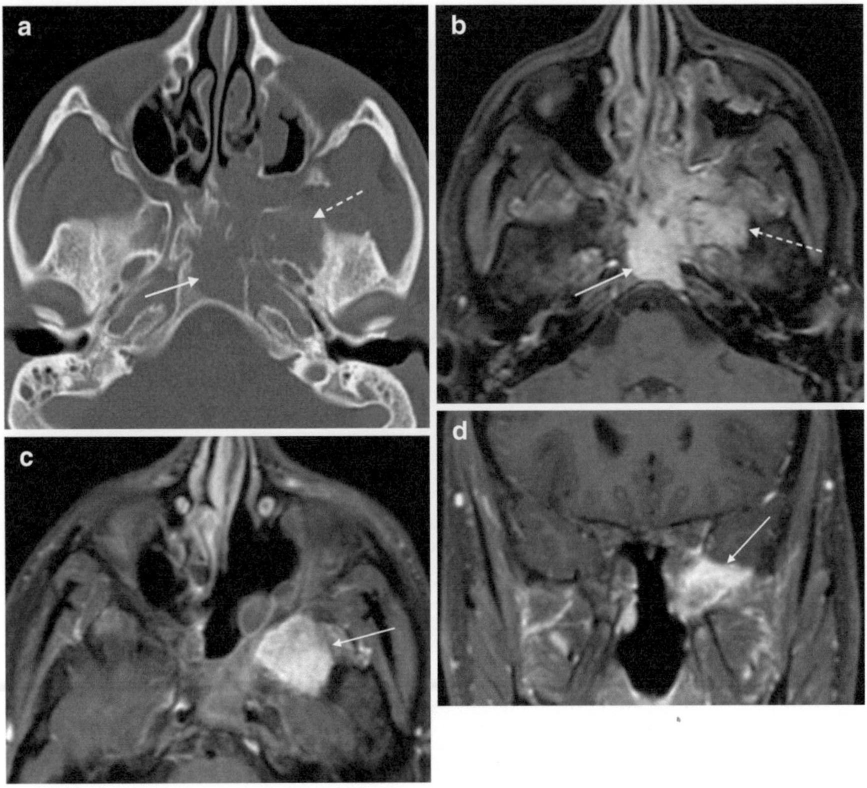

Fig. 7.25 Postsurgical surveillance. Preoperative CT (**a**) and MRI (**b**) in a 20-year-old patient with a posterior, lateral and superior growth pattern. Note the erosion of the marrow of the clivus posteriorly (*white arrow*) and the erosion of the floor of the middle cranial fossa into the extra-axial space (*broken arrow*). These anatomical sites of extension are markers for areas of possible residual/recurrent disease. Axial (**c**) and coronal (**d**) MRI T1 post-gadolinium at 6 months following surgery show residual disease in the middle cranial fossa (*arrow*). The posterior component of the JA has been successfully excised

(d) If on the 6-month scan the enhancing lesion has increased in size, then further treatment is initiated as this almost certainly represents recurrent disease.
(e) If on the 6 month scan the lesion is stable or involuting or enhancing less, then the chances are that it does not represent JA, and a further 6-month scan is performed.
(f) Patients are followed up to 4 years after treatment. Occasionally, further imaging may be performed years after treatment if there is concern regarding another pathology or a complication of treatment (Fig. 7.27).
Malignant transformation of JA is discussed in Chap. 22.

In our centre patients with small apparent residuals are watched serially with MRI without necessarily requiring surgical intervention.

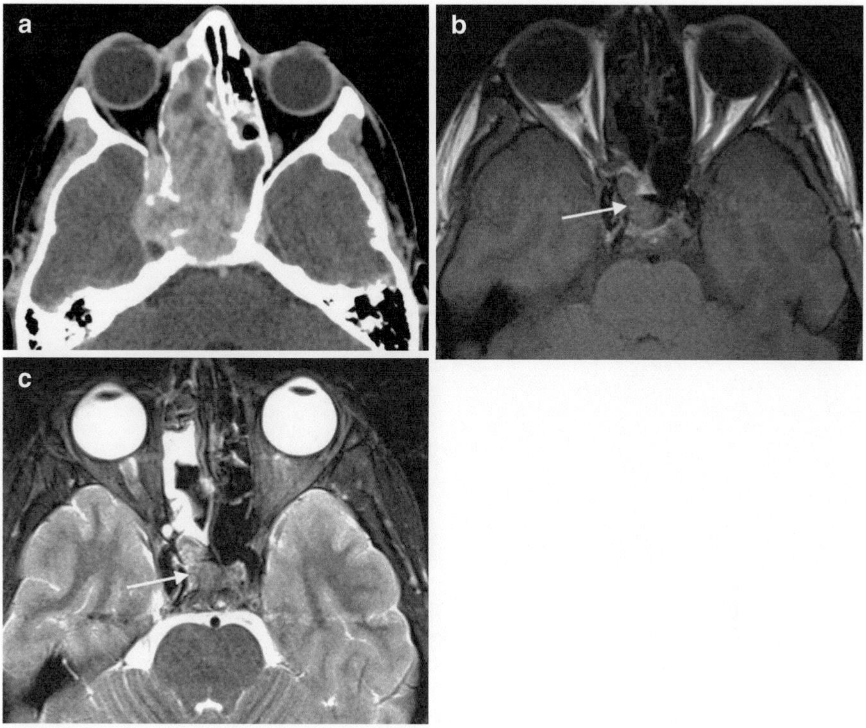

Fig. 7.26 Postsurgical surveillance. Preoperative CT (**a**) in a 13-year-old demonstrates a JA involving the marrow of the clivus and also within the inferior orbital fissure on the right. 3 years after surgery, a surveillance MRI with axial T1 (**b**) and T2fs (**c**) sequences demonstrates residual/recurrent tumor within the clivus (*arrow*)

Extranasopharyngeal Angiofibromas

Extranasopharyngeal angiofibromas (ENA) are rare with around 100 cases described in the literature [35]. They occur in an older age group with a mean age of presentation at 22 years but have been described in young children. Females constitute 25–26 % of all cases. The tumors have been described arising from the maxillary sinus, nasal septum, ethmoid sinus, nasal cavity, larynx, sphenoid sinus, cheek, conjunctiva, oropharynx, retromolar triangle, turbinates, external nose, hard palate, external ear, lachrymal sac, carotid bifurcation, esophagus, facial nerve, middle cranial fossa and infratemporal fossa.

The ENAs are a histologically heterogenous group of lesions and therefore do not always share the characteristic radiological features of JAs (Fig. 7.28). Some of the lesions may not enhance as intensely as a JA. They share a similar type of growth pattern spreading locally and extending through foramina and fissures. Angiographically, they may not always be supplied by the internal maxillary

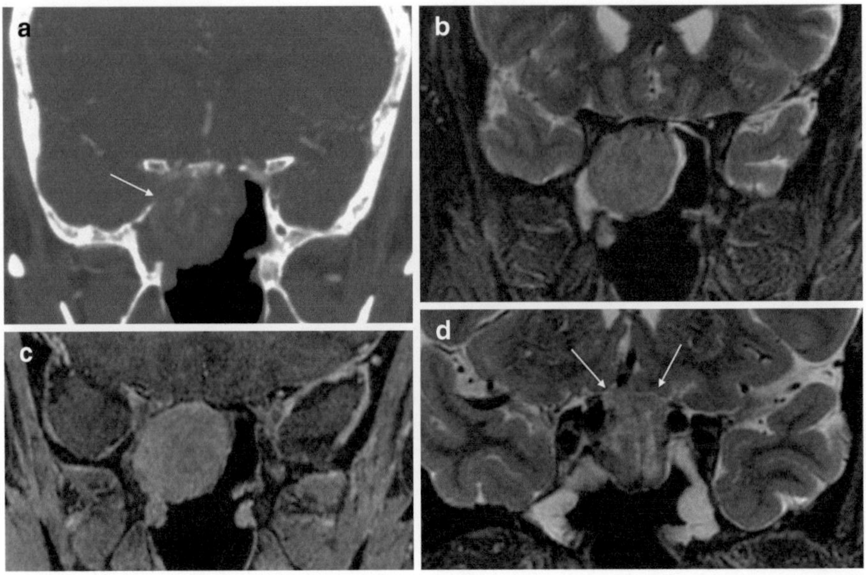

Fig. 7.27 Long-term complication of radiation therapy for JA. A 57-year-old man presented with a blocked nose and intermittent nosebleeds more than 30 years after surgery and radiation treatment for a JA. Post-contrast CT (**a**) showing a mass attached to the undersurface of the planum sphenoidale eroding bone (*arrow*). Coronal T2 (**b**) and coronal T1 post-gadolinium (**c**) MRI showing a spherical mass that is virtually identical in signal to a JA. It is slightly T2 hyperintense and enhancing homogenously. At surgery the lesion could not be completely removed. Histology revealed an aggressive fibrous tumor. At a 12-month follow-up (**d**), the lesion had extended intracranially to lie between the frontal lobes (*arrows*). It was still thought to be extra-axial but closely applied to dura

artery depending upon their location. The ENAs are treated similarly, with surgical excision, with low recurrence rates [35]. The ENAs are described in details in Chap. 21.

Summary

The imaging of JAs is performed with CT and MRI. CT aids in defining the extent and patterns of bony destruction and remodelling. MRI defines the relationship of the tumor to vital soft tissues including the carotid arteries, the dura and the optic nerves. Time-resolved MR angiography may also help define the vascular supply of the tumor and provide a road map for preoperative embolisation. Both modalities define the extent of tumor and in doing so help in differentiating this condition from other entities. The infiltration of the central skull base and in particular the sphenoid is a marker for possible recurrent tumor after surgery. Both modalities have a role in

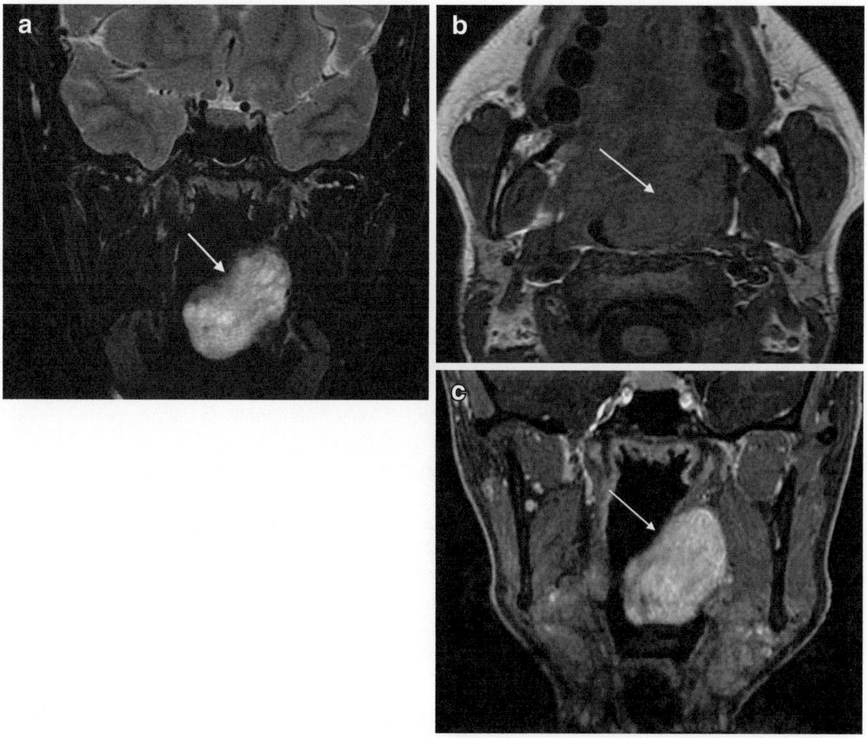

Fig. 7.28 Extranasopharyngeal angiofibroma. Coronal T2 (**a**), axial T1 (**b**) and post-gadolinium coronal T1 with fat sat (**c**) in a 24-year-old lady with oropharyngeal mass arising from the left palatine tonsil (*arrows*). The lesion is T2 hyperintense, T1 isointense and enhancing intensely following IV contrast

post-operative surveillance with the persistence of enhancing tissue at the surgical resection margins and an increase in size being key factors in the diagnosis of a recurrence.

Acknowledgements We would like to acknowledge the work of the radiographers at Queensland X-Ray and the Princess Alexandra Hospital, Brisbane. We would also like to thank Dr. SP Dubey, Dr. Mark Walsh, Dr. Andrew Lomas, Dr. James Earnshaw and Dr. Ben Panizza for sharing their cases with us.

References

1. Sessions RB, Wills PI, Alford BR, Harrell JE, Evans RA. Juvenile nasopharyngeal angiofibroma: radiographic aspects. Laryngoscope. 1976;86:2–18.
2. Lloyd G, Howard D, Phelps P, Cheesman A. Juvenile angiofibroma: the lessons of 20 years of modern imaging. J Laryngol Otol. 1999;113:127–34.

3. Tapia Acuna R. Juvenile nasopharyngeal fibroma. Ann Otol Rhinol Laryngol. 1981;90(5 Pt 1): 420–2.
4. Liston R. Tumour of the upper jaw bone: excision and recovery. Lancet. 1841;1:67–68.
5. Chelius MJ. A system of surgery. London: Renshaw; 1847.
6. Gosselin L. Fibrome ou polype fibreux nasophayngien. Clin Chirugicable De Hopital de la Charite (Paris). 1873;1:92–116.
7. Chauveau C. Histoire des Maladies du Pharynx. Paris: J.B. Balliere et Fils; 1906.
8. Friedberg SA. Vascular fibroma of the nasopharynx (nasopharyngeal fibroma). Arch Otolaryngol. 1940;31:313–26.
9. Holman CB, Miller W. Juvenile nasopharyngeal fibroma – roentgenologic characteristics. AJR Am J Roentgenol. 1965;94:292–8.
10. Weinstein MA, Levine H, Duchesneau PM, Tucker HM. Diagnosis of juvenile angiofibroma by computed tomography. Radiology. 1978;126:703–5.
11. Bryan RN, Sessions RB, Horowitz BL. Radiographic management of juvenile angiofibromas. AJNR Am J Neuroradiol. 1981;2:157–66.
12. Duckert LG, Carley RB, Hilger JA. Computerized axial-tomography in the preoperative evaluation of an angiofibroma. Laryngoscope. 1978;88:613–8.
13. Gonsalves CG, Briant TD. Radiologic findings in nasopharyngeal angiofibromas. J Can Assoc Radiol. 1978;29:209–15.
14. Lloyd GA, Phelps PD. Juvenile angiofibroma: imaging by magnetic resonance, CT and conventional techniques. Clin Otolaryngol Allied Sci. 1986;11:247–59.
15. Wu EC, Chark DW, Bhandarkar ND. Bilateral juvenile nasopharyngeal angiofibroma: report of a case. Int Forum Allergy Rhinol. 2014;4:603–6.
16. Schick B, Kahle G. Radiological findings in angiofibroma. Acta Radiol. 2000;41:585–93.
17. Weprin LS, Siemers PT. Spontaneous regression of juvenile nasopharyngeal angiofibroma. Arch Otolaryngol Head Neck Surg. 1991;117:796–9.
18. Gullane PJ, Davidson J, O'Dwyer T, Forte V. Juvenile angiofibroma: a review of the literature and a case series report. Laryngoscope. 1992;102:928–33.
19. Sessions RB, Zarin DP, Bryan RN. Juvenile nasopharyngeal angiofibroma. Am J Dis Child. 1981;135:535–7.
20. Sennes LU, Butugan O, Sanchez TG, Bento RF, Tsuji DH. Juvenile nasopharyngeal angiofibroma: the routes of invasion. Rhinology. 2003;41:235–40.
21. Szymanska A, Szymanski M, Czekajska-Chehab E, Szczerbo-Trojanowska M. Invasive growth patterns of juvenile nasopharyngeal angiofibroma: radiological imaging and clinical implications. Acta Radiol. 2014;55:725–31.
22. Szymanska A, Szymanski M, Czekajska-Chehab E, Szczerbo-Trojanowska M. Two types of lateral extension in juvenile nasopharyngeal angiofibroma: diagnostic and therapeutic management. Eur Arch Oto-Rhino-Laryngol: 2015;272:159–66.
23. Danesi G, Panizza B, Mazzoni A, Calabrese V. Anterior approaches in juvenile nasopharyngeal angiofibromas with intracranial extension. Otolaryngol Head Neck Surg: 2000;122:277–83.
24. Danesi G, Panciera DT, Harvey RJ, Agostinis C. Juvenile nasopharyngeal angiofibroma: evaluation and surgical management of advanced disease. Otolaryngol Head Neck Surg. 2008;138:581–6.
25. Wu AW, Mowry SE, Vinuela F, Abemayor E, Wang MB. Bilateral vascular supply in juvenile nasopharyngeal angiofibromas. Laryngoscope. 2011;121:639–43.
26. Uslu C, Yildirim M, Uslu H, Sutbeyaz Y, Varoglu E, Seven B, et al. 99mTc-labelled red blood cell single-photon emission computed tomography for the diagnosis and follow-up of juvenile nasopharyngeal angiofibroma. Nucl Med Commun. 2006;27:489–94.
27. Arslan H, Bozkurt M, Sakarya ME, Poyraz N. Power Doppler findings in nasopharyngeal angiofibroma. Clin Imaging. 1998;22:86–8.
28. Som PM, Cohen BA, Sacher M, Choi IS, Bryan NR. The angiomatous polyp and the angiofibroma: two different lesions. Radiology. 1982;144:329–34.
29. Howard DJ, Lloyd G, Lund V. Recurrence and its avoidance in juvenile angiofibroma. Laryngoscope. 2001;111:1509–11.

30. Herman P, Lot G, Chapot R, Salvan D, Huy PT. Long-term follow-up of juvenile nasopharyngeal angiofibromas: analysis of recurrences. Laryngoscope. 1999;109:140–7.
31. Bleier BS, Kennedy DW, Palmer JN, Chiu AG, Bloom JD, O'Malley Jr BW. Current management of juvenile nasopharyngeal angiofibroma: a tertiary center experience 1999–2007. Am J Rhinol Allergy. 2009;23:328–30.
32. Tyagi I, Syal R, Goyal A. Staging and surgical approaches in large juvenile angiofibroma – study of 95 cases. Int J Pediatr Otorhinolaryngol. 2006;70:1619–27.
33. Kania RE, Sauvaget E, Guichard JP, Chapot R, Huy PT, Herman P. Early postoperative CT scanning for juvenile nasopharyngeal angiofibroma: detection of residual disease. AJNR Am J Neuroradiol. 2005;26:82–8.
34. Chagnaud C, Petit P, Bartoli J, Champsaur P, Gaubert J, Dessi P, et al. Postoperative follow-up of juvenile nasopharyngeal angiofibromas: assessment by CT scan and MR imaging. Eur Radiol. 1998;8:756–64.
35. Szymanska A, Szymanski M, Morshed K, Czekajska-Chehab E, Szczerbo-Trojanowska M. Extranasopharyngeal angiofibroma: clinical and radiological presentation. Eur Arch Oto-Rhino-Laryngol: 2013;270:655–60.

Chapter 8
Staging Systems and Their Use

Zixiang Yi and Chang Lin

Abstract Staging of juvenile angiofibroma is essential for treatment, surgical decision-making, and prediction of lesion recurrence and prognosis. Classification depends primarily on factors such as tumor location, degree of invasion, biological behavior, extension route, and recurrence sites. With advances in radiographic imaging, embolization, and nasal endoscopy, tumor staging systems for juvenile angiofibroma have changed constantly over the past 30 years. Some newer staging systems have been developed to determine the risk of persistent disease, choose the appropriate surgical method, and maintain uniformity. The Sessions system is the first standardized juvenile angiofibroma classification system. The Radkowski system and either the Fisch system or the Andrews–Fisch system were the most popular in use. These systems have been recognized as the comprehensive, practical, and applicable guide to surgical approach and prediction of outcome. UPMC system is based on current advances in surgical technique and imaging; its applicability needs to be ascertained in the future.

Keywords Staging system • Juvenile angiofibroma

Introduction

Staging systems for juvenile angiofibroma (JA) are important to standardize evaluation, management, and prognosis. Cumulative factors that influence surgical decisions include the extent and size of the tumor and the risks of residual and recurrent disease.

Z. Yi, MD (✉) • C. Lin, MD
Department of Otolaryngology–Head & Neck Surgery, First Affiliated Hospital of Fujian Medical University, Fuzhou, Fujian Province, China, 350005
e-mail: yizixiang@sina.com

S.P. Dubey, B. Schick (eds.), *Juvenile Angiofibroma*,
DOI 10.1007/978-3-319-45343-9_8

Commonly Used Classifications

In 1981, Sessions et al. [1] proposed a staging system for JA based on computerized tomographic findings. It was considered to be the first staging system to more accurately reflect the unique behavior of JA. Its creators aimed to eliminate confusion among institutions with regard to surgical approaches, morbidity, and cure rates. The following staging designations were developed:

Stage IA, tumor limited to posterior nares and/or nasopharyngeal vault, with no paranasal sinus extension
Stage IB, same as IA but with extension into one or more paranasal sinuses
Stage IIA, minimal lateral extension through the sphenopalatine foramen, into and including a minimal part of the medial-most part of the pterygomaxillary fossa (PMF)
Stage IIB, full occupation of the PMF with forward displacement of the posterior wall of the maxillary antrum and lateral and/or anterior displacement of the branches of the maxillary artery (superior extension may occur, eroding the orbital bones)
Stage IIC, extension through the PMF into the cheek and temporal fossa
Stage III, intracranial extension

This system of classification represents the variety of extension of these tumors; in general, the number of anatomic sites involved, rather than the actual tumor size, complicates treatment. The authors believe that tumor extension, rather than size, determines the stage and the surgical approach to tumor clearance. However, this system is based on nasopharyngeal carcinoma staging and thus may result in inaccurate findings (Table 8.1).

Due to the insufficient classification of this protean tumor, surgical management of juvenile angiofibroma is confusing. Large case series have failed to clarify the situation. In 1983, Fisch [2] presented a staging system for juvenile angiofibroma based on his rich experience in skull base surgery. The classification was as follows: type I, tumor limited to the nasopharynx and nasalcavity, with no bone destruction; type II, tumor invading the PMF and the maxillary, ethmoid, and sphenoidal sinuses, with bone destruction; type III, tumor invading the infratemporal fossa, orbit, and parasellar region, remaining lateral to the cavernous sinus; and type IV, massive invasion of the cavernous sinus, optic chiasmal region, or pituitary fossa. In 1989, Andrews et al. [3] modified the system based on the growth pattern of this tumor to help surgeons choose access procedures. The modified staging system was named the Andrews–Fisch classification and became the most widely used staging system. The classification is as follows:

Class I, tumor confined to the site of origin at the sphenopalatine foramen, may extend unimpeded into the nasopharynx and nasal cavity
Class II, involvement of the pterygopalatine fossa or the regional paranasal sinuses (the next major sequence of invasion)

Table 8.1 Some of the staging systems of juvenile angiofibroma

	Sessions	Fisch	Andrews	Radkowski	UMPC	Yi Zixiang
Type/stage	1981	1983	1989	1996	2010	2013
I	IA Limited to nose and/or nasopharyngeal vault IB One or more sinuses	Limited to nasopharynx and nasal cavity	Limited to nasopharynx; bone destruction negligible or limited to sphenopalatine foramen	Ia, limited to nose or nasopharynx; Ib, as in stage Ia, with extension into ≥1 sinus	Nasal cavity, medial pterygopalatine fossa	Localized in nasal cavity, nasopharynx, sinus, pterygomaxillary fossa. Minimal extension in infratemporal fossa, orbit, or cranial fossa
II	IIA Minimal ext. into pterygomaxillary fossa IIB Full occupation of pterygomaxillary fossa with or without erosion of orbital bones IIc Infratemporal fossa with or without cheek	Pterygomaxillary fossa, maxillary, ethmoidal, and sphenoidal sinuses	Invading pterygomaxillary fossa or maxillary, ethmoid or sphenoidal sinus with bone destruction	IIa, minimal extension through sphenopalatine foramen and into medial pterygomaxillary fossa; IIb, full occupation of pterygomaxillary fossa, displacing posterior wall of maxilla forward, orbit erosion, displacement of maxillary artery branches; IIc, infratemporal fossa, cheek, posterior to pterygoid plates	Paranasal sinuses, lateral pterygopalatine fossa; no residual vascularity	Localized in infratemporal fossa, cheek, deep or minimal anterior cranial fossa extension, minimal middle cranial fossa extension. With or without cavernous sinus and internal carotid artery compression, but dura mater intact

(continued)

Table 8.1 (continued)

	Sessions	Fisch	Andrews	Radkowski	UMPC	Yi Zixiang
Type/stage	1981	1983	1989	1996	2010	2013
III	III Intracranial extension	Infratemporal fossa, orbit and parasellar region remaining lateral to cavernous sinus	Invading infratemporal fossa or orbital region: IIIa: no intracranial IIIb: extradural (parasellar) involvement	Erosion of skull base: IIIa: minimal intracranial extension IIIb: extensive intracranial extension ± cavernous sinus	Skull base erosion, orbit, infratemporal fossa; no residual vascularity	From pterygomaxillary fossa and superior orbital fissure, extending into middle cranial fossa as a large gourd-shaped lobe
IV		Cavernous sinus, optic chiasm, or pituitary fossa region	Intracranial, intradural tumor: IVa: without IVb: with cavernous sinus, pituitary or optic chiasm infiltration		Skull base erosion, orbit, infratemporal fossa; residual vascularity	
V					Intracranial extension, residual vascularity; M, medial extension; L, lateral extension	

Class III, involvement of the infratemporal fossa or orbital region (class IIIa refers to extracranial tumors and class IIIb refers to tumors that have expanded into the parasellar region while remaining extradural)
Class IV, intracranial spread (the next sequence of invasion; class IVa is without cavernous sinus, pituitary or optic chaisma infiltration, and class IVb includes the most aggressive tumors, which have grown into the cavernous sinus, pituitary, or optic chiasm)

Andrews and Fisch described the growth pattern of JA. The tumor originates at the superior margin of the sphenopalatine foramen, at the junction of the sphenoid process of the palatine bone and the pterygoid process of the sphenoid bone. The tumor grows into the nasopharyngeal and nasal cavities anteriorly and posteriorly. It also spreads laterally to the pterygopalatine fossa and from there into the infratemporal fossa and orbit through the inferior orbit fissure; the tumor can also spread into the middle cranial fossa through the foramina lacerum and ovale. Description of the characteristics of tumor growth and invasion, especially the analysis of extension at the skull base, makes this staging system a practical guide to the surgical approach. For example, the type C infratemporal fossa approach permits complete resection of all class III and IVa and some IVb tumors. Remnants of class IVb tumors infiltrating the cavernous sinuses should be irradiated or eradicated via a secondary neurosurgical procedure. However, as this staging system does not incorporate advances in radiological imaging and surgical techniques, evaluation of the cure rate, incidence of complications, and local residual and recurrence rates is difficult.

In 1996, through the review of 23 cases of JA based on the revision of Sessions' staging protocol, and combined with the advantages of the other systems, Radkowski et al. [4] proposed a new staging system. The authors believe that the proposed revised staging system allows accurate preoperative tumor assessment, evaluation of risk of tumor recurrence, appropriate surgical planning, and interinstitutional comparison of treatment results. They first reported tumor extension posterior to the pterygoid plates into the region of the medial and lateral pterygoid muscles, a conformation that places the angiofibroma within a muscular bed similar to that of the infratemporal fossa and greatly complicates complete surgical excision. The revised staging system differentiates isolated skull base erosion with minimal intracranial spread (stage IIIA) from a more extensive intracranial tumor with possible spread into the dural folds of the cavernous sinus (stage IIIB). The tumor stage at the time of diagnosis is the primary factor affecting recurrence. This staging system takes into account the choice of surgical approach and the risk of recurrence and thus is cited widely.

With the widespread adoption of endoscopic techniques, preoperative image evaluation, and preoperative vascular embolization, tumor size and the extent of sinus disease are less important in predicting complete tumor removal with endonasal surgical techniques. The University of Pittsburgh Medical Center (UPMC) proposed a new staging system for JA that reflects changes in surgical approaches (endoscopic), route of intracranial extension, and extent of vascular supply from the internal carotid artery (ICA) [5]. Embolization is performed 1 day before surgery using standard techniques, with a combination of small particles for the tumor bed and coils for the proximal feeding vessels. Pre-embolization and post-embolization angiograms are reviewed for evidence of residual vascularity from the ICA. Stage I includes the smallest tumors, with no significant extension beyond the site of origin, which remain medial to the midpoint of the pterygopalatine space. Stage II tumors extend into the paranasal sinuses and lateral to the midpoint of the pterygopalatine space. Together, stages I and II can be considered to describe minimal tumors. In this staging system, cases of all but the smallest tumors are presumed to involve preoperative embolization of the internal maxillary artery and other contributing branches of the external carotid arterial system to devascularize the tumor and facilitate surgery. Tumors that are locally advanced, with skull base erosion or extension to additional extracranial spaces, including the orbit and infratemporal fossa, but have no residual vascularity following embolization, are classified as stage III. Technically, surgical treatment of a stage III tumor requires greater access and is more challenging, but is not hampered by excessive bleeding. The tumor usually has a well-defined margin and is separated from the dura, periorbital region, and/or muscle fascia. Stage IV and V tumors are characterized by residual vascularity from the intracranial circulation following embolization. True intracranial extension (stage V) is subdivided into medial (medial cavernous sinus) and lateral (middle fossa) routes of extension, as this distinction has significant implications for surgical access, potential morbidity, and risk of residual disease. The UPMC staging system for juvenile angiofibroma accounts for two important prognostic factors – the route of cranial base extension and vascularity – and is applicable to endoscopic and open approaches. Compared with other staging systems, the UPMC system more effectively predicts immediate morbidity (including blood loss and the need for multiple operations) and tumor recurrence.

Other Proposed Classifications

Based on knowledge of presumed site of origin of most if not all of tumors and their growth patterns, Chandler et al. [6] in 1984 proposed a staging system similar to that proposed by the American Joint Committee: stage I tumor confined to nasopharynx; stage II tumor extending into the nasal cavity and/or sphenoidal sinus; stage III tumor extending into one or more of the following: antrum, ethmoid sinus, pterygomaxillary and infratemporal fossae, orbit, and/or cheek; and stage IV tumor extending into cranial cavity. The surgical procedure chosen should permit optimum exposure of the tumor through the antrum, behind the antrum, in the nasopharynx, through the nasal cavity, and wherever else extension is demonstrated by the clinical and/or radiological examination.

This system has been found to be useful in making decisions about the approach and management of JA by some surgeons. However, it failed to consider the complexity of intracranial extension and did not differentiate extranasopharyngeal sites, except the sphenoidal sinus and intracranial cavity.

Advances in radiographic imaging, embolization, and surgical methods, particularly endoscopes, made it necessary to devise more appropriate classification. By 2006, Onerci et al. [7] proposed a revised staging system for determining the risk of persistent disease, for choosing the appropriate surgical methods, and for maintaining uniformity. Stage I tumor extension to the nose, nasopharyngeal vault, and sphenoidal sinus. This stage indicates low possibility of persistent disease by endoscopic/microscopic approach. Stage II tumor extension to maxillary sinus or anterior cranial fossa, full occupation of the PMF, limited extension to infratemporal fossa, or the pterygoid plates posteriorly. This stage requires more extensive surgery, such as combining Caldwell–Luc or additional endonasal drilling. Stage III tumor deep extension into cancellous bone at the base of the body and the greater wing of sphenoid, significant extension to the infratemporal fossa or pterygoid plates posteriorly or orbit region, and obliteration of cavernous sinus. This stage represents a high possibility of persistent disease and more extensive surgery. Stage IV tumor intracranial extension between the pituitary gland and internal carotid artery, extension posterolateral to the internal carotid artery, and extensive intracranial extension. These stage tumors should be managed via combined extensive (intracranial) surgery. However, this system has been cited in only one study.

In 2008, by comparing with other staging systems, Carrillo et al. [8] proposed a novel and simple staging system (INCan system) based on an objective analysis of invasion patterns and tumor size. Stage I tumors locate in the nasopharynx, nasal fossae, maxillary antrum, anterior ethmoid cells, and sphenoidal sinus; stage IIa tumors invade to pterygomaxillary fossae or infratemporal fossae anterior to pterygoid plates, with major diameter <6 cm. Stage IIb tumors invade to pterygomaxillary fossae or infratemporal fossae anterior to pterygoid plates, with major diameter ≥6 cm. Stage III tumors invade to infratemporal fossae posterior to pterygoid plates or posterior ethmoid cells. Stage IV tumors have extensive skull base invasion >2 cm or intracranial invasion. Stage I and stage IIA can be managed via an endoscopic approach and stage IIB and stage III via a combined endoscopic and open approach. Stage IV tumor can be managed via a combined anterolateral skull base approach.

Based on our experience, we reviewed 51 cases in 2013 and proposed a clear and simplified classification system for juvenile angiofibroma that divides JNAs into three revised types [9].

Type I includes juvenile angiofibromas fundamentally localized to the nasal cavity, paranasal sinus, nasopharynx, or pterygopalatine fossa (Fig. 8.1).

Type II includes juvenile angiofibromas extending into the infratemporal fossa, cheek region, or orbital cavity, with anterior and/or minimal middle cranial fossa extension, but intact dura mater (Fig. 8.2). Before operation, the surgeon must pay attention to change in the dura mater and choice of reliable surgical treatment [10].

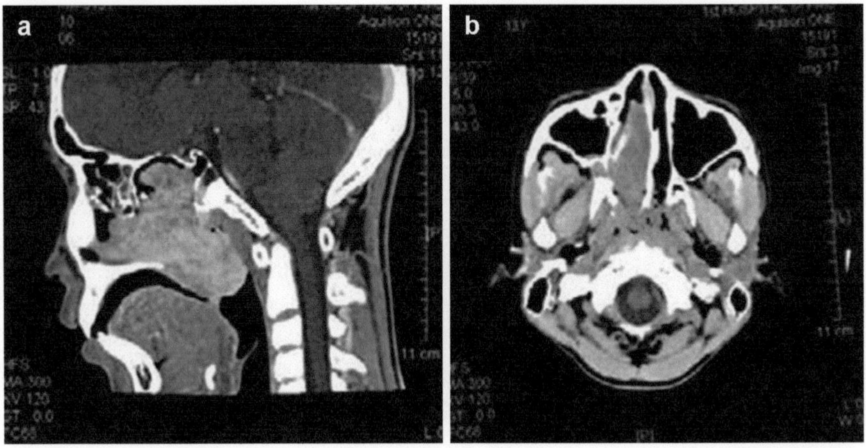

Fig. 8.1 (**a**, **b**) Shows the tumor in the nasal cavity, nasopharynx, and pterygopalatine fossa

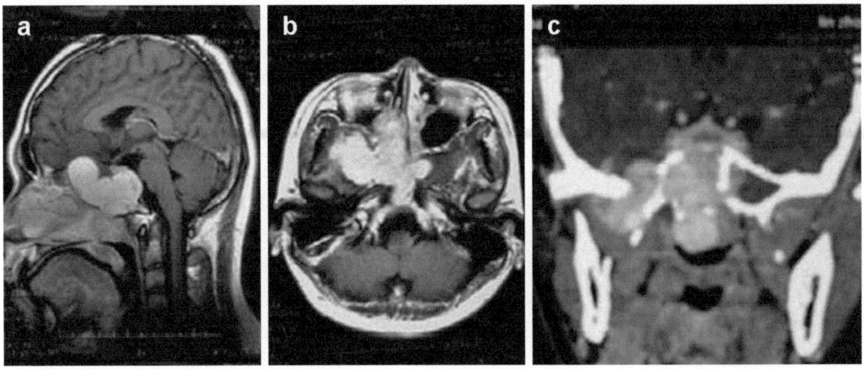

Fig. 8.2 (**a**–**c**) Shows a huge lobulated tumor extending into the anterior and middle cranial fossa and infratemporal fossa, with intact dura mater

Type III is a huge tumor with a calabash-like lobe extending into the middle cranial fossa (Fig. 8.3).

Useful treatments for the three types of juvenile angiofibroma are the transnasal cavity approach with endoscopic guidance that is suitable for type I juvenile angiofibroma resection and the combined transantral–infratemporal fossa–nasal cavity approach that is reliable for resection of type II juvenile angiofibroma that extends into the deep anterior cranial fossa and/or minimally into the middle cranial fossa, with intact dura mater. A combined intra- and extracranial approach is used for the removal of type III juvenile angiofibromas. If tumor residue remains in the middle cranial fossa, approximately 40-Gy radiotherapy affords a good outcome [11].

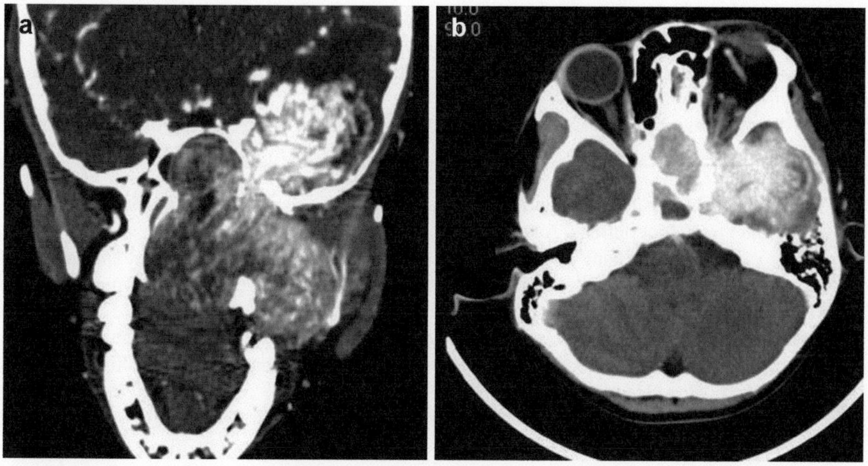

Fig. 8.3 (**a**, **b**) Shows a huge tumor with a calabash-like lobe extending into the middle cranial fossa through the supraorbital fissure

In 2015, Al Sheikh and Eleftheriadou [12] reviewed 32 articles describing the staging and treatment of juvenile angiofibroma. However, a new universal standardized staging system requires more clinical verification.

Conclusion

The Radkowski system was based on modification of the Sessions system. Either the Fisch system or the Andrews–Fisch system has been recognized as the comprehensive, practical, and applicable guide to surgical approach and prediction of outcome. These systems were the most popular used by surgeons. In 2013, the author and his team proposed a clear and simplified classification system and the related surgical managements. It is useful for clinical application.

References

1. Sessions RB, Nick Bryan R, Naclerio RM, et al. Radiographic staging of Juvenile Angiofibroma. Head Neck Surg. 1981;3:279–83.
2. Fisch U. The infratemporal fossa approach for nasopharyngeal tumors. Laryngoscope. 1983;93:36–44.
3. Andrews JC, Fisch U, Aeppli U, et al. The surgical management of extensive nasopharyngeal angiofibromas with the infratemporal fossa approach. Laryngoscope. 1989;99:429–37.
4. Radkowski D, Mcgill T, Healy GB, et al. Angiofibroma: changes in staging and treatment. Arch Otolaryngol Head Neck Surg. 1996;122:122–9.
5. Snyderman CH, Pant H, Carrau RL, et al. A new endoscopic staging system for angiofibromas. Arch Otolaryngol Head Neck Surg. 2010;136:588–94.

6. Chandler JR, Richard Goulding R, Lee Moskowitz L, Quencer RM. Nasopharyngeal Angiofibromas: staging and management. Ann Otol Rhinol Laryngol. 1984;93(4 Pt 1):322–9.
7. Onerci M, Oğretmenoğlu O, Yücel T. Juvenile nasopharyngeal angiofibroma: a revised staging system. Rhinology. 2006;44:39–45.
8. Carrillo JF, Maldonado F, Albores O, et al. Juvenile Nasopharyngeal Angiofibroma: clinical factors associated with recurrence, and proposal of a staging system. J Surg Oncol. 2008;98: 75–80.
9. Yi Z, Fang Z, Lin G, et al. Nasopharyngeal angiofibroma: a concise classification system and appropriate treatment options. Am J Otolaryngol. 2013;34:133–41.
10. Yi Z, Li Z, Cheng J, Zhang R, Lin C, Zhou A, Fang Z. Huge nasopharyngeal angiofibroma with intracranial extension: change in the dura mater and choice of surgical management. J Laryngol Otol. 2007;121:1108–12.
11. Zixiang Y, Jianmin H, Lin C, Lin C, Lin G, Zhichun L, Zhang H, Aidong Z, Shuzhan L. The modern radiation therapy for residual after resection of nasopharyngeal angiofibroma. Chin J Otolaryngol Head Neck Surg. 2010;45:427–8.
12. Alshaikh NA, Eleftheriadou A. Juvenile nasopharyngeal angiofibroma staging: an overview. Ear Nose Throat J. 2015;94:E12–22.

Chapter 9
Embolization of Juvenile Angiofibromas

Anton Valavanis and G. Baltsavias

Abstract Embolization is recognized as an established endovascular interventional neuroradiologic technique for the preoperative devascularization of juvenile angiofibromas. The goal of preoperative embolization of juvenile angiofibromas is the selective obliteration of the intratumoral abnormal arteriolocapillary bed, leading to tumor devascularization, with preservation of the normal arterial supply to surrounding tissues followed by ischemic transformation and some size reduction of the tumor. These embolization-induced changes improve the surgical conditions and contribute to radical tumor removal with minimal intraoperative blood loss. Appropriately performed embolization based on detailed knowledge of the local functional vascular anatomy carries a minimal risk for permanent neurologic morbidity and no mortality. To achieve this goal, a thorough pretherapeutic tumor evaluation by imaging techniques, a detailed angiographic workup, and the application of appropriate embolization techniques, which are described in detail, are necessary.

Keywords Juvenile angiofibroma • Embolization • Interventional neuroradiology

Introduction

Juvenile angiofibroma (JA) is a rare, histologically benign, fibrovascular, nonencapsulated, submucosally growing tumor of the nasopharynx with the potential for locally aggressive behavior. The great majority occurs in young males around puberty [1]. The treatment of choice is surgical tumor removal and in selected cases radiotherapy. Embolization is recognized as an established endovascular interventional neuroradiologic technique for the preoperative devascularization of JAs [2–5]. The goal of preoperative embolization of JAs is the selective obliteration of the intratumoral abnormal arteriolocapillary bed, leading to tumor devascularization with preservation of the normal arterial supply to surrounding tissues. To achieve

A. Valavanis, MD (✉) • G. Baltsavias, MD
Department of Neuroradiology, Clinical Neuroscience Center, University Hospital of Zurich, Zurich, Switzerland
e-mail: Antonios.Valavanis@usz.ch

S.P. Dubey, B. Schick (eds.), *Juvenile Angiofibroma*,
DOI 10.1007/978-3-319-45343-9_9

this goal, a thorough pretherapeutic tumor evaluation by imaging techniques, a detailed angiographic workup, and the application of appropriate embolization techniques are necessary [6].

This chapter is based on a previous contribution of the first author on the application of interventional neuroradiological techniques on the treatment of JAs [7] and summarizes the experience of the authors obtained from the preoperative embolization of 73 consecutive cases of JA performed between 1978 and 2015.

Most commonly the tumor originates from the sphenopalatine foramen. In its early stages of development, the tumor occupies the nasopharynx eccentrically and the ipsilateral posterior nasal fossa [8]. From here the tumor may secondarily extend into the paranasal sinuses, the infratemporal fossa, the central and paracentral middle cranial fossa, and finally intracranially and into the orbit [9]. Presenting symptoms of JA are nasal obstruction and variable degrees of epistaxis. Depending on the specific pattern of tumor extension, further symptoms may develop and include sinusitis, otitis, temporal swelling, exophthalmos, and cranial nerve palsies [10]. The modality of choice for the management of JAs is preoperative embolization followed by radical surgical tumor removal. High-resolution CT and multiplanar, T1-weighted, gadolinium-DTPA-enhanced MRI are essential imaging modalities for planning the angiographic workup and the embolization procedure and for selecting the appropriate surgical approach [8, 11].

In 1982 Fisch introduced a detailed topographic classification of JAs, which has proved useful in planning the angiographic workup and in selecting the appropriate operative approach for a given case of JA [12, 13]. This classification is derived from the evaluation of tumor extension and associated bone destruction as seen on MRI and CT, respectively. According to this classification, JAs are subdivided into the following classes:

Class I: Tumors limited to the nasopharynx and nasal cavity without significant bone destruction
Class II: Tumors invading the maxillary, ethmoid, sphenoid sinuses with significant bone destruction
Class IIIa: Tumors invading the pterygopalatine fossa, the infratemporal fossa, and the orbit
Class IIIb: Tumors with additional intracranial extradural extension lateral to the cavernous sinus
Class IVa: Tumors with extension into the cavernous sinus
Class IVb: Tumors with intracranial intradural, pituitary fossa or suprasellar extension

Angiographic Evaluation of JAs

Bilateral angiography of the common, external, and internal carotid arteries provides essential information on the specific arterial supply, the degree and pattern of vascularization, and the venous drainage of the tumor. Angiographically, the tumor has a typical appearance and can be differentiated from other nasopharyngeal and nasal cavity hypervascular lesions such as angiomatous polyp, hemangioma, hemangiopericytoma, angiosarcoma, and extracranial meningioma. The supplying arteries arising from the external (ECA) and internal carotid artery (ICA) are only minimally dilated. The tumor blush is intense but slightly inhomogeneous; it appears during the arterial phase but persists until the late venous phase of the angiogram. In frontal angiographic projection, the tumoral blush is always in a paramedian, not in a median location. The intensity and homo- or inhomogeneity of the tumoral blush depends on the underlying histologic composition of the individual tumor. JAs with high capillary density and dominance of the vascular component over the fibrous stromal component will exhibit an intense and mostly homogenous tumoral blush as opposed to tumors with low capillary density and dominance of the fibrous, stromal component over the vascular component which will exhibit less intense and inhomogeneous tumoral blush. The draining veins appear during the later part of the venous phase. The venous drainage of JAs occurs primarily through the pterygoid plexus. Depending on tumor extension, further veins such as the retromandibular vein, the facial vein, the cavernous sinus, and the ophthalmic veins may be involved. Only exceptionally may JAs exhibit intratumoral arteriovenous shunting, and in these cases there is early appearance of the draining veins. As a general rule, angiographic exploration of a given case of angiofibroma should be performed according to an individual protocol derived from the CT and MRI appearance of the tumor. Besides a detailed evaluation of the potential supplying branches of the ipsilateral ECA and ICA, the contralateral ECA should be explored in all cases, which reach the midline or extend beyond it [8, 10, 14].

Vascular Supply of JAs

Depending on their size and extension, JAs are supplied by several specific arteries (Fig. 9.1). Initially, the tumor occupies the anterior nasopharynx unilaterally and the ipsilateral posterior nasal cavity. Therefore, the distal internal maxillary artery, with its nasopharyngeal and nasal cavity branches, is the first arterial system to provide supply to a developing JA and represents therefore the exclusive arterial supply of class I JAs. While the recruitment of further arteries in the supply of the tumor depends variably on its pattern of extension, the distal internal maxillary system represents anatomically a constant, always present and hemodynamically the dominant arterial supply of all classes (I–IVb) of JAs. The distal internal maxillary artery branches supplying JAs are the sphenopalatine, the pterygovaginal, and frequently also the vidian arteries. The sphenopalatine artery supplies the nasal portion of the tumor, while the pterygovaginal artery supplies its nasopharyngeal portion. The sphenopalatine artery is an anterior branch of the distal internal maxillary artery and has a lateral to medial course. Upon reaching the posterior nasal cavity, it divides into a medial branch for the septum and a lateral trunk for the conchae. It is this lateral conchal branch which supplies the JAs in the initial stages of their evolution. The medial,

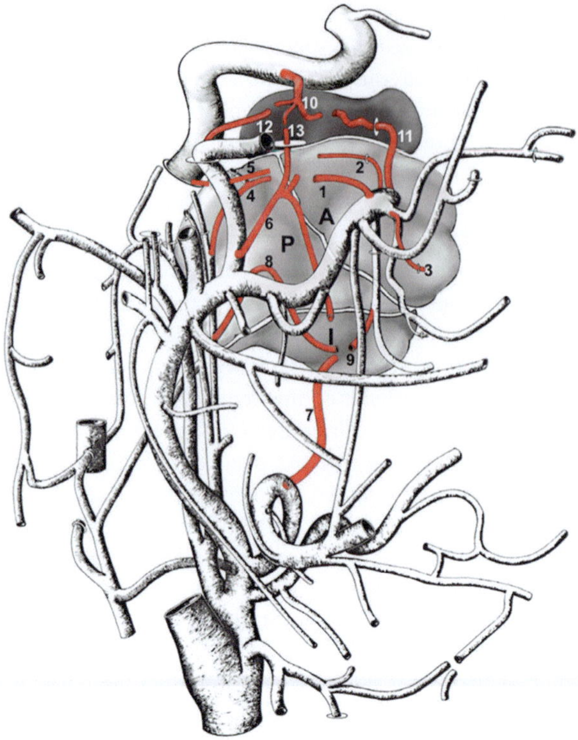

Fig. 9.1 Schematic drawing summarizing the arterial supply of JAs (Modified from Garcia-Monaco et al. [49]). The arteries providing supply to JAs are represented in *red* color. The three extracranial tumor compartments are reproduced in *light gray* color and separated by *white lines* (*A* anterior compartment, *P* posterior compartment, *I* inferior compartment). The intracranial extension is reproduced in *deep gray* color. *1* pterygovaginal a., *2* vidian a., *3* sphenopalatine a., *4* superior pharyngeal a., *5* mandibular a. *6* accessory middle meningeal a., *7* ascending palatine a., *8* middle pharyngeal a., *9* descending palatine a., *10* inferolateral trunk, *11* recurrent artery of the foramen rotundum, *12* cavernous branch of the middle meningeal a., *13* cavernous branch of the accessory middle meningeal artery

septal branch is involved in the supply of the tumor later, when it has reached the midline. The pterygovaginal artery is a recurrent branch of the distal internal maxillary artery. It courses within the pterygovaginal canal, supplies the lateral portions of the roof of the nasopharynx, and curves finally inferiorly to end near the orifice of the Eustachian tube. Here the pterygovaginal artery anastomoses with the inferomedially directed eustachian branch of the accessory meningeal artery, with the superior pharyngeal branch of the ascending pharyngeal artery, and inconstantly with the mandibular branch of the ICA [1]. The vidian artery is also frequently involved into the supply of the tumor. It is a small artery, which has also a recurrent course after its origin from the distal internal maxillary artery. It runs parallel and above the pterygovaginal artery within the pterygoid or vidian canal to enter the foramen lacerum, where it anastomoses with the vidian branch of the petrous internal carotid artery.

Larger tumors with extensions into the sphenoid sinus, the pterygopalatine fossa, the infratemporal fossa, or the parapharyngeal space receive additional supply from the accessory meningeal, the ascending pharyngeal, and the ascending palatine arteries [10].

The accessory meningeal artery represents an important source of supply to JAs of classes II–IV. The origin of this vessel depends on the course of the internal maxillary artery, i.e., in cases with a deep course of the internal maxillary artery, the accessory meningeal artery originates directly from the internal maxillary artery, whereas in cases with a superficial course of the internal maxillary artery, the accessory meningeal artery originates as a main branch of the extracranial segment of the middle meningeal artery. In cases where the middle meningeal artery originates from a system other than the internal maxillary artery, e.g., from the ophthalmic artery, the accessory meningeal artery originates always directly from the internal maxillary artery, irrespective of its course [1]. The accessory meningeal artery supplies with its extracranial branches the posterolateral and superior extracranial extensions of JAs. These branches anastomose with the other arteries participating in the supply of the area, i.e., the superior pharyngeal branch of the ascending pharyngeal artery, the pterygovaginal artery, the ascending palatine artery, and the mandibular artery. This again underlines the necessity of distal embolization, because occlusions proximal to the anastomotic points will result in reconstitution of the supply to the tumor. In addition to these extracranial branches and their anastomoses, the accessory meningeal artery also has a transcranial branch, which courses through either the foramen ovale or the foramen of Vesalius and anastomoses with the inferolateral trunk (ILT) of the ICA. While the two systems are usually in a hemodynamic balance, in some cases one of them is dominant [1].

If the accessory meningeal artery is hypoplastic, the ILT will be dominant and will supply with its posterior branch most of the tumor portion located in the territory of the accessory meningeal artery. In these cases angiography of the ICA will opacify through the dilated ILT the extracranial tumor compartment, which – in a balanced situation – would be supplied by the extracranial branches of the accessory meningeal artery. This may provide the erroneous impression of intracranial tumor extension. Careful analysis of the angiogram and correlation with CT/MRI help in the correct identification of the position of the tumor blush [10].

The ascending pharyngeal artery participates via its superior pharyngeal branch in the supply of the posterior and posteromedial portions of JAs. This branch anastomoses with the accessory meningeal, the pterygovaginal, and the mandibular arteries. Furthermore, it gives off the carotid branch, which courses through the foramen lacerum and anastomoses with the inferolateral trunk as well as the recurrent artery of the foramen lacerum, arising from the cavernous segment of the ICA [1].

The inferior extension of JAs toward the soft palate receives its supply from the terminal segment of the ascending palatine artery. The ascending palatine artery usually arises from the first, i.e., mandibular segment of the facial artery, but it may also arise directly from the external carotid trunk, the middle pharyngeal branch of the ascending pharyngeal artery, or even the accessory meningeal artery. The terminal segment of the ascending palatine artery anastomoses with the descending palatine artery, which, in cases of proximal embolization of the ascending palatine artery, may reconstitute the supply to the inferior portion of the tumor.

Extensions into the sphenoid sinus receive their supply from sphenoidal branches of the vidianmandibular anastomotic system and should be distinguished from intracranial, extradural, parasellar extensions. Extensions into the ethmoid sinus receive their supply from anterior and posterior ethmoidal branches of the ophthalmic artery and should be distinguished from true intraorbital extensions [10]. Intraorbital extensions occur mainly through the inferior orbital fissure and may receive their supply directly from the ophthalmic artery branches or the infraorbital artery. If the intraorbital extension occurs through the superior orbital fissure, then the anteromedial branch of the ILT will also be involved in the supply of the tumor [10].

Intracranial extradural tumor extensions into the middle cranial fossa and into the cavernous sinus occur through the basal foramina (ovale, rotundum, and lacerum) or after destruction of the sphenoid sinus walls and/or the greater wing of the sphenoid bone. The arterial supply is mainly provided by the branches of the ILT, which are in a hemodynamic balance with the transcranial branches of the internal maxillary artery and with the recurrent branches of the ophthalmic artery. If there is dominance of the internal maxillary system over the ILT, the intracranial extradural tumor extension will be mainly opacified during internal maxillary angiography. This represents a favorable hemodynamic condition for embolization of the intracranial extradural extension through the accessory meningeal artery and/or the artery of the foramen rotundum and/or the carotid branch of the superior pharyngeal branch of the ascending pharyngeal artery. In cases with a balanced supply between the ILT and the accessory meningeal artery, temporary occlusion of the ILT with a balloon inflated within the C4 portion of the ICA will induce increased flow through the transcranial branch of the accessory meningeal artery toward the intracranial portion, thus enabling embolization of the intracranial extradural tumor extension.

Intracranial intradural extensions are rare. They occur at the temporobasal area and are supplied by cortical branches of the temporopolar and/or anterior temporal arteries arising from the middle cerebral artery. Currently available microcatheters usually allow distal catheterization of these temporal branches of the middle cerebral artery and thus enable safe embolization of these rare intradural tumor extensions [15].

Compartmental Composition of JAs

Superselective angiographic investigation of JAs and correlation of the individual superselective angiograms with the selective ECA and ICA angiograms show that similar to other hypervascular tumors of the skull base, JAs are composed of multiple vascular compartments. The extracranial portion of the tumor is composed, in order of appearance during the evolution of the tumor, of three compartments, an anterosuperior, a posterosuperior, and an inferior compartment (Fig. 9.1). Each compartment has its own, distinct arterial supply. The anterosuperior compartment is supplied by the sphenopalatine, pterygovaginal, and vidian arteries, all arising from the distal internal maxillary artery. It is always the largest compartment of a JA. The posterosuperior compartment is supplied by the superior pharyngeal branch of the ascending pharyngeal artery and by the Eustachian tube branch of the accessory meningeal artery. The inferior compartment is supplied by the distal, horizontally oriented palatine branch of the ascending palatine artery, the inferior palatine branch of the accessory middle meningeal artery, the middle pharyngeal branch of the ascending pharyngeal artery, and the pterygoid branch of the descending palatine artery. The intracranial portion of the tumor, if present, may be composed of up to five compartments, depending on the pattern of intracranial extension of the tumor. The intracranial compartments are the parasellar-extradural compartment, the cavernous sinus compartment, the intraorbital compartment, the intra-suprasellar compartment, and the intradural compartment. The arterial supply of the different intracranial extensions of the tumor has been described above.

The intrinsic vascular network of each compartment is connected with the vascular network of the adjacent compartments. These intercompartmental communications allow reaching and filling an adjacent compartment with a fluid polymerizing embolic material injected from the principal artery of one compartment.

Endovascular Protocol for the Angiographic Evaluation and Transarterial Embolization of JAs

Below, a brief protocol is outlined for the endovascular exploration and embolization of JAs of classes III, IVa, and IVb:

1. Contralateral common carotid (CCA) injection in frontal projection with manual compression of the ipsilateral ICA for identification of contralateral supply and first evaluation of circle of Willis
2. Ipsilateral CCA injection for angiographic assessment of tumor extent and identification of ECA supply
3. Ipsilateral ICA injection for identification of ICA supply to: (a) extracranial tumor portions (mandibular artery, recurrent artery of foramen lacerum, ILT), (b) ethmoidal extension (ethmoid branches of ophthalmic artery), (c) orbital extension (ophthalmic artery), (d) intracranial extradural extension (ILT), and (e) intracranial intradural extension (temporopolar and anterior temporal branches of the middle cerebral artery) as well as evaluation of the wall of the cavernous, C4, and C3 portions of the ICA
4. Ipsilateral distal internal maxillary injection for identification of supplying arteries (sphenopalatine, pterygovaginal, descending palatine arteries), dangerous anastomoses with ICA (vidian artery, artery of foramen rotundum), or ophthalmic artery (ethmoidal arteries, infraorbital artery) and for embolization of tumor compartment through feeding arteries

5. Ipsilateral proximal internal maxillary injection for identification of supplying arteries (accessory meningeal and middle meningeal arteries)
6. Ipsilateral accessory meningeal superselective injection for identification of extracranial supplying branches, dangerous anastomoses with ICA (transcranial branch, mandibular artery), and transcranial supply to intracranial extradural extension and for embolization of tumor compartment(s)
7. Ipsilateral ascending pharyngeal superselective injection for identification of supplying arteries (superior pharyngeal branch) and dangerous anastomoses (carotid branch) and for embolization of tumor compartment
8. Ipsilateral ascending palatine superselective injection (variable origin: facial artery, external carotid trunk, middle pharyngeal artery) for identification of supplying artery (soft palate branch) and embolization of tumor compartment
9. Ipsilateral CCA injection for confirmation of devascularization of entire ECA supply and identification of persisting ICA supply to the tumor
10. Ipsilateral ICA injection and potential embolization of ICA branches supplying the tumor (mandibular artery, ILT, ophthalmic artery)
11. Ipsilateral CCA injection for final ipsilateral postembolization control
12. Contralateral CCA injection for identification of persisting contralateral supply. Continuation as with steps 4–8 described above

Techniques of Transarterial Embolization of JAs

Proximal occlusion of the extratumoral segments of the supplying arteries without previous obliteration of the intratumoral microvasculature is mostly ineffective regarding devascularization of the tumor and is expected to stimulate the development of collateral supply. This collateral supply may arise from unusual vessels and possibly less easily accessible by surgery, thus rendering the removal of the tumor technically more difficult.

Aspects of embolization technique depend also on the embolic material. The embolic materials used in transarterial embolization of JAs include both particles and fluid materials. Microparticles of polyvinyl alcohol (PVA) are available in different sizes ranging from 45 to 1,000 μ [16, 17]. Gelfoam powder, an alternative to PVA [18], is more rapidly reabsorbable, a factor which should be taken into consideration when planning postembolization surgical removal of the tumor. With the use of PVA, a delay of more than 4 weeks between embolization and operation should be avoided. Among the fluid materials, N-butyl-2-cyanoacrylate (NBCA) [19] has been used for transarterial tumor embolization. Addition of oily iodinated contrast material can delay the polymerization time of NBCA and a small amount of tantalum powder made it radiopaque [20]. NBCA is considered a dangerous material because it can penetrate distally into vascular territories and thus cause ischemia of vital tissues, or it may polymerize rapidly, thus gluing the catheter tip within the arterial lumen [21]. As a general rule, we advocate the use of microparticles (Contour, Boston Scientific Corporation, Natick, MA) in preoperative tumor embolization. They are easier and safer to use and, if properly sized, can reach the intratumoral microvasculature. In most cases the use of the smallest available size, 45–150 μ, is indicated.

From a technical point of view, there are three principal factors that determine the success of intratumoral deposition of the embolic material: (a) the degree of catheterization selectivity, (b) the choice of the embolic material, and (c) the absence of spasm in the arteries to be embolized. In order to avoid vasospasm in the territory of the ECA, the guiding catheter is positioned either just proximal to the origin of the ECA or in the very proximal ECA, and both the advancement of the microcatheters and the insertion of the microguidewire into branches of the ECA are performed in a slow and gentle manner. For PVA embolization, the selective catheterization of the terminal feeding artery is equally essential as the requirement for preservation of the free flow and avoidance of vasospasm. For embolization of ECA branches, ophthalmic artery, dural branches of the vertebral artery flow-guided microcatheters are preferable for atraumatic and distal catheterization. For embolization through small ICA branches as the ILT and medial and lateral clival arteries, selective catheterization with a microcatheter shaped appropriately under steam and embolization with microparticles should be attempted [21]. If this fails, embolization can be performed after temporary balloon occlusion of the ICA immediately distal to the origin of the ILT followed by injection of microparticles through a microcatheter placed proximal to the origin of the ILT. These techniques are also used for embolization of the mandibular artery [7, 10].

Permanent Balloon Occlusion of the ICA

Permanent preoperative balloon occlusion of the ICA should be considered in the rare class IVb and in some class IVa JAs exhibiting extensive invasion of the cavernous sinus and encasement of the cavernous portion of the ICA [8, 22]. Permanent balloon occlusion of the ICA should be performed after the transarterial embolization and following a balloon occlusion test of the ICA. For that purpose, a nondetachable microballoon is inflated in the horizontal cavernous segment of the ICA proximal to the origin of the ophthalmic artery and followed by angiographies of (1) the CCA in lateral projection to confirm occlusion of the ICA and to evaluate the flow conditions within the ophthalmic artery, (2) the contralateral ICA in frontal projection to evaluate the adequate filling of the cerebral hemisphere ipsilateral to the occluded ICA through the anterior communicating artery, and (3) the dominant vertebral artery in lateral projection to evaluate the contribution of the posterior communicating artery to the cerebral hemisphere ipsilateral to the occluded ICA. Tolerance to ICA occlusion is confirmed if the balloon test occlusion of the ICA shows synchronous filling of both cerebral hemispheres throughout the late venous phase or a minimal delay in filling of less than 2 s of the ipsilateral hemisphere as compared to the contralateral hemisphere. For permanent balloon occlusion of the ICA, a latex detachable microballoon is inserted coaxially through the guiding catheter into the ICA and advanced toward the cavernous segment of the ICA. The balloon is inflated with isotonic iodinated contrast material until the lumen of the ICA is occluded. Preferably the balloon is positioned between the origins of the ILT and ophthalmic artery. This will prevent anterograde thromboembolism from thrombus formed distal to the balloon and dislodged by inflow through the ILT [22]. Complete occlusion of the ICA is confirmed by a lateral carotid angiogram performed through the guiding catheter. The balloon is then detached. The procedure is terminated by detaching a second balloon within the proximal ICA. This will prevent distal migration of the first balloon in case it should deflate prematurely, and it also prevents extensive thrombus formation within the proximal ICA, which is known to carry the risk of ophthalmic artery embolism through the ECA system [10]. Following the procedure the patient should be closely monitored for at least 12 h in an intensive care unit. During this time special care is taken to avoid a fall in blood pressure below the systolic level of 100 mm/Hg because this may cause ischemia in the cerebral hemisphere ipsilateral to the occluded ICA [15].

Effects of Transarterial Embolization

The intratumoral deposition of the embolic material through a transarterial approach leads to intratumoral ischemia, which can be minimal, moderate, significant, or complete (Fig. 9.2a–g). The degree of intratumoral ischemia is always assessed by postembolization contrast-enhanced MR or CT (Fig. 9.2h). In our series of 73 patients of JA who underwent transarterial embolization, significant ischemic transformation of the tumor was achieved in 66 %, moderate ischemic transformation in 21 %, and minimal ischemic transformation in 8 % of the cases. In 5 % of the cases, no ischemic transformation was seen on postembolization MR despite an

Fig. 9.2 (**a**) T1-weighted contrast-enhanced sagittal MR shows strongly, slightly inhomogenously enhancing class IIIa JA. (**b**) Common carotid artery angiography in lateral projection shows the hypervascular, class IIIa JA. (**c**) Internal carotid artery angiography in lateral projection shows the contribution of the mandibular artery (*arrow*), arising from the ICA at the level of the foramen lacerum to the supply of the tumor. (**d**) Superselective angiography of the pterygovaginal artery (*arrow*) in late arterial phase and lateral projection showing the large, dominant compartment of the tumor prior to its embolization with PVA microparticles of 45 μm. (**e**) Selective angiography of the ventral division (*arrow*) of the ascending pharyngeal artery in frontal projection showing supply of the posterosuperior compartment of the tumor (*double arrow*). This compartment was embolized with PVA microparticles of 45 μm. (**f**) Selective angiography in lateral projection of the ascending palatine artery (*bold arrow*) arising from the proximal facial artery showing supply of the small inferior compartment of the tumor from two palatine branches (*arrows*). This compartment was embolized with PVA microparticles of 45 μm. (**g**) Final common carotid angiography in lateral projection at the end of the embolization showing complete devascularization of the tumor with preservation of all branches of the external carotid artery. Notice regression of the mandibular artery (*arrow*). (**h**) Sagittal, contrast-enhanced CT following embolization showing extensive ischemic transformation and some size decrease of the tumor

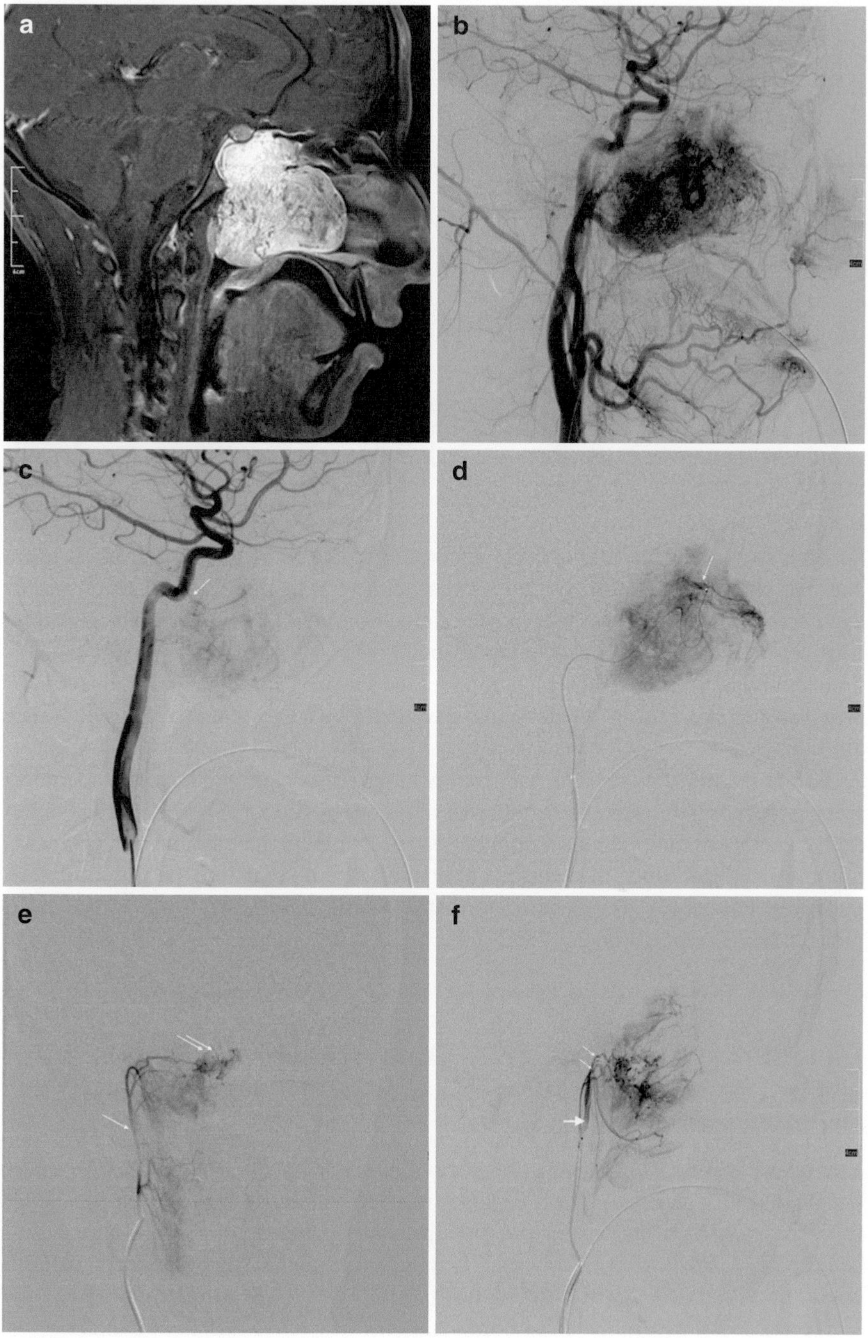
a
b
c
d
e
f

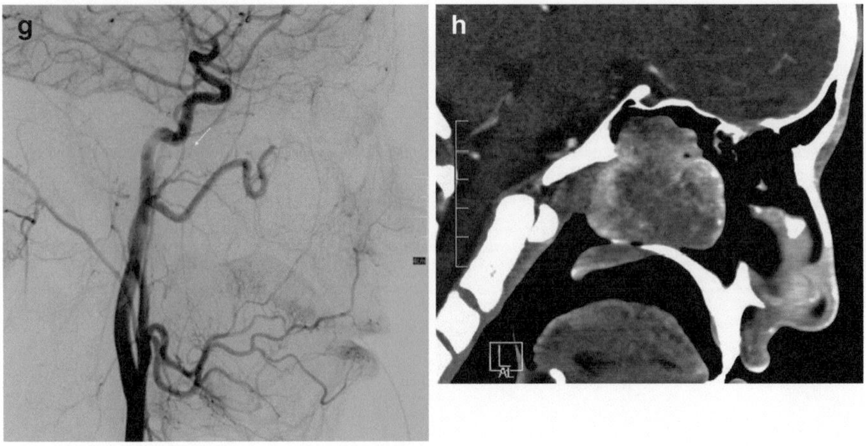

Fig. 9.2 (continued)

apparently successful embolization according to the immediate postembolization angiography. In cases with a significant ischemic transformation, moderate shrinkage of the tumor is observed on postembolization imaging. Furthermore, during a time period of several weeks, the tumor undergoes ischemic changes and some volume reduction, phenomena, which improve the surgical conditions for radical tumor removal and corroborate to delaying the operative removal for 2–3 weeks after embolization.

Before the routine application of preoperative embolization, patients who underwent surgery for JAs were at distinct risk of exsanguination [23]. The average blood replacement without previous embolization is reported in the literature to be approximately 2,000 cc. Since the routine application of embolization, the risk of exsanguination has almost disappeared, and the blood loss during surgery has been reduced to less than 1,000 cc [24, 25].

Dangers and Complications of Transarterial Embolization of JAs

Embolization itself, if properly performed after precise evaluation of the superselective angiograms, carries today a very low risk [26]. In the authors' series consisting of 73 cases, which underwent preoperative embolization, only one complication leading to permanent partial visual loss occurred following permanent balloon occlusion of the ICA, corresponding to a morbidity of 1.3 % and a mortality of 0 %.

Nevertheless, several types of complications may occur during embolization of JAs and have been reported in the literature, the most serious being cerebral stroke, blindness, and cranial nerve palsies [26–28]. Cerebral stroke may occur rarely when there is a reflux of embolic material from the ECA into the ICA or when embolic material refluxes from superselectively catheterized ILT branches of the ICA into the main stem of these vessels. Reflux can be avoided by injecting the embolic material very carefully and synchronously with the heartbeat and thereby during the systolic pulse wave of the arterial bloodstream. Embolization of ICA small branches should be interrupted as soon as the blood flow is significantly decreased but before it ceases [29]. Exceptionally protection of the cerebral circulation with a temporarily inflated balloon can be applied. Stroke may also occur when embolic material passes anterogradely through arterio-arterial anastomoses between the ECA and the ICA. Blindness may occur when embolic material passes through anastomoses between the distal internal maxillary artery and the ophthalmic artery. Such anastomoses may be present but functionally inactive and therefore invisible on the pre-embolization angiogram. During embolization and with increasing pressure within the embolized vessel such an inactive anastomosis may become functionally active. Therefore good knowledge of these anastomoses is a prerequisite and special care is necessary in order to detect fluoroscopically their appearance during embolization [29]. As a general rule, timely detection and avoidance of fluid embolic materials inadvertent passage into the cerebral circulation in comparison to microparticles is more difficult.

Cranial nerve palsies may occur when branches of the ICA or ECA known to supply the transcranial course of the cranial nerves, as the ILT, are completely occluded. Depending upon the type of embolic material and on the presence or absence of collateral supply, such cranial nerve palsies may be permanent or transient. With the use of PVA and with care to avoid occlusion of nerve supplying branches, the risk of inducing permanent cranial nerve palsy during embolization is very low. Other complications as skin necrosis have been also reported, but remain exceptional. Side effects as fever, local pain, and other non-neurological symptoms have been also reported and they are transient [28].

Since embolization of tumors is a preoperative measure to be followed by surgical removal, every effort and caution should be undertaken to minimize the morbidity to nearly zero, because otherwise the patient has to face two management risks, i.e., an endovascular risk followed by a surgical risk.

Direct Intratumoral Embolization of JAs

In 1994, the direct intratumoral embolization (DIE) of JAs as an alternative technique to endovascular embolization was proposed [30, 31]. The technique of percutaneous embolization has been developed since years for the treatment of accessible hypervascular lesions of the head and neck using liquid embolic materials as alcohol and NBCA [32]. An important motivation for seeking techniques alternative to endovascular approach was the, at the time widely used, proximal external carotid ligation for the treatment of intractable bleedings [31]. Since then, several case reports and small series of JA direct embolization have been published, using NBCA in the first years [30–32, 34, 43] and increasingly Onyx in the recent years [35–42,

45–47]. The procedure is carried out under general anesthesia, and the first step is the diagnostic selective angiography of bilateral internal and external carotid arteries. Transnasal or percutaneous (precondylar, transzygomatic, transbuccal, etc.) puncture of the tumor with a long needle is obtained under biplane fluoroscopy using transarterial road map or bone landmarks. Correct needle position is verified by continuous slow blood reflux. A parenchymography of the tumor is then obtained by contrast agent injection. Then, under fluoroscopy, the liquid embolic material is injected through one or more needle punctures until the tumoral vascular bed is obliterated. The extent of devascularization is documented with postembolization arteriography [31, 35, 45].

The main arguments for a direct approach regardless embolic material are the following: (1) In high-grade (Fisch III, IV) or in recurrent tumors with supply through small branches of the internal carotid, a direct approach obviates the challenge and risk of their superselective catheterization. (2) Especially in low-grade tumors, getting access directly to the vasculature of the tumor is safer than the endovascular approach because you stay away from dangerous IC-EC anastomoses. (3) The risk of cranial nerve damage is less with direct than endovascular embolization through vessels supplying cranial nerves. (4) Based on the authors' experience, with direct approach, one can obtain more extensive devascularization by overcoming the limitations of transarterial embolization (small arterial feeders, vessel tortuosity, vasospasm). (5) More extensive devascularization leads to less blood loss during surgery and also facilitates less invasive approaches, as endoscopic surgery. (6) The consistency and especially the staining of the tumor with the embolic material facilitate complete resection. (7) Direct embolization is possible even after proximal ligation of the feeding vessels. (8) The direct embolization requires less radiation times and less contrast medium in comparison to embolization with PVA. Recently, Onyx largely replaced NBCA in DIE due to its properties and namely the slower precipitation properties of Onyx, thereby allowing deep penetration within the tumor vasculature and the possibility of interruption of the injection during the procedure to allow assessment of the embolization pattern and early recognition of dangerous vascular anastomoses.

Despite the above arguments and developments, Elhammady et al. [37], in a review of case series published between 1990 and 2011 comparing transarterial embolization of JAs with DIE, reported similar safety and efficacy of the two methods. Presumably, this is because DIE can lead to severe complications despite the above tenable-sounding arguments. Casasco et al. in a series of 29 cases reported on one patient with postoperative middle cerebral artery (MCA) infarct and subsequent death as well as one patient with blindness (3.5 % morbidity and 3.5 % mortality) [33]. Other smaller and more recent studies reported zero morbidity-mortality [37, 39, 43, 44]. Cases of inadvertent liquid embolic material migration to the cerebral vasculature prompted the use of balloon protection of the large intracranial arteries (carotid, vertebral), which already makes the procedure of an extracranial tumor more complicated [33, 35] since manipulations of the cerebral vasculature are preventively involved for a questionably increased safety [45]. Some authors also noticed that progressive increase of the dense Onyx cast makes the distinction of a small reflux to the cerebral vasculature difficult [35]. Unusual complications or risks are also linked to the use of Onyx for preoperative embolization as the release of trigeminocardiac reflex with asystole during injection of dimethyl sulfoxide (DMSO) [38, 40] as well as sparking and self-contained combustion of Onyx with bipolar or monopolar electrocautery during surgery [41].

However, the most important aspect to consider when reviewing the literature is the fact that the DIE is predominantly compared with a type of transarterial embolization, which invalidates or vitiates the advantages of endovascular technique. For instance, the standard described technique of transarterial embolization (which subsequently was declared as inferior to the DIE) used relatively large PVA particles (above 100 or even 300 μ) and the referred target of the procedure was the "feeder embolization" [43] and not the intratumoral embolization, which has the potential of tumor necrosis and shrinkage. This explains the charges about "coalescence of PVA and occlusion of the microcatheters, necessitating recatheterization of feeding arteries" [37]. The arguments that the particles "dissipate over time allowing revascularization of the tumor" or "collaterals tend to be recruited to feed the tumor" except of inexplicable (since the authors advocate and apply immediate postembolization surgery) are also pointless since they attack the above type of transarterial embolization technique, which is linked to such weaknesses by definition. The same applies with the use of relatively large and stiff guide- and microcatheters, which may explain exaggerated vasospasm during endovascular navigation [37, 42, 43, 45]. Regarding the difference in intraoperative blood loss between patients embolized by DIE and transarterial PVA embolization, it did not reach statistical significance in a relatively small series of patients [8], whereas it was found to be statistically significant in a larger and more recent series [45]. However, comparable low intraoperative blood loss has been reported also in series with PVA embolization [48].

The technique of DIE is certainly an alternative of intra-arterial embolization in cases of proximal arterial ligation and lack of endovascular access. Last but not least, the issue of costs and extremely high price of Onyx in comparison to PVA and whether this may be justified after comparing surgical operative times, blood loss, transfusion requirements, and complications needs further investigation.

References

1. Lasjaunias P, Berenstein A. Surgical neuroangiography, vol I: functional anatomy of craniofacial arteries. Berlin/Heidelberg/New York: Springer; 1987.
2. Ballah D, Rabinowitz D, Vossough A, Rickert S, Dunham B, Kazahaya K, et al. Preoperative angiography and external carotid artery embolization of juvenile nasopharyngeal angiofibromas in a tertiary referral paediatric centre. Clin Radiol. 2013;68:1097–106.
3. Chan KH, Gao D, Fernandez PG, Kingdom TT, Kumpe DA. Juvenile nasopharyngeal angiofibroma: vascular determinates for operative complications and tumor recurrence. Laryngoscope. 2014;124:672–7.
4. Parikh V, Hennemeyer C. Microspheres embolization of juvenile nasopharyngeal angiofibroma in an adult. Int J Surg Case Rep. 2014;5:1203–6.
5. Giavroglou C, Constantinidis J, Triaridis S, Daniilidis J, Dimitriadis A. Angiographic evaluation and embolization of juvenile nasopharyngeal angiofibroma. HNO. 2007;55:36–41.

6. Schick B, Kahle G. Radiological findings in angiofibroma. Acta Radiol. 2000;41:585–93.
7. Valavanis A. Embolization of juvenile nasopharyngeal angiofibromas. In: Valavanis A, editor. Interventional neuroradiology. Berlin/Heidelberg: Springer; 1993. p. 77–83.
8. Valavanis A, Fisch U. Juvenile nasopharyngeal angiofibroma: imaging, classification and embolization. In: Fisch U, Valavanis A, Yasargil MG, editors. Neurological surgery of the ear and skull base. Amsterdam: Kugler and Ghedini; 1989. p. 235–44.
9. Szymańska A, Szymański M, Czekajska-Chehab E, Szczerbo-Trojanowska M. Two types of lateral extension in juvenile nasopharyngeal angiofibroma: diagnostic and therapeutic management. Eur Arch Otorhinolaryngol. 2015;272:159–66.
10. Lasjaunias P, Berenstein A. Surgical neuroangiography, vol II: endovascular treatment of craniofacial lesions. Berlin/Heidelberg/New York: Springer; 1987.
11. Wu AW, Mowry SE, Vinuela F, Abemayor E, Wang MB. Bilateral vascular supply in juvenile nasopharyngeal angiofibromas. Laryngoscope. 2011;121:639–43.
12. Fisch U, Fagan P, Valavanis A. The infratemporal fossa approach for the lateral skull base. Otolaryngol Clin N Am. 1987;17:513–22.
13. Andrews JC, Fisch U, Valavanis A. The infratemporal fossa approach for extensive nasopharyngeal angiofibromas. In: Fisch U, Valavanis A, Yasargil MG, editors. Neurological surgery of the ear and skull base. Amsterdam: Kugler and Ghedini; 1989. p. 249–55.
14. Griauzde J, Srinivasan A. Imaging of vascular lesions of the head and neck. Radiol Clin N Am. 2015;53:197–213.
15. Valavanis A. Interventional neuroradiology for head and neck surgery. In: Cummings CW, Fredrickson JM, Harker LA, Krause CJ, Schuller DE, editors. Otolaryngology – head and neck surgery. Update II. St. Louis: Mosby Year Book; 1990. p. 206–23.
16. Jack Jr CR, Forbes G, Dewanjee MK, Brown ML, Earnest FN. Polyvinyl alcohol sponge for embolotherapy: particle size and morphology. AJNR. 1985;6:595–7.
17. Kerber CW, Bank WO, Horton JA. Polyvinyl alcohol foam: prepackaged emboli for therapeutic embolization. AJR Am J Roentgenol. 1978;130:1193–4.
18. Berenstein A, Russell E. Gelatin sponge in therapeutic neuroradiology: a subject review. Radiology. 1981;141:105–12.
19. Brothers MF, Kaufmann JCE, Fox AJ, Deveikis JP. N-Butyl-2-cyanoacrylate: substitute for IBCA in interventional neuroradiology-histopathologic and polymerization time studies. AJNR. 1989;10:777–86.
20. Spiegel SM, Vinuela F, Glodwasser MJ, Fox AJ, Pelz DM. Adjusting polymerization time of isobutyl-2-cyanoacrylate. AJNR. 1986;7:109–12.
21. Dion JE. Principles and methodology. In: Vinuela F, Halbach VV, Dion JE, editors. Interventional neuroradiology: endovascular therapy of central nervous system. New York: Raven; 1992. p. 1–15.
22. Valavanis A, Fisch U. Balloon-occlusion of the internal carotid artery in extensive skull base tumors. In: Fisch U, Valavanis A, Yasargil MG, editors. Neurological surgery of the ear and skull base. Amsterdam: Kugler and Ghedini; 1989. p. 81–6.
23. Cummings BJ. Relative risk factors in the treatment of juvenile nasopharyngeal angiofibroma. Head Neck Surg. 1980;3:21–6.
24. Davis KR, Debrun GM. Embolization of juvenile nasopharyngeal angiofibromas. Semin Interv Radiol. 1987;4:309–20.
25. Moulin G, Chagnaud C, Gras R, Gueguen E, Dessi P, Gaubert JY, et al. Juvenile nasopharyngeal angiofibroma: comparison of blood loss during removal in embolized group versus nonembolized group. Cardiovasc Intervent Radiol. 1995;18:158–61.
26. Lasjaunias P. Nasopharyngeal angiofibromas. Hazards of embolization. Radiology. 1980;136:119–23.
27. Onerci M, Gumus K, Cil B, Eldem B. A rare complication of embolization in juvenile nasopharyngeal angiofibroma. Int J Pediatr Otorhinolaryngol. 2005;69:423–8.
28. Ogawa AI, Fornazieri MA, da Silva LV, Pinna FR, Voegels RL, Sennes LU, et al. Juvenile angiofibroma: major and minor complications of preoperative embolization. Rhinology. 2012;50:199–202.

29. Valavanis A. Preoperative embolization of the head and neck: indications, patient selection, goals and precautions. AJNR. 1986;7:943–52.
30. Piérot L, Boulin A, Castaings L, Chabolle F, Moret J. Embolization by direct puncture of hypervascularized ORL tumors. Ann Otolaryngol Chir Cervicofac. 1994;111:403–9. French.
31. Tranbahuy P, Borsik M, Herman P, Wassef M, Casasco A. Direct intratumoral embolization of juvenile angiofibroma. Am J Otolaryngol. 1994;15:429–35.
32. Casasco A, Herbreteau D, Houdart E, George B, Tran Ba Huy P, Deffresne D, et al. Devascularization of craniofacial tumors by percutaneous tumor puncture. AJNR Am J Neuroradiol. 1994;15:1233–9.
33. Casasco A, Houdart E, Biondi A, Jhaveri HS, Herbreteau D, Aymard A, et al. Major complications of percutaneous embolization of skull-base tumors. AJNR Am J Neuroradiol. 1999;20:179–81.
34. Liang Y, Wang D, Huang W, Ling F, Liu Y, Lü F. Direct intratumoral embolization of hypervascular tumors of the head and neck. Chin Med J (Engl). 2003;116:616–9.
35. Lehmann M, Ulrich S, Reineke U, Hamberger U, Dietrich U, Sudhoff H. Intratumoral Onyx embolisation in the management of juvenile nasopharyngeal angiofibroma. HNO. 2010;58:853–7.
36. Herman B, Bublik M, Ruiz J, Younis R. Endoscopic embolization with onyx prior to resection of JNA: a new approach. Int J Pediatr Otorhinolaryngol. 2011;75:53–6.
37. Elhammady MS, Johnson JN, Peterson EC, Aziz-Sultan MA. Preoperative embolization of juvenile nasopharyngeal angiofibromas: transarterial versus direct tumoral puncture. World Neurosurg. 2011;76:328–34; discussion 263–5.
38. Puri AS, Thiex R, Zarzour H, Rahbar R, Orbach DB. Trigeminocardiac reflex in a child during pre-Onyx DMSO injection for juvenile nasopharyngeal angiofibroma embolization. A case report. Interv Neuroradiol. 2011;17:13–6.
39. Gemmete JJ, Chaudhary N, Pandey AS, McHugh JB, Marentette LJ. Complete devascularization of a juvenile angiofibroma by direct percutaneous embolization with only ethylene vinyl alcohol copolymer (Onyx) through a single needle placement. J Neurointerv Surg. 2011;3:191–3.
40. Potti TA, Gemmete JJ, Pandey AS, Chaudhary N. Trigeminocardiac reflex during the percutaneous injection of ethylene vinyl alcohol copolymer (Onyx) into a juvenile nasopharyngeal angiofibroma: a report of two cases. J Neurointerv Surg. 2011;3:263–5.
41. Hira A, Chao K. Direct endoscopic intratumoral injection of Onyx for the preoperative embolization of a recurrent juvenile nasal angiofibroma. Interv Neuroradiol. 2011;17:477–81.
42. Gemmete JJ, Patel S, Pandey AS, Sullivan SE, McKean EL, Marentette LJ, et al. Preliminary experience with the percutaneous embolization of juvenile angiofibromas using only ethylene-vinyl alcohol copolymer (Onyx) for preoperative devascularization prior to surgical resection. AJNR Am J Neuroradiol. 2012;33:1669–75.
43. Lv MM, Fan XD, Su LX, Chen D. Preoperative direct puncture embolization of advanced juvenile nasopharyngeal angiofibroma in combination with transarterial embolization: an analysis of 22 consecutive patients. Cardiovasc Intervent Radiol. 2013;36:111–7.
44. Jang HU, Kim TH, Park CM, Kim JS. Direct intratumoral embolization of intranasal vascular tumors. Auris Nasus Larynx. 2013;40:103–5.
45. Gao M, Gemmete JJ, Chaudhary N, Pandey AS, Sullivan SE, McKean EL, et al. A comparison of particulate and onyx embolization in preoperative devascularization of juvenile nasopharyngeal angiofibromas. Neuroradiology. 2013;55:1089–96.
46. Lutz J, Holtmannspötter M, Flatz W, Meier-Bender A, Berghaus A, Brückmann H, et al. Preoperative embolization to improve the surgical management and outcome of Juvenile Nasopharyngeal Angiofibroma (JNA) in a single center: 10-year experience. Clin Neuroradiol. 2015. doi:10.1007/s00062-015-0374-2
47. Borota L, Mahmoud E, Nyberg C, Ekberg T. Combined percutaneous and transarterial devascularisation of juvenile nasopharyngeal angiofibroma with protection of internal carotid artery: a modification of the technique. Interv Neuroradiol. 2015;21:390–6.

48. Nicolai P, Villaret AB, Farina D, Nadeau S, Yakirevitch A, Berlucchi M, et al. Endoscopic surgery for juvenile angiofibroma: a critical review of indications after 46 cases. Am J Rhinol Allergy. 2010;24:e67–72.
49. Garcia-Monaco R, Lasjaunias P, Alvarez H, Rodesch G. Embolization of vascular lesions of the head and neck. In: Valavanis A, editor. Interventional neuroradiology. Berlin/Heidelberg: Springer; 1993. p. 1–22.

Part III
Management

Chapter 10
Anesthesia and Management of Intraoperative Bleeding

Alexander Izakson and Tiberiu Ezri

Abstract Anesthesia for resection of juvenile angiofibroma (JA) imposes numerous challenges for the anesthesiologist. These include but are not limited to detection of preoperative complications associated with embolization of the vessels feeding the tumor and radiotherapy and avoiding aspiration of blood and secretions during induction of anesthesia and recovery from anesthesia and extubation of the patient's trachea. Intracranial extension of JA necessitates special anesthetic considerations.

A special consideration is accorded to intraoperative bleeding which occasionally may be massive and life threatening, to the blood and blood product replacement, and to the prevention and management of coagulopathy. Blood conservation strategies are described including deliberate hypotension. Both the risk of massive bleeding and the use of deliberate hypotension dictate continuous invasive monitoring of the hemodynamic state of the patient.

Since bleeding may continue after surgery, close surveillance of the patient and intensive treatment should be undertaken postoperatively, in a milieu of a high dependency unit, such as postanesthesia care unit or intensive care unit.

Keywords Juvenile angiofibroma • Resection • Anesthetic considerations • Bleeding • Blood transfusion • Coagulopathy

---

A. Izakson, MD
Lecturer, Head, Department of Anesthesia, Rebecca Sieff Medical Center, Galil Medical Faculty, Bar Ilan University, Safed, Israel
e-mail: izaksondoc@gmail.com

T. Ezri, MD (✉)
Associate Professor, Head, Department of Anesthesia, Wolfson Medical Center, Sackler Medical School, Tel Aviv University, 62 Halochamim Street, Holon 58100, Israel

Outcomes Research Consortium, Cleveland, OH, USA
e-mail: tezri@bezeqint.net

S.P. Dubey, B. Schick (eds.), *Juvenile Angiofibroma*,
DOI 10.1007/978-3-319-45343-9_10

Preanesthetic Concerns

Advances in radiological imaging, better preoperative identification of the feeding vessels of the tumor, and angiographic embolization performed before surgery, together with using deliberate hypotension techniques and blood conservation strategies, have revolutionized the surgical management of JA.

During the preoperative, pre-anesthetic visit, the anesthesiologist must be aware of the preoperative preparative treatment modalities related to JA with their side effects and complications.

Complications associated with preoperative embolization of the vessels supplying JA include the potential for cerebrovascular accident if one of the carotid arteries is affected or blindness if the ophthalmic artery is embolized [1]. Other authors reported numbness and mild pain on the ipsilateral hemiface and difficulty in opening the mouth for up to 1 week. These transient phenomena have to be taken into consideration prior to anesthesia and are presumed to be caused by the temporarily reduced blood supply, sometimes causing spasm of the masseter muscles [2].

Radiation therapy as an adjuvant to surgical resection may lead to complications such as growth retardation, temporal lobe radionecrosis, keratopathy, and potential carcinogenic side effects [3–5]. Prior radiation therapy makes laryngoscopy difficult owing to tissue fibrosis causing a noncompliant submandibular space and can lead to significant postoperative edema owing to obliteration of the lymphatic vessels. Patients on radiotherapy are more susceptible to infection and bleeding during airway manipulation if they suffer from oral mucositis [6].

The main goals of anesthesia for JA resection are prevention of aspiration of blood and nasopharyngeal secretion, continuous hemodynamic monitoring and control, minimizing blood loss during surgery, along with blood and blood products replacement if necessary, and prevention of airway obstruction in the postoperative period owing to the edema produced by surgical manipulation and further bleeding.

Induction and Maintenance of Anesthesia

Rapid sequence induction of anesthesia with cricoid pressure may be preferred in patients with active epistaxis. After securing the airway, a throat pack is inserted as an additional measure to prevent aspiration and should be removed at the end of surgery, before extubation of the trachea to prevent airway obstruction [7]. Maintenance of anesthesia is tailored to facilitate deliberate hypotension and may be provided with either a balanced anesthetic technique based on an inhaled anesthetic or total intravenous anesthesia (TIVA) [7–10].

Anesthetic Management of Intracranial Involvement of Juvenile Angiofibroma

As the tumor grows, tumor extension can occur to the infratemporal fossa through the pterygomaxillary space and onto the middle cranial fossa via the superior or inferior orbital fissures.

Preoperative assessment of patients with intracranial extension of JA should include the evaluation of the level of consciousness, neurological deficits, and the occurrence of seizures. Symptoms and signs of raised intracranial pressure (ICP), such as persistent headache, vomiting, and papilledema, may be present [11].

The specific anatomic involvement and the planned procedure should be discussed between the anesthesiologist and the surgeon. The presence of increased ICP implies special anesthetic management considerations. Smooth induction of anesthesia, invasive monitoring including beat-to-beat blood pressure measurement through an indwelling arterial cannula, and promotion of moderate hyperventilation are crucial measures to be taken [11].

The cerebral perfusion pressure (CPP), defined as the difference between mean arterial pressure and ICP, should be kept in the range of pressures where autoregulation of the brain is preserved (60–150 mmHg), although there may be individual variability in the CPP [12]. To maintain a normal or near-normal ICP and CPP, moderate arterial CO_2 reduction by hyperventilation is advised, along with avoidance of potent vasodilators and the use of anesthetic agents known to decrease cerebral metabolic rate and oxygen consumption. Thiopental, propofol, and inhaled anesthetics may have beneficial effects by decreasing the cerebral metabolic rate in contrast to ketamine which tends to increase it.

Patient Monitoring

In addition to standard, routine monitoring (ECG, pulse oximetry, noninvasive blood pressure, core temperature and capnography measurements), invasive hemodynamic monitoring is essential in providing safe hypotensive anesthesia by beat-to-beat blood pressure measurement and for frequent blood sampling for blood gases, CBC, coagulation profile, and chemistry analyses. Since the access to the neck veins is limited, either the basilic or cephalic, or subclavian or femoral vein can be cannulated for central venous pressure (CVP) monitoring. In one study, cubital fossa veins were used for CVP measurements [10]. However, Ezri et al. [7] have used internal jugular catheterization in all their patients.

Lower limb veins may be preferred for venous access because they are accessible intraoperatively, as upper limbs are kept by the patient's side and are under the surgical drapes. Proper extension tubing should be connected if upper limb veins are employed. Either the radial artery or dorsalis pedis artery can be used for invasive, continuous blood pressure monitoring.

Intraoperative Blood Loss and Blood Replacement

Since blood loss may be significant during JA resection, several therapeutic strategies are employed to decrease intraoperative blood loss and the need for blood and blood product transfusion. These include but are not limited to performing preoperative procedures aimed to decrease the tumor's vascular supply, improving surgical technique, and using deliberate hypotension during surgery.

Preoperative selective arterial embolization of the feeding vessels significantly decreased intraoperative blood loss and facilitated the resection of larger tumors [2, 13]. Preoperative embolization is generally undertaken 24–72 h prior to surgical resection. The rationale for this is that occluding the feeding arteries of the JA will decrease intraoperative blood loss and may even decrease the tumor's size to augment resectability.

When comparing the endoscopic with the open surgical approaches, the endoscopic approach was associated with significantly less surgical bleeding [3, 14, 15]. The endoscopic approach reportedly reduced the intraoperative blood loss, length of hospital stay, and recurrence rate [3]. Furthermore, there have been reports of endoscopic tumor resection, without significant bleeding, even in the absence of preoperative embolization [15, 16]. The use of endoscopic bipolar cautery by the surgeon is another effective adjuvant technique in reducing blood loss [17].

Ezri et al. [7] reported a case series of ten patients who underwent resection of JA in a teaching hospital. Patients' age was 11–29 years. Eight tumors were resected via a lateral rhinotomy and two were resected endoscopically (after embolization of the tumor's feeding vessels). The duration of surgery was approximately 6 h for both surgical approaches. Due to the risk of blood/secretion aspiration, anesthesia was induced in a rapid-sequence manner. Arterial and central venous catheters were placed in all patients. The mean arterial pressure was targeted to 55–65 mmHg by deliberate hypotension with isoflurane. Patients in the open surgery group lost $4,800 \pm 1,600$ mL of blood, while the two endoscopic resection cases lost 600 and 1,500 mL, respectively. In another report [10], endoscopic surgical resection was associated with a median blood loss of 500 mL, which is significantly less than that reported during open surgery [7]. The open surgical approach is associated with significant intraoperative and postoperative morbidity because of massive blood loss and the need for massive blood and blood product transfusion. Patients fulfilling the criteria for massive blood loss and massive transfusion (transfusion of ≥ 10 red blood cell units [RBC], which approximates the total blood volume [TBV] of an average adult patient, within 24 h, or transfusion of four RBC units in 1 h with anticipation of continued need for blood product support, or replacement of 50 % of the TBV by blood products within 3 h) should be managed according to established massive blood transfusion strategies [18].

Apart from preoperative embolization and endoscopic surgery, other strategies aimed at reducing blood loss may be employed, such as placing the operating table with the patient in reverse Trendelenburg position (head-up 15–30°) and deliberate hypotension. The reverse Trendelenburg position deviates the blood away from the surgical field by gravity and thus decreases blood loss [7, 17]. It also facilitates better surgical exposure. The lower limbs should be elevated and the knees kept at the heart level to ensure optimal venous return. One major concern with the head-up position is the risk of venous air embolism (VAE), which occurs with an incidence of 6–30 % in the semi-sitting position [17]. Euvolemia should be maintained, and the surgical field should be flushed by the surgeon frequently with saline solution to prevent VAE. A sudden drop in end-tidal carbon dioxide value, measured by capnography, may be an early sign of air embolism.

In order to minimize intraoperative bleeding and oozing and to maintain a dry surgical field, deliberate hypotension (DH) is frequently employed in these patients. DH consists of maintaining a systolic blood pressure of 85–90 mmHg and a mean arterial pressure (MAP) of 50–65 mmHg during the procedure [19, 20]. Techniques which use the "natural" hypotensive effects of the anesthetic agents themselves and maintain an appropriate anesthetic depth or analgesia, without producing toxic metabolites, are preferred [7, 8].

Inhalational anesthetics, vasodilators, and beta-blockers have been employed effectively to produce deliberate hypotension. The chosen vasodilators should be short acting and easy to titrate to the desired effect. The literature does not support the use of any particular single agent over another for this purpose. A recently proposed technique was using a combination of remifentanil, with either propofol or an inhalational agent (isoflurane, desflurane, or sevoflurane), in concentrations routinely employed in the clinical practice [8]. Total intravenous anesthesia with propofol and remifentanil was found to provide a drier surgical field than balanced general anesthesia (consisting of an inhaled anesthetic and an opiate) plus esmolol, in children undergoing functional endoscopic sinus surgery. However, both techniques were safe and effective in producing deliberate hypotension [9]. Traditionally, vasodilators such as sodium nitroprusside (SNP) and nitroglycerine (NTG) have been used for providing hypotensive anesthesia [8, 19]. Though still in use, they may have side effects such as reflex tachycardia and toxic metabolites with SNP and tachyphylaxis with NTG. Calcium channel blockers or beta-blockers are also used as adjuvants to achieve a target blood pressure [19]. Additionally, dexmedetomidine and magnesium have also been found to be effective. These two drugs may also decrease intraoperative anesthetic agent requirement, postoperative pain, shivering, and nausea and vomiting in adult patients undergoing functional endoscopic sinus surgery and middle ear surgery [20, 21]. Following a systematic review of the relevant publications, Choi and Samman [22] concluded that the benefits of hypotensive anesthesia were a significant decrease of blood loss, a significant decrease in transfusion rate, and a significant reduction in operation time. There were no significant cerebral, cardiovascular, renal, and hepatic complications compared to the control groups. However, a scrutinous patient selection is mandatory, since patients with significant coexisting diseases may not tolerate even short periods of hypotension.

Intra- and postoperatively, the patient's coagulation profile should be checked frequently and corrected if necessary [7].

Prevention and Management of Intraoperative Coagulopathy

Life-threatening bleeding in patients undergoing JA resection is usually caused by a combination of vascular injury and coagulopathy. While bleeding from vascular injury can usually be repaired surgically, coagulopathy-related bleeding is often more difficult to manage and may also mask the site of vascular injury. The causes of coagulopathy in patients with severe bleeding are multifactorial, including consumption and dilution of platelets and coagulation factors, as well as dysfunction of platelets and the coagulation system. The interplay between hypothermia, acidosis, and progressive coagulopathy, referred to as the "lethal triad," often results in exsanguination [23].

Implementation of blood conservation strategies (see next topic) may prevent or significantly reduce the risk of coagulopathy.

Additionally, pharmacological agents including antifibrinolytics like tranexamic acid or epsilon aminocaproic acid are frequently used to prevent and/or manage coagulopathies.

Epsilon aminocaproic acid inhibits fibrinolysis via inhibition of plasminogen inhibitors and, to a lesser degree, through antiplasmin activity. Tranexamic acid is similar to epsilon aminocaproic acid, but it is approximately ten times more potent [24].

Recombinant activated factor VII is a recombinant coagulation factor concentrate, specifically approved for patients with factor deficiencies (hemophilia), but because it is also known to enhance thrombin generation, it has been suggested to provide hemostasis in various other clinical situations. The major categories of off-label use included closed-space (including intracranial) bleeding, surgical bleeding, and other bleeding causes [25]. Preserving normothermia and a normal pH as well as normal ionized calcium levels are prerequisites for a normal coagulation process.

Thromboelastometry is a sensitive monitor of various coagulation factors and may help in prevention and management strategy [26]. Well-designed institutional strategies are necessary for successful management of major transfusion and prevention and/or treatment of ensuing coagulopathies [18]. Early replacement of clotting factors and using fibrinogen concentrate is the first-line treatment [27, 28] as preventive and management tools of intraoperative coagulopathy.

Blood Conservation Strategies

Blood conservation strategies encompass a series of measures taken to reduce the need for allogeneic blood transfusion.

Tissue oxygenation requires adequate hemoglobin concentration and a well-preserved tissue perfusion. Massive intraoperative hemorrhage may lead to hypotension and organ hypoperfusion, along with a sudden decrease in hemoglobin level. Prolonged tissue oxygen deprivation will result in anaerobic metabolism, a significant reduction in tissue energy reserves, and profound tissue acidosis. Therefore in such a scenario, the need for red blood cells (RBCs) transfusion is almost inevitable.

Transfusion of allogeneic blood components affects patient outcome in a dose-related fashion – the larger the number of allogeneic blood components transfused, the higher the rate of transfusion-related complications such as dilutional coagulopathy (which may cause a vicious circle of rebleeding and more blood requirement), infections, respiratory distress syndrome, or other organ dysfunction [29–31].

Blood transfusion requirement may be reduced by several blood conservation strategies.

In the setting of JA, where the intervention is scheduled days or weeks ahead, blood conservation strategies may be planned to avoid massive blood transfusion in case of major bleeding.

Such strategies may include minimizing surgical bleeding, erythropoietin administration followed by autologous blood collection [32], and application of restrictive transfusion strategies.

The following discussion refers to blood conservation strategies that may be employed in patients undergoing JA resection.

Minimizing Surgical Bleeding

(a) *Preoperative embolization* of the vessels feeding the tumor usually decreases the vascularity sufficiently to make resection easier and without major blood loss [33, 34]. However, large tumors may still bleed, owing to incomplete embolization or by the presence of nonembolized branches from the internal carotid artery system.

(b) *Controlled hypotension* has been demonstrated to reduce surgical bleeding and facilitate surgical hemostasis [35]. See details about controlled hypotension earlier in this chapter.

(c) *Techniques and pharmacological agents that preserve hemostasis* during surgical removal of JA include the use of adequate surgical hemostasis, appropriate patient positioning, maintaining a normal pH, temperature and acceptable calcium levels, and correction of coagulation disturbances by administration of blood products (platelets, frozen plasma, cryoprecipitate), antifibrinolytic agents, desmopressin, and, rarely, recombinant activated factor VII. See detailed discussion earlier in this chapter.

The use of an intratumoral injection of fibrin glue has been described in a few case reports [17].

Pharmacological Treatment

Erythropoietin may reduce the amount of transfusion of allogeneic blood in special cases such as patient's transfusion refusal, chronic anemia or renal failure [36].

EPO represents a good alternative to autotransfusion when this is not feasible. One should however take into consideration the cost-benefit ratio of using EPO [37].

Perioperative iron administration has been suggested to mitigate perioperative anemia [38].

Autologous Blood Transfusions

Autologous blood is the safest means of blood transfusion [39]. Various autologous transfusion techniques have been developed with the aim of reducing the rate of allogeneic transfusions including pre-deposit of autologous blood, acute normovolemic preoperative hemodilution, and collection of intraoperative and postoperative blood. Preoperative donations, generally combined with the intravenous administration of iron, generally start 1 month before the surgery with an interval of 3–4 days between donations and a final interval of 7 days before surgery [40]. Baseline hemoglobin levels should be measured since the presence of anemia may contraindicate the use of autologous blood donation.

Intraoperative Blood Salvage

Techniques of autologous transfusion include collecting intraoperative blood with the technique of washing the red blood cells [41]. Like preoperative normovolemic hemodilution, intraoperative blood collection with a cell saver has the advantage of being independent from the planned date of surgery and can also be used in emergency surgery.

Red blood cell salvage is commonly used for procedures in which major blood loss is anticipated. However, its use for endonasal surgeries is controversial because the site of surgery and blood collection can be contaminated by the nasal flora [42].

Restrictive Transfusion Strategy

In the past, a Hb concentration of less than 10 g/dL was considered a threshold for blood transfusion; however, several studies have shown that in most patients, far lower Hb levels are well tolerated [32].

Studies have shown that a minimum tolerable Hb value, in normovolemic, normoxic patient, without severe heart or carotid disorders, may be as low as 6–7 g/dL [43, 44].

The adherence to a restrictive (at a Hb of 7–8 g/dL) rather than a liberal blood transfusion strategy has been recommended; however, choosing a strict number may not be appropriate [45] since the decision to transfuse depends on many factors including the patient's coexisting diseases and the presence of ongoing bleeding.

Extubation of the Trachea and Postoperative Management

At the end of surgery, a decision to extubate the trachea should be taken only after consulting the surgeon. Massive blood loss and transfusion, extensive surgical dissection, suspicion of residual tumor, uncontrolled oozing of blood from the surgical site, and leaving in situ postnasal packs are conditions that preclude safe extubation. In such cases, the endotracheal tube is left in place for at least 24 h, with continuous monitoring of the airway control and of the hemodynamic status. Endoscopic resection of NA causes less intraoperative bleeding and less extensive surgical trauma. Hence, after endoscopic resection, there is more chance for safe tracheal extubation in the operating room, immediately after surgery. In a study by Khanna et al. [10], extubation was delayed in only 50 % of the patients after endoscopic surgery. In another series [7] where the majority of patients had open surgeries, all were deliberately sedated and ventilated for 8–24 h after surgery, to ensure safe extubation of the patients' trachea.

The patient's trachea is extubated after ensuring hemostasis and conducting a positive leak test around the deflated endotracheal tube's cuff. The cuff leak test helps to identify patients at risk of developing post-extubation stridor due to laryngeal or supraglottic edema. However, the discriminatory power of the cuff leak test is highly variable. While the presence of a cuff leak predicts successful extubation, a failed cuff leak test is not an accurate predictor of post-extubation stridor and, if used as a criterion for extubation, may lead to unnecessarily prolonged intubation or to needless tracheostomy [46, 47].

Bleeding can occur during removal of the pack, and it is advisable to conduct the procedure under general anesthesia or sedation with the airway secured and with resuscitation equipment immediately available.

Since bleeding may continue after surgery, close surveillance of the patient and the intensive treatment should be continued postoperatively in a milieu of high dependency unit, such as postanesthesia care unit or intensive care unit [7].

In conclusion, anesthesia for resection of NA is challenging and should focus on multiple purposes that include but are not limited to avoiding aspiration of blood and secretions during induction of anesthesia and emergence, decreasing intraoperative bleeding, timely replacement of blood and blood products, and a safe extubation of the patient's trachea along with postoperative close surveillance.

References

1. Casasco A, Houdart E, Biondi A, Jhaveri H, Herbreteau D, Aymard A, Merland JJ. Major complications of percutaneous embolization of skull-base tumors. AJNR Am J Neuroradiol. 1999;20:179–81.
2. Li J, Qian J, Shan X, Wang L. Evaluation of the effectiveness of preoperative embolization in surgery for nasopharyngeal angiofibroma. Eur Arch Otorhinolaryngol. 1998;255:430–32.
3. Blount A, Riley K, Woodworth B. Juvenile nasopharyngeal angiofibroma. Otolaryngol Clin N Am. 2011;44:989–1004.
4. Garca M, Yuca S, Yuca K. Juvenile nasopharyngeal angiofibroma. Eur J Gen Med. 2010;7:419–25.

5. Lee J, Chen P, Safa A, Juillard G, Calcaterra T. The role of radiation in the treatment of advanced juvenile angiofibroma. Laryngoscope. 2002;112:1213–20.
6. Lefor AT. Perioperative management of patient with cancer. Chest. 1999;115(5 Suppl): 165S–71S.
7. Ezri T, Roth Y, Geva D, Konichezky S, Marshak G, Halperin D. Anesthetic management of juvenile nasopharyngeal angiofibroma resection. J Cardiothorac Vasc Anesth. 2003;17: 622–24.
8. Degoute C. Controlled hypotension: a guide to drug choice. Drugs. 2007;67:1053–76.
9. Ragab S, Hassanin M. Optimizing the surgical field in pediatric functional endoscopic sinus surgery: a new evidence-based approach. Otolaryngol Head Neck Surg. 2010;142:48–54.
10. Khanna P, Ray B, Sinha R, Kumar R, Sikka K, Singh A. Anaesthetic management of endoscopic resection of juvenile nasopharyngeal angiofibroma: our experience and a review of the literature. S Afr J Anaesth Analg. 2013;19:314–20.
11. Goma H (2011). Anesthetic considerations of brain tumor surgery, diagnostic techniques and surgical management of brain tumors. In: Abujamra AL, editor. ISBN: 978-953-307-589-1, InTech. Available from: http://www.intechopen.com/books/diagnostic-techniques-and-surgical-management-of-brain-tumors/anesthetic-considerations-of-brain-tumor-surgery.
12. Dagal A, Lam AM. Anesthesia for neurosurgery. In: Barash P, Cullen B, Stoelting R, Cahalan M, Stock M, Ortega R, editors. Clinical anesthesia. 7th ed. Philadelphia: Wolters Kluver – Lippincott Williams and Wilkins; 2013. p. 998–9. Chapter 36.
13. Siniluoto T, Luotonen J, Tikkakoski T, Leinonen A, Jokinen K. Value of pre-operative embolization in surgery for nasopharyngeal angiofibroma. J Laryngol Otol. 1993;107:514–21.
14. Renkonen S, Hagström J, Vuola J, Niemelä M, Porras M, Kivivuori SM, Leivo I, Mäkitie AA. The changing surgical management of juvenile nasopharyngeal angiofibroma. Eur Arch Otorhinolaryngol. 2011;268:599–607.
15. Andrade N, Pinto J, Nóbrega Mde O, Aguiar J, Aguiar T, Vinhaes E. Exclusively endoscopic surgery for juvenile nasopharyngeal angiofibroma. Otolaryngol Head Neck Surg. 2007; 137:492–6.
16. Borghei P, Baradaranfar M, Borghei S, Sokhandon F. Transnasal endoscopic resection of juvenile nasopharyngeal angiofibroma without preoperative embolization. Ear Nose Throat J. 2006;85:740–3.
17. Romani R, Tuominen H, Hernesniemi J. Reducing intraoperative bleeding of juvenile nasopharyngeal angiofibroma. World Neurosurg. 2010;74:497–500.
18. Pham H, Shaz B. Update on massive transfusion. Br J Anaesth. 2013;111(S1):i71–82.
19. Tobias J. Controlled hypotension in children: a critical review of available agents. Paediatr Drugs. 2002;4:439–53.
20. Elsharnouby N, Elsharnouby M. Magnesium sulphate as a technique of hypotensive anesthesia. Br J Anaesth. 2006;96:727e31.
21. Ryu J, Sohn I, Do S. Controlled hypotension for middle ear surgery: a comparison between remifentanil and magnesium sulphate. Br J Anaesth. 2009;103:490–5.
22. Choi W, Samman N. Risks and benefits of deliberate hypotension in anaesthesia: a systematic review. Int J Oral Maxillofac Surg. 2008;37:687–703.
23. Lynn M, Jeroukhimov I, Klein Y, Martinowitz U. Updates in the management of severe coagulopathy in trauma patients. Intensive Care Med. 2002;28:S241–7.
24. Shakur H, Roberts I, Bautista R, Caballero J, Coats T, Dewan Y, et al. Effects of tranexamic acid on death, vascular occlusive events, and blood transfusion in trauma patients with significant haemorrhage (CRASH-2): a randomised, placebo-controlled trial. Lancet. 2010;376:23–32.
25. Shander A, Goodnough L, Ratko T, Matuszewski K, Cohn S, Diringer M, et al. Consensus recommendations for off-label use of recombinant human factor VIIa (Novoseven) therapy. P&T. 2005;30:644–58.

26. Schochl H, Nienaber U, Hofer G, Voelckel W, Jambor C, Scharbert G, et al. Goal-directed coagulation management of major trauma patients using thromboelastometry (ROTEM)-guided administration of fibrinogen concentrate and prothrombin complex concentrate. Crit Care. 2010;14:R55.
27. Rourke C, Curry N, Khan S, Taylor R, Raza I, Davenport R, et al. Fibrinogen levels during trauma hemorrhage, response to replacement therapy, and association with patient outcomes. J Thromb Haemost. 2012;10:1342–51.
28. Nienaber U, Innerhofer P, Westermann I, Schochl H, Attal R, Breitkopf R, et al. The impact of fresh frozen plasma vs coagulation factor concentrates on morbidity and mortality in trauma-associated haemorrhage and massive transfusion. Injury. 2011;42:697–701.
29. Dzik W. Fresh blood for everyone? Balancing availability and quality of stored RBCs. Transfus Med. 2008;18:260–5.
30. Ranucci M, Carlucci C, Isgrò G, Boncilli A, De Benedetti D, De la Torre T, et al. Duration of red blood cell storage and outcomes in pediatric cardiac surgery: an association found for pump prime blood. Crit Care. 2009;13:R207.
31. Vandromme MJ, McGwin GJ, Weinberg JA. Blood transfusion in the critically ill: does storage age matter? Scand J Trauma Resusc Emerg Med. 2009;17:35.
32. Zimrin AB, Hess JR. Current issues relating to the transfusion of stored red blood cells. Vox Sang. 2009;96:93–103.
33. Nicolai P, Berlucchi M, Tomenzoli D, Cappiello J, Trimarchi M, Maroldi R, et al. Endoscopic surgery for juvenile angiofibroma : when and how. Laryngoscope. 2003;113:775–82.
34. Li JR, Qian J, Shan XZ, Wang L. Evaluation of the effectiveness of preoperative embolization in surgery for nasopharyngeal angiofibroma. Eur Arch Otorhinolaryngol. 1998;255:430–2.
35. Dhariwal D, Gibbons A, Kittur M, Sugar A. Blood transfusion requirements in bimaxillary osteotomies. Br J Oral Maxillofac Surg. 2004;42:231–5.
36. Apfelbaum JL, Nuttall GA, Connis RT, Harrison CR, Miller RD, Nickinovich DG, et al. Practice guidelines for perioperative blood management. An updated report by the American Society of Anesthesiologists Task Force on perioperative blood management. Anesthesiology 2015;122:241–75.
37. Deutsch A, Spaulding J, Marcus RE. Preoperative epoetin alfa vs autologous blood donation in primary total knee arthroplasty. J Arthroplasty. 2006;21:628–35.
38. Hallet J, Hanif A, Callum J, Pronina I, Wallace D, Yohanathan L, et al. The impact of perioperative iron on the use of red blood cell transfusions in gastrointestinal surgery: a systematic review and meta-analysis. Transfus Med Rev. 2014;28:205–11.
39. Borghi B, Pignotti E, Montebugnoli M, et al. Autotransfusion in major orthopaedic surgery: experience with 1785 patients. Br J Anaesth. 1997;79:662–4.
40. Goodnough L. Autologous blood donation. Crit Care. 2004;8 suppl 2:S49–52.
41. Friederichs MG, Mariani EM, Bourne MH. Perioperative blood salvage as an alternative to predonating blood for primary total knee and hip arthroplasty. J Arthroplasty. 2002;17:298–303.
42. Anderson S, Panizza B. Are cell salvage and autologous blood transfusion safe in endonasal surgery? Otolaryngol Head Neck Surg. 2010;142(3 Suppl 1):S3–6.
43. Spahn DR. Perioperative transfusion triggers for red blood cells. Vox Sang. 2000;78 suppl 2:163–6.
44. Isbister JP. Decision making in perioperative transfusion. Transfus Apher Sci. 2002;27:19–28.
45. Vincent JL. Indications for blood transfusions: too complex to base on a single. Ann Intern Med. 2012;157:71–2.
46. Fisher M, Raper R. The 'cuff-leak' test for extubation. Anaesthesia. 1992;47:10–2.
47. Kriner E, Shafazand S, Colice G. The endotracheal tube cuff- leak test as predictor for post-extubation stridor. Respir Care. 2005;50:1632–8.

Chapter 11
Endoscopic Surgery of Juvenile Angiofibroma

Ahmad Safadi, Alberto Schreiber, and Piero Nicolai

Abstract Surgery is considered the gold standard for the treatment of juvenile angiofibroma (JA), and preoperative embolization has provided significant reduction of complications and intraoperative bleeding with minimal risk of residual disease. The advent of endoscopic surgery has revolutionized the management of JA, which was traditionally based on a wide array of external approaches. Endonasal endoscopic resection is currently adopted as a safe and effective technique for the removal of small- and intermediate-sized JAs. Endoscopic removal of large and invasive JAs is feasible even in selected cases but should only be performed by experienced teams with expertise also in external approaches. Recurrent or more appropriately residual lesions are commonly diagnosed within 3 years from surgery.

Keywords Juvenile angiofibroma • Endoscopic surgery • Surgical treatment of juvenile angiofibroma

Introduction

Surgical treatment of juvenile angiofibroma (JA) is challenging in view of the rich vascularity of the lesion, the complex anatomy of the skull base, and the young age of patients. Although preoperative embolization has largely decreased intraoperative bleeding and facilitated surgical resection [1], control of bleeding is still a major problem in managing JA, especially when consistent vascularization from internal carotid artery (ICA) is present. Because children and adolescents

A. Safadi, MD
Department of Otorhinolaryngology – Head and Neck Surgery and Maxillofacial Surgery, Tel Aviv Sourasky Medical Center, Sackler School of Medicine, Tel Aviv University, Tel Aviv, Israel

A. Schreiber, MD • P. Nicolai, MD (✉)
Department of Otorhinolaryngology – Head and Neck Surgery, Spedali Civili of Brescia, University of Brescia, Brescia, Italy
e-mail: pieronicolai@virgilio.it

S.P. Dubey, B. Schick (eds.), *Juvenile Angiofibroma*,
DOI 10.1007/978-3-319-45343-9_11

have a small intravascular blood volume compared with adults, they have a reduced tolerance to operative blood loss. Additionally, in young patients, the potential for osteotomies to affect facial growth should be considered when planning the surgical approach [2].

Although external approaches have been the mainstay of surgical treatment for decades, they were associated with a high rate of morbidity. Apart from the already mentioned risks related to severe blood loss and need for osteotomies, there are complications which are typical of specific approaches. Cerebrospinal fluid leak, facial and infraorbital nerve damage, lacrimal dysfunction, facial deformities, and dental malocclusion have been reported with transfacial approaches [3, 4]. The lateral approach via the infratemporal fossa may result in trismus, hypoesthesia, and conductive hearing loss [5].

The Rise and Evolution of Endoscopic Surgery in the Management of JA

In 1996, Kamel [6] first reported a case of JA limited to the right posterior nasal cavity, nasopharynx, and pterygopalatine fossa that was operated transnasally under endoscopic control, with the intent to propose a "minimal invasive" alternative to external approaches. The lesion was completely excised and the patient was free of tumor after 2 years of follow-up. Kamel [6] stated that "In limited lesions, the option of a transnasal endoscopic approach could be cautiously considered by experienced surgeons." One year later, the Pittsburgh group [7] reported their experience with 16 cases of JA, 3 of which were operated by a transnasal endoscopic approach. They considered an endoscopic approach to be appropriate for small tumors limited to the nasopharynx, nasal cavity, ethmoid, and sphenoid sinuses and may be attempted in tumors with limited pterygopalatine fossa extension. Additionally, preoperative embolization was considered essential due to the limited access, which makes visualization of the surgical field suboptimal in case of extensive bleeding.

A review of case series published during the first years following the introduction of endoscopic approach for resection of JA shows that exclusive endoscopic surgery was restricted to early stage JAs, which were confined to the nasal cavity, nasopharynx, ethmoid, and sphenoid sinuses with limited pterygopalatine fossa extension (Radkowski et al. [4] stages Ia to IIb, Andrew et al. (modified Fisch) [5] stages I–II) [3, 8–17]. Although Carrau et al. [17] in 2001 considered that lesions extending to the pterygopalatine and infratemporal fossa could be treated by endoscopic surgery alone, most authors agreed that significant involvement of these spaces was a contraindication for an exclusively endoscopic resection. Relapse rates were comparable to those achieved with external approaches or even more favorable (0–15 % [4, 7, 18]).

The low recurrence rates and minimal morbidity associated with an endoscopic approach encouraged many surgeons to extend the indications to more advanced lesions. In 2002, Roger et al. [19] reported a retrospective series of 20 patients with JAs classified according to the system of Radkowski et al. [4] and followed for an average of 3.75 years. Ten patients had advanced disease, one had involvement of the infratemporal fossa (stage IIC), and nine had erosion of the skull base (stage IIIA). Major blood loss occurred in stage IIIA cases compared with stage I and II cases, but none of the patients required blood transfusion. A residual lesion was left in the infratemporal fossa and in the apex of the orbit in a stage IIC and IIIA JA, respectively, but in neither case was progression on scans at 18 and 20 months observed. In 2003, Nicolai et al. [20] reported the outcome of a series of 15 patients with JA that were resected endoscopically, where the lesions were staged according to the system described by Andrews et al. [5], and patients were followed for a mean of 50 months. Four JAs were advanced (stage III a or b), with three invading the infratemporal fossa and one the parasellar region. All lesions were successfully resected without blood transfusion. The single patient who had persistence in the floor of the sphenoid sinus had a stage I tumor. In this series, 46.6 % of lesions received feeding vessels from the ICA. However, this did not preclude endoscopic resection and did not correlate with intraoperative blood loss. Despite the excellent results achieved with these four advanced JAs, the authors suggested that only extremely limited stage IIIa and IIIb lesions (infratemporal fossa with or without parasellar invasion) should be selected for an endoscopic approach. In the same year, Onerci et al. [21] reported on a series of 12 patients staged according to the system of Radkowski [4]. Four patients had stage IIIA disease with limited intracranial penetration. Intraoperative blood loss was significantly higher in these four patients compared with the other eight who had smaller JAs (1,500 ml vs. 1,000 ml). Two of the four patients had residual disease around the cavernous sinus, but there was no progression of these remnants over a follow-up of 2 years by MRI. Wormald et al. [22] reported on a series of seven patients with JAs, one with invasion of the infratemporal fossa. All patients had complete macroscopic clearance, and none had recurrence after a mean follow-up of 3.75 years. Pasquini et al. [23] reported only one recurrence after endoscopic resection of six cases of JA, one of which involved the infratemporal fossa. The recurrence was treated endoscopically and the patient remained free of recurrence at 25 months after the last procedure.

Despite the successful resection of some advanced lesions in these early reports, the overall number of patients treated was limited, and therefore the validity of endoscopic surgery was still considered questionable. The advantages of an endoscopic approach can be easily identified in the avoidance of facial incisions, osteotomies, and bone plating, which do not expose young patients to the risk of craniofacial alterations. In addition, the magnified field of view and angled view "behind the corner" may be associated with more complete inspection of the resection cavity and the shorter hospitalization time. However, a few limitations of endoscopic surgery remained to be addressed: the potential of extensive bleeding to obscure a restricted surgical field, the difficulty of one hand dissection especially in separating the lesion from soft tissues, the limitation in accessing far lateral infratemporal extension, the inability to directly control the ICA and optic nerve, and the difficulty in controlling intracranial and cavernous sinus invasion.

In order to overcome some of these limitations, many technical refinements have been adopted during the last decade. Advancements in preoperative embolization resulted in significant reduction in intraoperative bleeding, and, despite some reports of safe resection without embolization [24, 25], it is considered the standard of care in most centers [19, 26, 27]. Some authors advocated the use of laser for the resection of JA in order to improve bleeding control. Nd:YAG laser was used to photocoagulate the lesion before it was safely resected with a microdebrider [28], an instrument which in our experience has limited indications in JA. Potassium titanyl phosphate (KTP) laser has also been used as an adjunct to endoscopic resection and resulted in less blood loss compared to monopolar electrocoagulation [29]. Radiofrequency coblation was also introduced to reduce blood loss [30, 31]. However, laser and coblation have not been used in large series, and hemostasis was successfully achieved mostly by early detection and control of the internal maxillary artery and other feeding vessels. Even in cases of feeding vessels from the ICA, which are not amenable to embolization, these tributaries can be coagulated in most cases [26, 27]. Additionally, when extensive bleeding is encountered, staging of the operation with delayed resection of the skull base component was suggested to allow patients to recover, equilibrate blood volume, and correct hemorrhage-induced coagulopathies before addressing the residual critical part of the lesion supplied by the ICA [27]. A subperiosteal and submucosal plane of dissection is also recommended to minimize bleeding.

The development of hemostatic materials dramatically improved control of venous bleeding from the cavernous sinus, pterygoid plexus, and basilar plexus. A second assistant can introduce a malleable suction device through the ipsilateral nostril, which helps in keeping the surgical field clear [19]. Since the introduction of three instruments through the same nostril is difficult and limits the angle of movements, Robinson and Wormald [32] introduced a two-surgeon transnasal approach for the resection of infratemporal space lesions, using a Killian incision in the septum of the contralateral side, elevation of mucoperichondrial flap, removing bony septum, and then performing a horizontal incision on the ipsilateral side. This allows a high-volume suction tip or instrument to be placed through the opposite nostril into the surgical field. While traction is placed on the tumor, the surgeon can follow the well-defined capsule, dissecting free lateral extensions that otherwise would be difficult to access. Four JAs have been successfully resected from the infratemporal fossa by using this technique. With a similar intent, to overcome the limitation of one hand dissection, surgeons frequently use posterior septectomy [27]. Combined approaches have also been used to better control far lateral and intracranial extension. El-Banhawy et al. [24] in 2006 reported a series of 20 patients with type III JA (according to Fisch classification [33]) who were successfully treated using a combined midfacial degloving and endoscopic approach without preoperative embolization. Khalifa et al. [34] reported a series of 16 patients with type III JA (infratemporal involvement) who were treated successfully using an endoscopic-assisted antral window approach.

Along with technical improvements, a better understanding of the disease and its patterns of spread have contributed to the development of endoscopic surgery for advanced JAs. First, JA has the tendency to invade the vidian canal and basisphenoid, and extensive drilling of these areas is an important tip to avoid recurrence [35]. This area is better approached by a median or paramedian skull base approach such as the transnasal endoscopic approach. Second, while intracranial involvement is not infrequent, dural invasion is very rare [36], which explains the very low risk of CSF leak during JA resection. This fact translates into the need to combine gentle movements of tumor traction and dissection from critical structures (i.e., ICA, cavernous sinus, dura) during skull base dissection and obviate the need for craniectomy and intradural dissection. Third, residual lesions in critical areas such as the cavernous sinus can be followed rather than aggressively approached, as they can remain asymptomatic or even spontaneously regress [21, 37, 38].

Accordingly, some experienced surgeons reported their experience with the resection of advanced JAs. Hackman et al. [27] presented a series of 17 patients with advanced JA, who were treated either by an exclusively endoscopic or an endoscopic plus limited external approach. Recurrences were noted in four patients (mean follow-up 4 years), all of which were successfully treated by a second endoscopic procedure. The authors favored the Caldwell-Luc or Denker approach as an adjunct to endoscopy to control infratemporal extension and proposed that for extensive skull base involvement, the intranasal component of the lesion has to be resected first and the skull base component at a later stage when the patient has been stabilized.

In 2010, Nicolai et al. [26] presented a series of 46 JAs who were treated exclusively by an endoscopic approach after vascular embolization. In this series, 17 of 46 (37 %) had Andrews et al. [5] stage IIIa or IIIb disease. Feeding vessels from the internal carotid artery (ICA) were reported in 14 (30 %) patients. Mean intraoperative blood loss was 580 ml. In four (8.7 %) cases, suspicious residual disease was detected by magnetic resonance imaging (MRI). All four residual lesions involved the root of pterygoid. In one patient, a residual lesion was successfully resected, while the other three lesions remained stable during MRI follow-up.

More recently, Cloutier at al. [38] compared their surgical outcomes based on a 10-year experience on 72 patients, which were divided into two groups based on year of resection; group 1 (2000–2005) and group 2 (2005–2010). The rate of endoscopic approach was significantly higher in group 2 than group 1 (82.9 % vs. 45 %). Around half of the cases had advanced disease (stage IIIA or higher according to Radkowski et al. [4]) with no significant difference between the two groups. The rate of recurrence was 8.3 % and did not differ between groups. While massive and large tumors were treated through an external approach during the earlier period, in the second period all tumors were addressed endoscopically, except in cases of middle cranial fossa invasion or optic nerve or internal carotid artery (ICA) encasement.

As the majority of studies reporting surgical outcomes of JAs are retrospective, single institutional investigations, and consist of a limited number of cases, true comparison between the outcomes of external versus endoscopic approaches is difficult. However, Boghani et al. [39] published a systematic review focusing on the outcomes of endoscopic, endoscopic-assisted, and open surgical approaches. A total of 85 studies comprising 1,047 surgical cases were identified. Studies were divided into groups depending on whether data were presented as individual patients (IPD) ($n = 345$) or the aggregate of all patients in the study (APD) ($n = 702$). These groups were analyzed separately for recurrence rates, intraoperative blood loss, and the impact of preoperative embolization on intraoperative blood loss. For the IPD cohort, recurrence rates for the three approaches were 10.8 %, 14.5 %, and 46.6 % for endoscopic, open, and endoscopic assisted, respectively. There was no significant difference between open and endoscopic techniques. Regarding blood loss, there was a significant difference between the endoscopic group (average of 544 mL) and the open group (average of 1,579.5 mL). In the endoscopic cases, patients with preoperative embolization had significantly lower blood loss (average of 406.7 mL) than non-embolized patients (average 828.3 mL). In the APD cohort, the recurrence rate was significantly lower for the endoscopic approach (4.7 %) compared to open (20.6 %) and endoscopic-assisted approaches (22.6 %). Huang et al. [40] recently reported a single institutional case series that compared outcomes between open and endoscopic approaches. The study included 162 patients, 96 treated by a transpalatal or transmaxillary approach, and 66 treated using transnasal endoscopic approach, with or without labiogingival incision. Approximately half of patients who were treated by open approach and 60 % of patients who were treated endoscopically had advanced lesions (Radkowski stages IIc, IIIa, and IIIb). Compared to the open surgery group, the endoscopic surgery group had a lower median blood loss as well as a lower number of complications. The overall recurrence rate was 31.4 %, with no significant difference between groups.

Indications and Contraindications for Endoscopic Surgery

JAs involving the nasal cavity, nasopharynx, sphenoid sinus, and pterygopalatine fossa can be easily resected through an endoscopic approach. Furthermore, lesions extended to the infratemporal fossa, orbit, and/or parasellar regions can be endoscopically managed according to the surgeon's expertise. External approaches should be considered in JAs with large invasion of the skull base, extensive vascular feeders from the ICA, or critical encasement of ICA. Advanced JAs, especially those with residual vascularity from ICA after embolization, can show massive intraoperative bleeding with a considerable increase of surgical risk and need for intraoperative transfusion. In such a situation, it is wise to consider the possibility of multistage treatment that should be preoperatively discussed with the patient. Another strategy for very advanced JAs with critical intracranial extension and unacceptable surgical hazard is to endoscopically resect the extracranial portion intentionally leaving residual disease and subsequently evaluate for "wait and see" monitoring or surgical treatment based on the rate of growth as demonstrated radiologically. The management of residual tumors involving critical areas or neurovascular structures (i.e., ICA, optic nerve, cavernous sinus, dura, cerebral arteries) should always be carefully discussed considering the need for external approaches due to the impact that adhesions could have on the possibility to perform a safe dissection. Finally, the indication for endoscopic treatment cannot ignore the availability of adequate and dedicated equipment as well as the support of interventional radiology, neurosurgery, and intensive care units.

Surgical Equipment

In addition to the experience of the surgeon, endoscopic surgery for JA requires the availability of surgical instruments and technological equipments which are critical for safe resection of such a tricky lesion.

The following are indispensable surgical equipments that should be available in the operative room for endoscopic treatment of JA:

- Endoscopic skull base set including angled and miniaturized instruments
- Powered endoscopic angled blades and burs
- Angled endoscopes with HD camera
- Laser or monopolar electrocautery with malleable tip
- Hemostatic agents (absorbable gelatin powder, sponge oxidized regenerated cellulose, microfibrillar collagen, or fibrin or synthetic sealants)
- Navigation system
- Endoscopic ultrasonic Doppler probe

Tips and Tricks

- Preoperative embolization 24–48 h before surgery.
- Exposure of the lesion as extensively as possible without manipulating its surface to minimize bleeding.
- Disassembling large-volume JAs by first removing the nasal-nasopharyngeal portion and subsequently addressing its peripheral projections.
- Use of a diode laser or electrocautery to minimize bleeding when sectioning the lesion.
- Use of a "four-hand two-nostril" technique to take advantage of the assistant's collaboration.
- Maintain a proper cleavage plain directly on the surface of the JA to facilitate the dissection of surrounding tissues.
- Early identification and clipping of the maxillary artery to prevent its accidental injury.
- Steady control of bleeding with warm water irrigation and hemostatic agents.

- Use of intraoperative navigation and Doppler to precisely identify the ICA and avoid its injury.
- Extensive drilling of the basisphenoid and other bony areas involved by the lesion to remove hidden microscopic nests.
- Anterior retraction of the soft palate to manage the posterior attachment and transorally remove the JA.

Surgical Technique

The key principle in the endoscopic approach to JA is to expose the lesion as extensively as possible without traumatizing its surface to minimize bleeding. As a minimum, ethmoidectomy, sphenoidotomy, and a large middle antrostomy extended posteriorly to expose the crucial area of the sphenopalatine foramen should be performed. JA always originates from the superior margin of the sphenopalatine foramen where the sphenoid process of the palatine bone meets the pterygoid base and the horizontal ala of vomer; from there it spreads in a submucosal plane and follows its typical patterns of spread (Fig. 11.1). The resection of large-volume lesions can rarely be achieved in a single bloc, and it is preferable to disassemble the JA by first

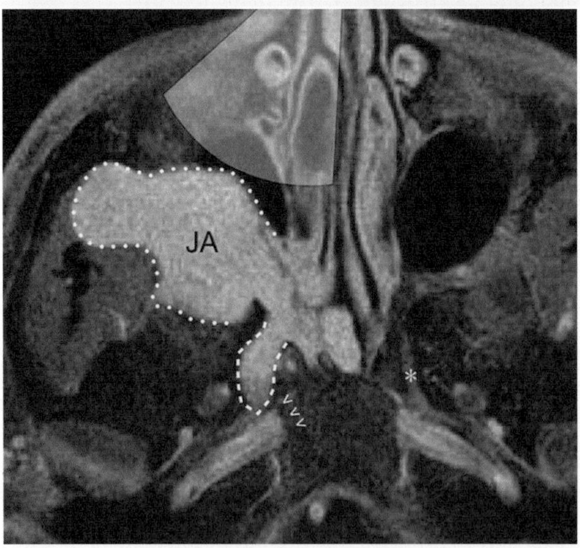

Fig. 11.1 Axial contrast-enhanced T1 image. Juvenile angiofibroma (JA) showing remodeling of posterolateral wall of the right maxillary sinus with wide lateral extension into the infratemporal fossa (*white dotted line*). Posteriorly, JA spreads into the vidian canal (*white dashed line*) reaching the foramen lacerum (*white arrowheads*). The *white asterisk* indicates the contralateral vidian nerve. Lateral exposure of its posterior wall can be effectively increased by sectioning the lacrimal duct and removing the medial part of the anterior maxillary wall with the so-called Sturman-Canfield (or endonasal Denker) operation (transparent *white cone*)

removing the nasal-nasopharyngeal portion and subsequently addressing the peripheral deepest projections. A diode laser or electrocautery with malleable tip is mandatory to minimize bleeding during this step (Fig. 11.2). Moreover, the resection of the posterior third of nasal septum allows exposure of the nasopharyngeal portion of the lesion and enables easier use of the "four-hand two-nostril" technique. In this way, the assistant helps the surgeon to maintain a proper cleavage plain by gentle traction on the lesion itself (Figs. 11.3 and 11.4). Steady control of

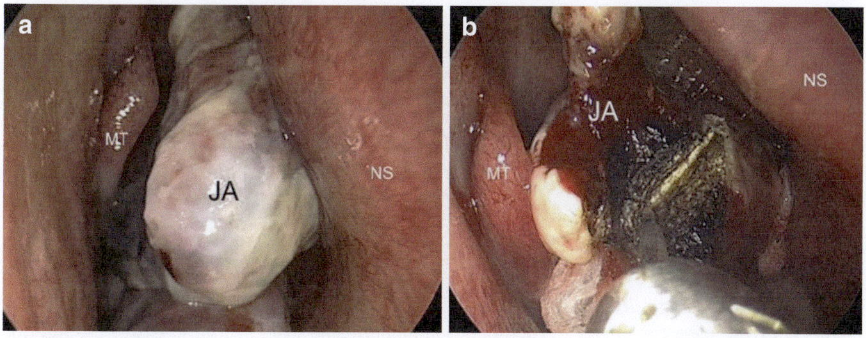

Fig. 11.2 (**a**) Endoscopic view of right nasal fossa juvenile angiofibroma (*JA*). (**b**) Diode laser allows removal of the nasal portion of the JA to minimize bleeding. *MT* middle turbinate, *NS* nasal septum

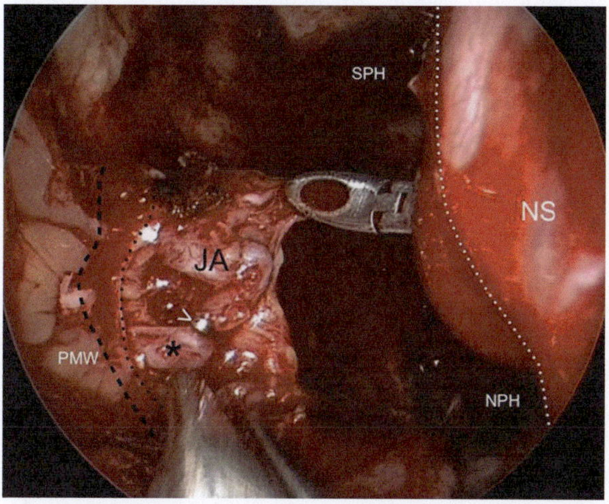

Fig. 11.3 Resection of the posterior third of nasal septum (*white dotted line*) allows using the "four-hand" and "two-nostril" technique. The second surgeon helps the surgeon by gentle traction on the juvenile angiofibroma (*JA*) from the contralateral fossa. The dissection plane is achieved by incising the periosteum (*black dotted line*) after removal of the posterior maxillary wall (*black dashed line*). The maxillary artery (*black asterisk*) is identified and clipped to prevent its accidental injury. *NPH* nasopharynx, *NS* nasal septum, *PMW* posterior maxillary wall, *SPH* sphenoid

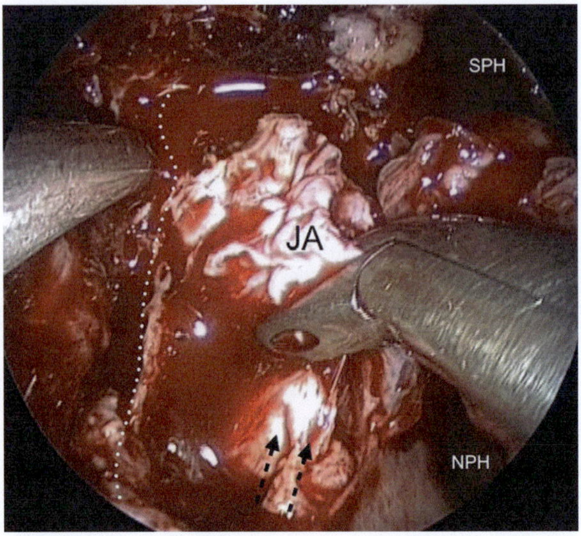

Fig. 11.4 Juvenile angiofibroma (*JA*) can inferiorly spread through the infratemporal fossa, nasopharynx, or the pterygoid fossa to the upper parapharyngeal space. In these cases, the inferior turbinate and medial wall of the maxillary sinus should be resected to the floor of the nasal cavity. The assistant helps the surgeon from the contralateral fossa by gentle traction upward (*black dashed arrows*). *White dotted line*: maxillary periosteum; *NPH* nasopharynx, *SPH* sphenoid

hemostasis with copious irrigation through the nasal cavities with warm water (40–45 °C) or using hemostatic agents for major bleeding is also crucial to optimize visualization of the surgical field.

JA often extends laterally to the pterygopalatine fossa, which is an important crossroad, from where the lesion can grow along different pathways. Anteriorly, it can displace the posterior wall of the maxillary sinus and, laterally, through the pterygomaxillary fissure, can expand into the infratemporal fossa, while extension into the hard palate through the descending palatine canal can be also observed. By modulating the opening of the meatal wall of the maxillary sinus, lateral exposure of its posterior wall can be effectively increased. Medial maxillectomy can be anteriorly enlarged by sectioning the lacrimal duct at the inferior limit of the lacrimal sac or also removing the medial part of the anterior maxillary wall with the so-called Sturman-Canfield (or endonasal Denker) operation (Fig. 11.1). Once the posterior wall of the maxillary sinus has been removed, a crucial point is the identification of the correct dissection plane of the lesion, which is achieved by incising the periosteum. It is noteworthy that the maxillary periosteum can be easily confused with the surface of the JA, leading the surgeon along a wrong surgical plane of dissection. Careful dissection and continuous gentle traction also allow to progressively pull out far lateral projections of the JA that extend to the infratemporal/temporal fossa. In order to minimize morbidity, special attention must be paid to identify the maxillary nerve. The dissection plane into the pterygopalatine fossa is posterior with respect to the palatine nerves; therefore, only in lesions with a small lateral extension can the nerves be preserved. Moreover, it is advisable to identify and clip the maxillary artery early, not only to reduce intraoperative bleeding but also to prevent its accidental damage during the procedure (Fig. 11.3).

Posteriorly, from its site of origin in the pterygopalatine fossa, JA typically extends into the cancellous bone and pterygoid root and, following the vidian canal, grows along the floor of the sphenoid sinus. Extension to the nasopharynx commonly occurs following the submucosal plane. By eroding the pterygoid process of the sphenoid bone, JA can also invade the pterygoid fossa and the upper parapharyngeal space. In this case, the inferior turbinate and the medial wall of the maxillary sinus should be resected to the floor of the nasal cavity to optimize exposure (Fig. 11.4). The surgical procedure should always include extensive drilling of the basisphenoid and other bony areas involved by the JA that are well beyond the apparent margin of infiltration to remove microscopic nests of the lesion that may not be visible and prevent their regrowth (Fig. 11.5). Even if the vidian nerve is sacrificed to ensure a radical resection at the site of origin of the JA, patients rarely complain of dry eye.

From the pterygopalatine fossa, the lesion may spread to the cavernous sinus via two pathways: (1) through the inferior orbital fissure, the orbit, and then the superior orbital fissure and (2) following the maxillary nerve. Although at primary treatment, JA does not commonly show tight adhesions with adjacent neurovascular structures, whenever a portion of JA is in close contact with the cavernous sinus or ICA, it should be addressed as a last step after achieving wide exposure of the critical area and possibly resecting the nasal-nasopharyngeal part of the lesion. The use of intraoperative navigation and Doppler is mandatory to precisely identify the artery and avoid its injury. The dissection of JA from ICA should be cautiously performed with the help of small cottonoids to avoid any direct traumatic pressure on the vessel. Until the intervention is completed, the presence of an interventional radiologist in the hospital who can manage uncontrolled ICA bleeding is another precautionary measure that should be considered. Intracranial extension may occur from the infratemporal fossa through the floor of the middle cranial fossa, from the pterygomaxillary fissure and infratemporal fossa into the superior and inferior orbital fissures, through direct erosion of the sphenoid sinus into the region of the sella turcica and cavernous sinus, or, more rarely, along the ethmoid fovea and cribriform plate into the anterior cranial fossa. Despite the high prevalence of skull base and intracranial invasion, true dural invasion is rare, allowing removal of the lesion endoscopically without the need to carry out complex skull base reconstruction techniques.

Identification of the posterior and inferior margin of the lesion within the nasopharynx at the end of the surgical procedure may be difficult due to several factors, including poor visualization in a bloody surgical field. The use of two rubber catheters passed transnasally to retract the palate anteriorly can be used to isolate the posteroinferior nasopharyngeal attachment of the JA and to effectively remove the mass from the mouth (Fig. 11.6).

Light packing is placed in the nasal cavities for 24–48 h, and third-generation cephalosporin is administered starting the day before surgery until nasal packing is

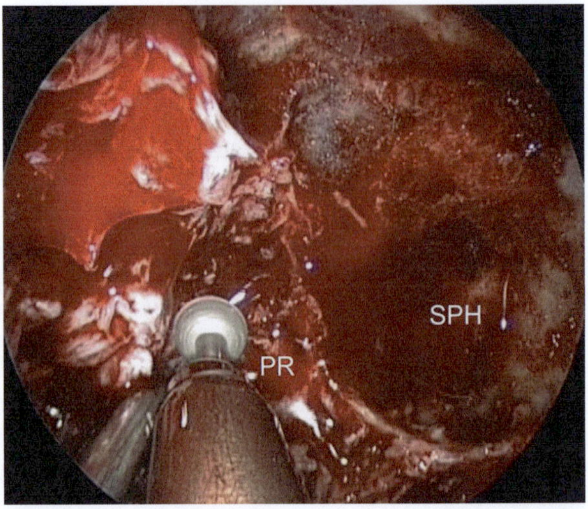

Fig. 11.5 Extensive drilling of the pterygoid root (*PR*) well beyond the apparent margin of infiltration to remove microscopic nests of the juvenile angiofibroma. *SPH* sphenoid

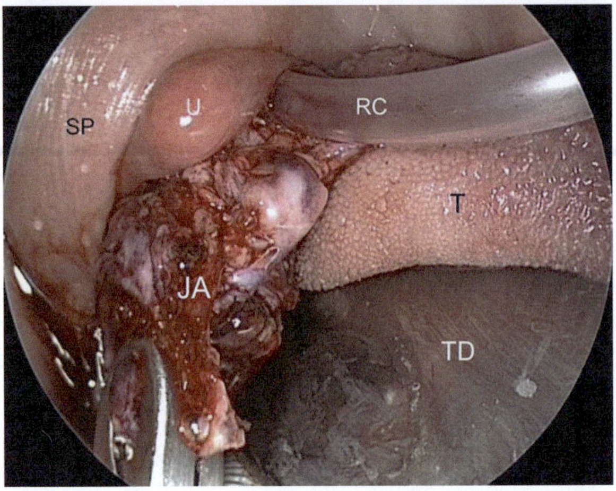

Fig. 11.6 Rubber catheter (*RC*) passed transnasally retracts the soft palate (*SP*) anteriorly. The juvenile angiofibroma (*JA*) is effectively extracted from the mouth. *T* tongue, *TD* tongue depressor, *U* uvula

removed. Cleaning of the surgical cavity is performed under endoscopic control to remove clots and fibrin, and the patient is instructed to perform daily irrigations of the sinonasal cavity with saline solution to moisten secretions and minimize crust formation.

Follow-Up

Imaging surveillance after surgery is always required because persistences or recurrences are typically localized submucosally and inaccessible to endoscopic evaluation. Moreover, postoperative MRI within 72 h after surgery has shown to be effective in differentiating vascularized nodules of persistence in the early

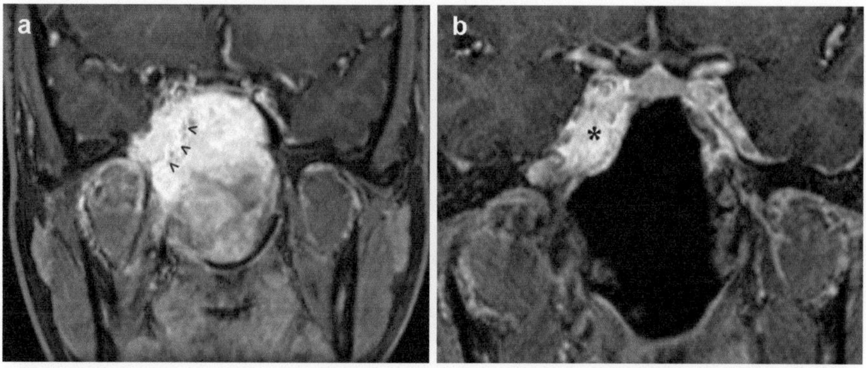

Fig. 11.7 (**a**) Coronal contrast-enhanced T1 image of a 23-year-old boy affected by Andrews IIIb juvenile angiofibroma (*JA*) with extensive cavernous sinus involvement (*black arrowheads*). Endoscopic resection was performed leaving intentionally the cavernous sinus component due to unacceptable surgical hazard. (**b**) The JA residue (*black asterisk*) was monitored with magnetic resonance that showed no progression of disease after 6 years of follow-up

postoperative period. Imaging should be performed every 6–8 months for at least 3 years after surgery. Persistent JAs, either intentionally unresected due to unacceptable surgical hazard or detected by routine follow-up scans, require close surveillance with contrast-enhanced MRI to assess its possible growth before establishing that treatment is actually required (Fig. 11.7).

Conclusions

Endoscopic surgery has revolutionized the treatment of small- and intermediate-sized JAs by showing that compared to external approaches, similar results in terms of disease control can be achieved but with less morbidity. Large and invasive JAs may also be managed endoscopically, but only by experienced teams. Traditional external techniques still play a role in the management of advanced lesions with critical relationships with the ICA or intracranial-intradural extent. JA residues should be adequately monitored with imaging techniques (preferably MRI) before embarking in treatments that may be associated with non-negligible morbidity.

References

1. Moulin G, Chagnaud C, Gras R, et al. Juvenile nasopharyngeal angiofibroma: comparison of blood loss during removal in embolized group versus nonembolized group. Cardiovasc Intervent Radiol. 1995;18:158–16.
2. Freihofer HP1, BjörkG JE, Kuijpers-Jagtman AM. Timing of facial osteotomies. A consensus conference. Oral Surg Oral Med Oral Pathol. 1994;78:432–6.

3. Herman P, Lot G, Chapot R, Salvan D, Huy PT. Long-term follow-up of juvenile nasopharyngeal angiofibromas: analysis of recurrences. Laryngoscope. 1999;109:140–7.
4. Radowski D, McGill T, Healy GB, et al. Angiofibroma: changes in staging and treatment. Arch Otolaryngol Head Neck Surg. 1996;122:122–9.
5. Andrews JC, Fisch U, Valavanis A, Aeppli U, Makek MS. The surgical management of extensive nasopharyngeal angiofibromas with the infratemporal fossa approach. Laryngoscope. 1989;99:429–37.
6. Kamel RH. Transnasal endoscopic surgery in juvenile nasopharyngeal angiofibroma. J Laryngol Otol. 1996;110:962–8.
7. Fagan JJ, Snyderman CH, Carrau RL, Janecka IP. Nasopharyngeal angiofibromas: selecting a surgical approach. Head Neck. 1997;19:391–9.
8. Zicot AF, Daele J. Endoscopic surgery for nasal and sinusal vascular tumours: about two cases of nasopharyngeal angiofibromas and one case of turbinate angioma. Acta Otorhinolaryngol Belg. 1996;50:177–82.
9. Tseng HZ, Chao WY. Transnasal endoscopic approach for juvenile nasopharyngeal angiofibroma. Am J Otolaryngol. 1997;18:151–4.
10. Mitskavich MT, Carrau RL, Snyderman CH, Weissman JL, Fagan JJ. Intranasal endoscopic excision of a juvenile angiofibroma. Auris Nasus Larynx. 1998;25:39–44.
11. Bernal-Sprekelsen M, Vazquez AA, Pueyo J, Carbonell Casasu J. Endoscopic resection of juvenile nasopharyngeal fibromas. HNO. 1998;46:172–4.
12. Nakamura H, Kawasaki M, Higuchi Y, Seki S, Takahashi S. Transnasal endoscopic resection of juvenile nasopharyngeal angiofibroma with KTP laser. Eur Arch Otorhinolaryngol. 1999;256:212–4.
13. Schick B, el Rahman el Tahan A, Brors D, Kahle G, Draf W. Experiences with endonasal surgery in angiofibroma. Rhinology. 1999;37:80–5.
14. Newlands SD, Weymuller Jr EA. Endoscopic treatment of juvenile nasopharyngeal angiofibroma. Am J Rhinol. 1999;13:213–9.
15. Jorissen M, Eloy P, Rombaux P, Bachert C, Daele J. Endoscopic sinus surgery for juvenile nasopharyngeal angiofibroma. Acta Otorhinolaryngol Belg. 2000;54:201–19.
16. Khalifa MA. Endonasal endoscopic surgery for nasopharyngeal angiofibroma. Otolaryngol Head Neck Surg. 2001;124:336–7.
17. Carrau RL, Snyderman CH, Kassam AB, et al. Endoscopic and endoscopic-assisted surgery for juvenile angio-fibroma. Laryngoscope. 2001;111:483–7.
18. Ungkanont K, Byers RM, Weber RS, Callender DL, Wolf PF, Goepfert H. Juvenile nasopharyngeal angiofibroma: an update of therapeutic management. Head Neck. 1996;18:60–6.
19. Roger G, Tran Ba Huy P, Froehlich P, et al. Exclusively endoscopic removal of juvenile nasopharyngeal angiofibroma; trend and limits. Arch Otolaryngol. Head Neck Surg. 2002;128:928–35.
20. Nicolai P, Berlucchi M, Tomenzoli D, et al. Endoscopic surgery for juvenile angiofibroma: when and how. Laryngoscope. 2003;113:775–82.
21. Onerci TM, Yucel OT, Ogretmenoglu O. Endoscopic surgery in treatment of juvenile nasopharyngeal angiofibroma. Int J Pediatr Otolaryngol. 2003;67:1219–25.
22. Wormald PJ, Van Hasselt A. Endoscopic removal of juvenile angiofibromas. Otolaryngol Head Neck Surg. 2003;129:684–91.
23. Pasquini E, Sciarretta V, Frank G, et al. Endoscopic treatment of benign tumours of the nose and paranasal sinuses. Otolaryngol Head Neck Surg. 2004;131:180–6.
24. El-Banhawy OA, Ragab A, El-Sharnoby MM. Surgical resection of type III juvenile angiofibroma without preoperative embolization. Int J Pediatr Otorhinolaryngol. 2006;70:1715–23.
25. El Sharkawy AA. Endonasal endoscopic management of juvenile nasopharyngeal angiofibroma without angiographic embolization. Eur Arch Otorhinolaryngol. 2013;270:2051–5.
26. Nicolai P, Villaret AB, Farina D, et al. Endoscopic surgery for juvenile angiofibroma: a critical review of indications after 46 cases. Am J Rhinol Allergy. 2010;24:e67–72.

27. Hackman T, Snyderman CH, Carrau R, Vescan A, Kassam A. Juvenile nasopharyngeal angiofibroma: the expanded endonasal approach. Am J Rhinol Allergy. 2009;23:95–9.
28. Mair EA1, Battiata A, Casler JD. Endoscopic laser-assisted excision of juvenile nasopharyngeal angiofibromas. Otolaryngol Head Neck Surg. 2003;129:454–9.
29. Scholtz AW, Appenroth E, Kammen-Jolly K, Scholtz LU, Thumfart WF. Juvenile nasopharyngeal angiofibroma: management and therapy. Laryngoscope. 2001;111(4 Pt 1):681–7.
30. Ye L, Zhou X, Li J, Jin J. Coblation-assisted endonasal endoscopic resection of juvenile nasopharyngeal angiofibroma. J Laryngol Otol. 2011;125:940–4.
31. Syed MI, Mennie J, Williams AT. Early experience of radio frequency coblation in the management of intranasal and sinus tumors. Laryngoscope. 2012;122:436–9.
32. Robinson S, Patel N, Wormald PJ. Endoscopic management of benign tumors extending into the infratemporal fossa: a two-surgeon transnasal approach. Laryngoscope. 2005;115:1818–22.
33. Fisch U. The infratemporal fossa approach for nasopharyngeal tumors. Laryngoscope. 1983;93:36–44.
34. Khalifa MA, Ragab SM. Endoscopic assisted antral window approach for type III nasopharyngeal angiofibroma with infratemporal fossa extension. Int J Pediatr Otorhinolaryngol. 2008;72:1855–60.
35. Howard DJ, Lloyd G, Lund V. Recurrence and its avoidance in juvenile angiofibroma. Laryngoscope. 2001;111:1509–11.
36. Danesi G, Panciera DT, Harvey RJ, et al. Juvenile nasopharyngeal angiofibroma: Evaluation and management of advanced disease. Otolaryngol Head Neck Surg. 2008;138:581–6.
37. Jones GC, DeSanto LW, Bremer JW, Neel HB. Juvenile angiofibromas: behavior and treatment of extensive and residual tumors. Arch Otolaryngol Head Neck Surg. 1986;112:1191–3.
38. Cloutier T, Pons Y, Blancal JP, Sauvaget E, Kania R, Bresson D, Herman P. Juvenile nasopharyngeal angiofibroma: does the external approach still make sense? Otolaryngol Head Neck Surg. 2012;147:958–63.
39. Boghani Z, Husain Q, Kanumuri VV, et al. Juvenile nasopharyngeal angiofibroma: a systematic review and comparison of endoscopic, endoscopic assisted, and open resection in 1,047 cases. Laryngoscope. 2013;123:859–69.
40. Huang Y, Liu Z, Want J, Sun X, Yang L, Wang D. Surgical management of juvenile nasopharyngeal angiofibroma: analysis of 162 cases from 1995 to 2012. Laryngoscope. 2014;124:1942–6.

Chapter 12
Endoscopic Excision of Advanced Tumor with Skull Base Involvement

Carl H. Snyderman, Paul A. Gardner, Juan C. Fernandez-Miranda, and Eric W. Wang

Abstract Advanced juvenile angiofibromas (JA) are challenging tumors to treat surgically due to the involvement of skull base structures and vascularity derived from the intracranial circulation. Tumor infiltration of the pterygoid base encompasses the pterygoid canal and derives blood supply from branches of the internal carotid artery (ICA), most commonly the vidian artery and branches from the cavernous segment. Large tumors may surround the petrous and cavernous segments of the ICA and increase the risk of vascular injury during surgery.

With proper planning, large juvenile angiofibromas with intracranial extension can be managed using endoscopic techniques. The biggest challenges are bleeding from tumor vessels derived from the intracranial circulation. The UPMC staging system is useful in devising a surgical strategy based on the degree of residual vascularity and the route of intracranial extension. A staged approach with excision of vascular territories of the tumor allows safe resection with minimal morbidity. There is a higher risk of residual tumor with advanced juvenile angiofibroma with skull base involvement, but not all patients require further surgery. Radiation therapy can be avoided with a comprehensive surgical strategy.

C.H. Snyderman, MD, MBA (✉)
Department of Otolaryngology, University of Pittsburgh School of Medicine, Pittsburgh, PA, USA

Department of Neurological Surgery, University of Pittsburgh School of Medicine, Pittsburgh, PA, USA

UPMC Center for Cranial Base Surgery, 200 Lothrop Street, EEI Suite 500, Pittsburgh, PA 15213, USA
e-mail: snydermanch@upmc.edu

P.A. Gardner, MD • J.C. Fernandez-Miranda, MD
Department of Neurological Surgery, University of Pittsburgh School of Medicine, Pittsburgh, PA, USA
e-mail: gardpa@upmc.edu; fernandezmirandajc@upmc.edu

E.W. Wang, MD
Department of Otolaryngology, University of Pittsburgh School of Medicine, Pittsburgh, PA, USA
e-mail: wangew@upmc.edu

S.P. Dubey, B. Schick (eds.), *Juvenile Angiofibroma*,
DOI 10.1007/978-3-319-45343-9_12

Keywords Angiofibroma • Internal carotid artery • Skull base • Staging

Introduction

Advanced juvenile angiofibromas (JA) are challenging tumors to treat surgically due to the involvement of skull base structures and vascularity derived from the intracranial circulation. Skull base involvement occurs to varying degrees and is not necessarily a reflection of tumor size. Erosion of the base of the pterygoid bone is a common feature of JA and predisposes to recurrence if all remnants of the tumor are not removed from the bone (Fig. 12.1) [1]. Tumor infiltration of the pterygoid base encompasses the pterygoid canal and derives blood supply from branches of the internal carotid artery (ICA), most commonly the vidian artery and branches from the cavernous segment [2]. Large tumors may surround the petrous and cavernous segments of the ICA and increase the risk of vascular injury during surgery.

Advanced JA erode the skull base and are often in contact with the dura (Fig. 12.2). Although true dural invasion is rare, JA can displace the dura and grow intracranially. There are two major pathways for intracranial spread of tumor:

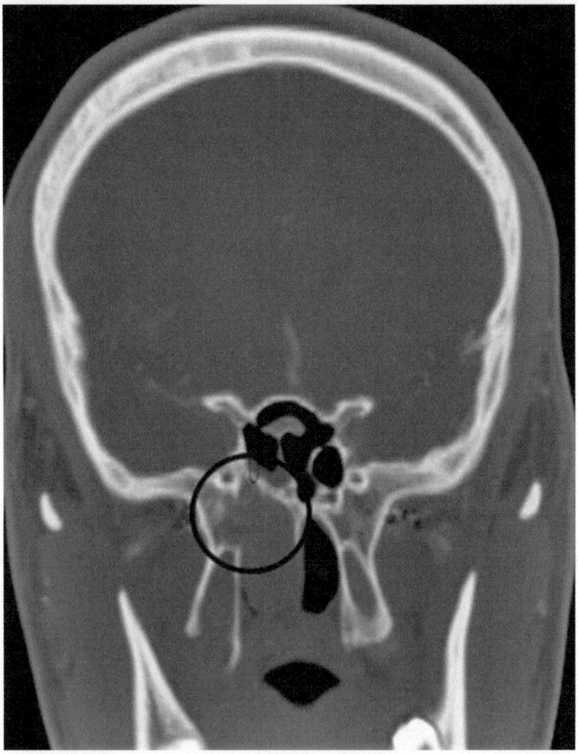

Fig. 12.1 Tumor erosion and infiltration of the pterygoid base (*circle*) increase the risk of recurrence unless all of the tumor-involved bone is drilled. The vidian nerve and vidian artery are often encased by tumor; the vidian artery is a major source of residual vascularity

medial and lateral to the orbital apex. Tumors that extend into the sphenoid sinus may erode the bone of the planum sphenoidale to gain access to the anterior cranial fossa, compress the optic nerve, and invade the medial cavernous sinus. Tumors that extend laterally typically gain access to the middle cranial fossa through the inferior orbital fissure, orbital apex, and superior orbital fissure. Direct erosion of the floor of the middle cranial fossa is also observed more laterally.

In the past, intracranial extension of JA was an indication for a transcranial approach in combination with a transfacial approach (endoscopic or open). With advances in endoscopic techniques and increased experience, even advanced JA with skull base involvement and intracranial extension can be completely resected using completely endoscopic or endoscopic-assisted approaches [3–5]. An anterior endoscopic approach has the advantage of providing access both medial and lateral to the cavernous ICA.

Principles of Endoscopic Surgery

The primary goal of surgery for JA is complete tumor excision with preservation of major neural and vascular structures. Secondary goals are to minimize morbidity related to blood loss or approach and avoid the need for radiation therapy in this

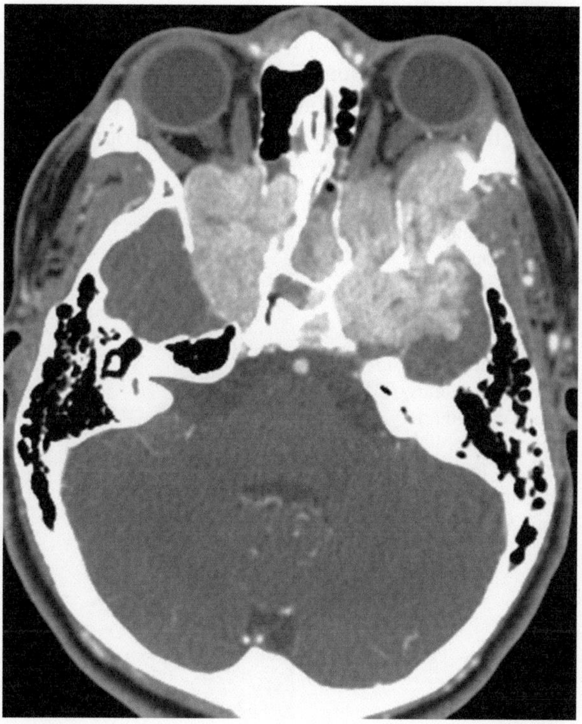

Fig. 12.2 This giant JA encompasses both internal carotid arteries and extends to the middle cranial fossa via the inferior orbital fissure. There is erosion of the cranial base both medial and lateral to the internal carotid artery. The patient presented with bilateral visual loss

young patient population. With advanced JA, complete tumor excision is not always possible and residual tumor may be left in proximity to nerves and vessels, especially when there is true cavernous invasion. Not all residual tumors will grow and a "wait and watch" policy is adopted, especially in late adolescence. If significant growth of the residual tumor is observed, treatment options include additional surgery or radiation therapy.

Surgery for advanced JA is skull base surgery and is best performed by an experienced team of skull base surgeons with proficiency in both endoscopic and open techniques. Team surgery has multiple benefits including superior visualization, greater operative efficiency (with decreased blood loss), and improved ability to deal with a crisis. These are advanced level procedures (training levels 4 and 5) [6] and the surgical team should have extensive experience working in the coronal plane in proximity to the ICA. It is difficult to achieve adequate surgical volume performing pediatric skull base surgery; as a result, the ideal team consists of both pediatric and adult skull base surgeons.

The major anatomic structure of the ventral skull base is the ICA (Fig. 12.3). The relationship of the tumor to the ICA and its vascular contributions dictates the surgical approach. Advanced JA are often bilateral and may derive significant vascularity from both ICA. It is important to understand the anatomical landmarks for the ICA and develop a surgical strategy for each patient's tumor based on the involvement of the ICA [2, 7]. Preoperative embolization is a critical step in the safe treatment of JA and can significantly decrease blood loss, but ICA contributions cannot be safely or easily embolized.

Large JA require multiple endoscopic corridors to reach the limits of the tumor and provide room for instrumentation [8]. Even though an open incision is used (anterior maxillotomy) in conjunction with an endonasal approach, all of the tumor dissection is done endoscopically. The surgical strategy is to

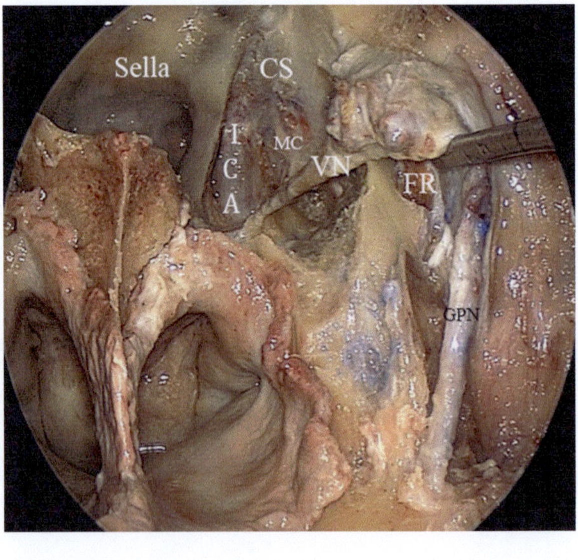

Fig. 12.3 The key anatomical landmarks of an endoscopic transpterygoid approach to the internal carotid artery and middle cranial fossa are shown here (*left side*). *CS* cavernous sinus, *ICA* internal carotid artery, *MC* Meckel's cave, *VN* vidian nerve, *FR* foramen rotundum, *GPN* greater palatine nerve

expose all of the margins of the tumor prior to manipulation since bleeding may be brisk. The simple addition of the anterior maxillotomy corridor provides access to the extensions lateral to the ICA and orbital apex as well as allowing the passage of larger instruments such as standard bipolar cautery forceps.

JA can be divided into surgical segments based on vascular territories (Fig. 12.4). With large tumors, the extracranial segment on each side is first resected. This is often necessary to create working space and provide visualization of the intracranial portion of the tumor. If blood loss is not excessive and the patient is not coagulopathic, the intracranial segment on each side is then addressed. It is not uncommon to stage surgeries to avoid excessive blood loss and avoid the additional morbidity of massive transfusions and associated coagulopathy, especially during intracranial surgery. Other reasons to stage surgery include the duration of surgery with attendant surgeon fatigue and inexperienced staff, and the need for repeat imaging.

With an experienced team, there are no absolute contraindications to endoscopic surgery for advanced JA. If there is a large infratemporal component, a lateral infratemporal skull base approach may facilitate removal of this portion of the tumor and provide superior access to the middle cranial fossa. However, these portions are usually not invasive; rather, they are lobular extensions of the tumor which can be retracted into the sinus cavity.

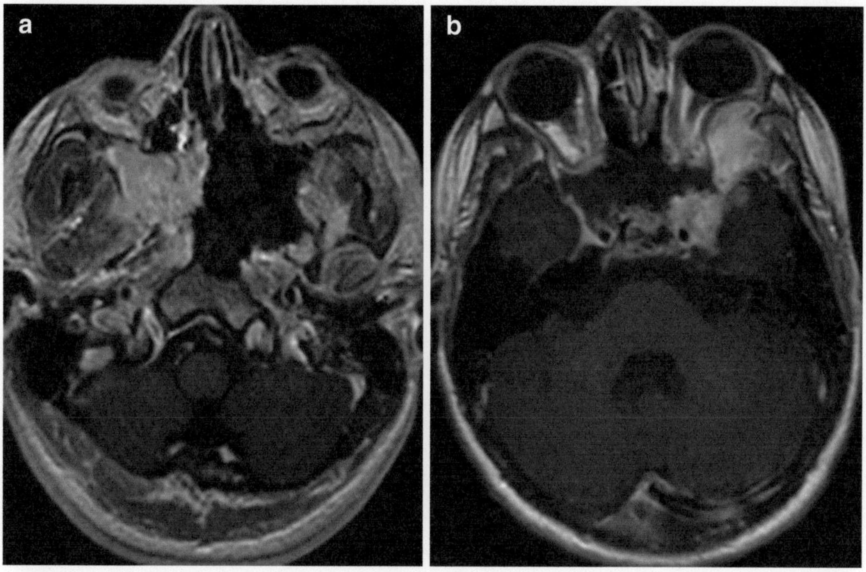

Fig. 12.4 (**a**) The left extracranial portion of the tumor shown in Fig. 12.2 was removed in the first operation. (**b**) Following removal of the extracranial portion on the right side, the residual intracranial tumor on the left side was removed at a third operation

Preoperative Assessment

The UPMC staging system [9–11] is preferred for advanced JA since it addresses two issues that other staging systems do not address: the vascularity of the tumor derived from intracranial circulation and the route of intracranial extension. All of these tumors are UPMC stage 4 or 5. Staging of the tumor is based on clinical assessment, radiologic examination, and angiography. Both computed tomography (CT) angiogram and magnetic resonance imaging (MRI) are obtained using a skull base protocol for navigation. They provide complementary information. The CT angiogram provides visualization of bony landmarks and the course and involvement of the ICA. The MRI provides superior visualization of the tumor itself as well as its interface with soft tissues and nerves. It is important to obtain imaging prior to embolization as embolic materials are all radio-opaque and can obliterate radiographic visualization of the embolized portion of the tumor and its adjacent margins.

Angiography is essential to examine the course of the ICA, assess collateral circulation through the circle of Willis, and identify branches of the ICA that contribute vascularity to the tumor [12, 13]. Residual vascularity following embolization of the tumor and all involved branches of the ECA is a good predictor of intraoperative hemorrhage (Fig. 12.5). Embolization of ICA branches is sometimes feasible but is usually not performed due to the increased risk of stroke. If there is tumor encasement of the ICA, the adequacy of collateral circulation can be further assessed with balloon test occlusion (BTO) of the artery. Awake BTO is usually not possible in children or even young adolescents due to cooperation, but MR spectroscopy or CT perfusion can provide information about areas at risk. In young patients, however, sacrifice of the ICA is rarely needed and usually well tolerated in the advent of an

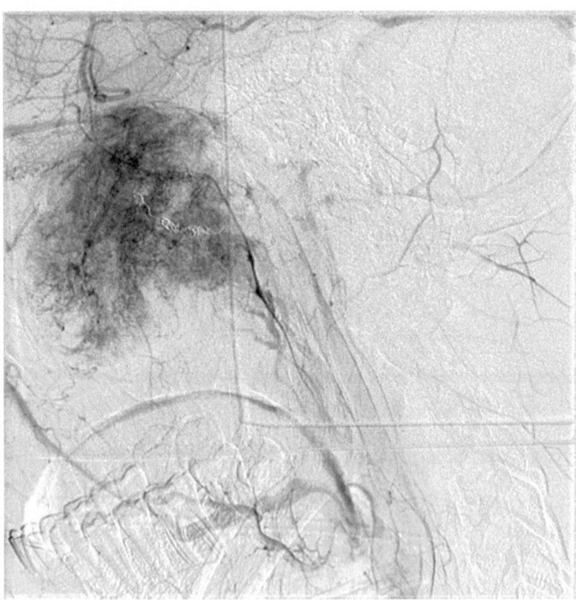

Fig. 12.5 UPMC stage 5 tumor with significant residual vascularity on angiography following embolization of branches of the external carotid artery. The coils in the main trunk of internal maxillary artery are visible

intraoperative injury, and routine testing is not necessary. Consideration may be given in recurrent or postradiation cases.

Particles and flowable embolics (e.g., Onyx) have both been used with great success [14]. Particles, if properly size matched, have little risk of distal embolization but may get somewhat better tumor penetration. However, distal embolization is always a potential concern with overaggressive treatment. Onyx provides very complete embolization of treated areas, but deep penetration into larger tumors may be limited as the glue polymerizes in proximal vessels. Finally, coils can be used in larger ECA branches.

Prior treatment may have an impact on the ability to achieve the goals of surgery. Past embolization may result in recruitment of new blood supply from the ICA and decrease the effectiveness of further preoperative embolization. Prior embolization and incomplete tumor resection contribute to scarring/tumor adherence and increase the risk of vascular or cranial nerve injury. The tumor may not dissect easily from the dura, resulting in a CSF leak, something that is very rare in virgin cases. Finally, discontinuity of the tumor predisposes to incomplete resection.

Intraoperative Preparation

The patient is positioned in a supine position with the head rotated slightly toward the surgeons. Reverse Trendelenburg position with 15° elevation helps to decrease venous pressure with resultant decrease in mucosal, tumor, and cavernous sinus bleeding. A Mayfield head holder is used to secure the head and facilitate registration of an image-based navigation system and fix the desired head position. If there is involvement of the ICA, the neck may be included in the surgical field in case proximal control of the ICA is needed.

Neurophysiological monitoring includes somatosensory evoked potentials (SSEP) for monitoring of cortical function and can provide a surrogate measure of global ischemia. Electromyographic (EMG) monitoring of the third division of the trigeminal nerve is helpful when tumor extends to foramen ovale or into the masticator space. If there is erosion of the middle clivus, EMG monitoring of sixth nerve function is also performed. If there is tumor extension into the cavernous sinus, the extraocular muscles (cranial nerves III, IV, and VI) are monitored.

Perioperative antibiotic prophylaxis consists of a third-generation cephalosporin with CSF penetration (e.g., ceftriaxone) in any case with risk of dural injury. Cottonoid pledgets soaked in 0.05% oxymetazoline solution are used to decongest the nasal cavity, taking care not to traumatize the tumor. The sublabial tissues are infiltrated with 0.5% xylocaine with 1:200,000 epinephrine for a transmaxillary approach.

Surgical Technique [8]

An anterior maxillotomy (Caldwell Luc approach) is performed on one or both sides to gain access to the lateral margin of the tumor, especially if there is tumor extending to the floor of the middle cranial fossa or lateral to the maxilla.

The alternative is to perform a Denker's (anteromedial) maxillotomy endonasally but this has a greater risk of cosmetic deformity and does not provide as large a corridor for passage of instruments. The infraorbital nerve is identified and preserved, although it can be difficult to identify the plane of dissection. The bone of the posterior maxillary wall is removed (if not already eroded) to expose the tumor and pterygopalatine contents, and the lateral margin of the tumor defined. The thin superficial periosteum of the pterygopalatine fossa typically overlies the actual tumor capsule and should be carefully opened to find the correct dissection plane. The descending palatine branch of the maxillary nerve (V2) is often displaced anteriorly and surrounded by tumor; preservation is often not possible. Patient and family should be properly counseled of the risk of permanent palatal numbness with large tumors. The consequence of this is minor, but the patient should be cautioned about the risk of palatal burns when eating hot food.

Endonasally, a medial maxillectomy is performed endoscopically on the side of the tumor. The nasolacrimal duct is sharply transected to prevent stenosis. The posterior septum is transected anterior to the tumor to provide binarial access. Bilateral ethmoidectomies are performed as needed to provide access superior to the tumor and tumor is bluntly dissected from the anterior cranial base. If possible, mucosal incisions are made in the nasopharynx with needle-tip electrocautery at the inferior tumor margin to facilitate later dissection, as this is often an area of firm attachment (to the basopharyngeal fascia). Binarial and anterior maxillary corridors should be expanded as widely as possible around the tumor prior to any tumor dissection, as bleeding from the tumor will limit further exposure.

The vascular contributions of the ICA to the tumor can be approached from medial or lateral, but the anatomy is generally more recognizable starting from the parasellar ICA and dissecting inferolaterally. Prior to dissection of tumor from the ICA, however, it is necessary to debulk large tumors by excising vascular segments. The extracranial component in the masticator space can be transected first, using bipolar electrocautery or an ultrasonic cauterization device (Harmonic scalpel) for hemostasis. There is often a natural cleavage plane in the tumor at the medial maxilla, as well as direct ipsilateral endonasal access for the Harmonic scalpel. It is generally wise to transect the tumor lateral to the pterygoid to avoid the most vascular core of the tumor around the ICA. The additional room afforded by the anterior maxillotomy allows more effective use of standard bipolar electrocautery forceps. Tumors that have been embolized with Onyx can be very firm and difficult to remove unless they are cut into smaller pieces with sinus scissors.

If tumor is filling the sphenoid sinus, it is helpful to dissect the portion of the tumor that does not involve the ICA to provide early visualization of key landmarks (Fig. 12.3). The surgical field is bounded by the planum sphenoidale and optic canals superiorly and by the carotid arteries laterally. There is usually a nice dissection plane between the tumor and the skull base/dura in this region and tumor is dissected from the planum to identify the sella and optic canals superiorly. The tumor is elevated from the clival recess and the nasopharyngeal component of the tumor is debulked as necessary. Bleeding from the sphenoid bone and dural surfaces is typically venous and can be packed off with flowable gelfoam (Surgifoam) or other similar hemostatic agents. As dissection proceeds laterally, tumor is peeled from the cavernous sinus wall and paraclival ICA (Fig. 12.6). This dissection must proceed slowly as bleeding from multiple feeders from the ICA is encountered and they must be individually localized and cauterized with bipolar electrocautery.

Continuing to work from medial to lateral, tumor is dissected from the orbital apex and Meckel's cave region. There is typically extensive infiltration of the base of pterygoid and small deposits of tumor are excavated from the recesses of the bone. The pterygoid canal with the vidian nerve and artery is an important landmark in this region (Fig. 12.3). The nerve courses superior to the petrous segment of the ICA and helps to define the depth of the artery. The vidian artery is often a major vascular source for the tumor and cauterization of this vessel can significantly decrease bleeding from the tumor. If the petrous or lacerum ICA is difficult to localize due to tumor invasion, coagulation and packing of this region with a subsequent lateral to medial dissection of the lateral portion of the tumor is an option at this point.

Tumor is then dissected along the orbital floor with preservation of the second division of the trigeminal nerve (Fig. 12.7). The infraorbital and maxillary nerves are displaced superiorly (often involved by tumor), while the mandibular nerve is displaced posteriorly (rarely involved by tumor). Working through the anterior maxillotomy and endonasally, tumor dissection continues inferior to the orbital apex to follow the course of the tumor to the middle cranial fossa (Fig. 12.8). Large tumors may grow lateral to the orbital apex and the lateral cavernous sinus, displacing and eroding Meckel's cave and the middle cranial fossa. Tumor in this region may be sharply dissected from the maxillary nerve and then bluntly dissected from the middle fossa, lateral aspect of the orbital apex, and superior orbital fissure. Dura can be preserved in most cases without a CSF leak.

These lateral or nasopharyngeal segments, which often have significant residual vascularity following endovascular embolization, can also be embolized intraoperatively by direct tumor puncture. However, this should be done with great care under fluoroscopic visualization and is probably best performed by an endovascular

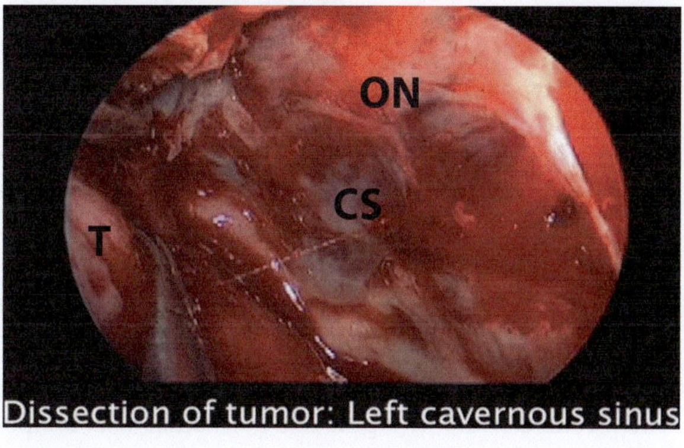

Fig. 12.6 Although there is erosion of bone over the left cavernous sinus, the tumor is extradural and dissects easily from the dura. *CS* cavernous sinus, *ON* optic nerve, *T* tumor

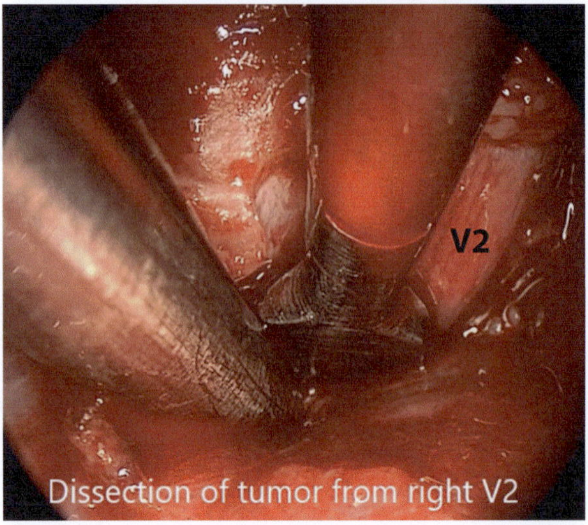

Fig. 12.7 Transmaxillary endoscopic view of tumor being dissected from the infraorbital nerve branch of the second division of the trigeminal nerve (V2)

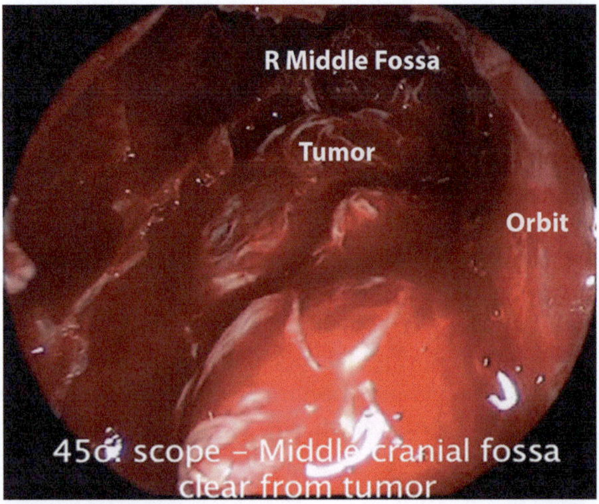

Fig. 12.8 Transmaxillary endoscopic view of the right (R) middle cranial fossa with extradural dissection of tumor lateral to the orbit

surgeon who has experience performing embolization procedures. Onyx is preferred due to its injection characteristics and low risk of distal embolization. Focal tumor bleeding, which can be profuse, can also be controlled with forceful hemostatic injection (e.g., Surgifoam). Both of these techniques should only be applied with some distance/separation from the ICA to avoid reflux into the intracranial vasculature and with neurophysiological monitoring.

Reconstruction of the surgical defect is not necessary in most cases. If there is exposure of middle fossa dura, an adipose tissue graft is used to fill the defect. Adipose tissue graft may also be used to cover an exposed ICA. The surgical field is then coated with fibrin glue and gelfoam. Nasal tampons (Merocel) may be placed for additional hemostasis.

Staging of Surgery

Staging of surgery is often necessary for large JA with residual vascularity (Fig. 12.4) [8]. The primary indication for staging surgery is excessive blood loss (greater than the patient's blood volume) and varies depending on the size of the patient, the vascularity of the tumor, and the quality of the dissection planes. It is best to avoid intracranial dissection if the patient is coagulopathic from excessive blood loss (will occur with less than half of their blood volume). Resultant subarachnoid hemorrhage can result in cerebral vasospasm and contributes to postoperative hydrocephalus. Once a prearranged blood loss limit is reached, the surgeon should finish the procedure by cauterizing all bleeding sites and packing the surgical cavity with Merocel tampons or similar packing. This limit should generally be set at approximately one-half of the patient's blood loss, as significant additional blood loss often occurs until complete hemostasis is achieved.

The optimal timing of the next stage depends on the physiological recovery of the patient and normalization of hematologic parameters, including platelet count, international normalized ratio (INR), partial thromboplastin time (PTT), and fibrinogen levels, which should be followed closely in the early postoperative period (with careful attention to signs of disseminated intravascular coagulopathy). Generally, a second stage is attempted within 4–7 days as these young patients recover rapidly. The nasal packing is left in place during this interval with continued antibiotic coverage. Repeat angiography and embolization is not necessary unless surgery is delayed for more than a few weeks.

Some large tumors will require multiple stages to achieve a complete resection (Fig. 12.9). Vascular segments of the tumor are resected sequentially, saving the intracranial portion for last.

Risks and Complications

The risks and complications are all related to dissection of tumor from the neural and vascular structures [5, 15]. Lack of hemostasis is probably the greatest risk factor for injury, interfering with visualization and identification of structures. A systematic approach without panicked attempts to achieve hemostasis helps prevent injury. In general, the majority of the dissection should be performed with the goal of avoiding transgression of the tumor except when planned for staging as detailed above. Dissection is greatly facilitated by team surgery. Other benefits of team surgery include dealing with a vascular injury and problem-solving during surgery.

Vascular Injury

Most carotid injuries occur in the region of foramen lacerum since this is where the tumor deeply infiltrates the bone and cartilage which is adherent to the ICA and brisk bleeding from the vidian artery may be encountered. Other risk factors include

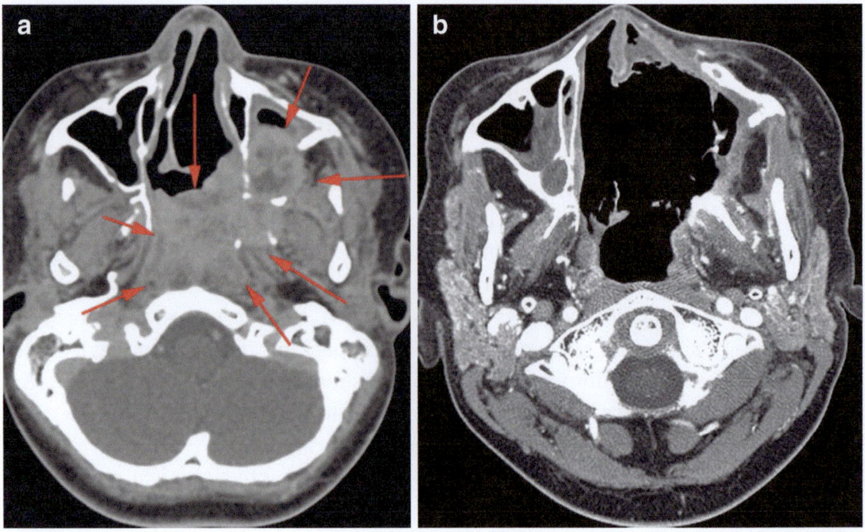

Fig. 12.9 (**a**) Previously irradiated "inoperable tumor" that required 4 staged operations. (**b**) An endoscopic anteromedial maxillotomy (Denker's approach) provided lateral access to the masticator space and middle cranial fossa to achieve a complete resection

prior embolization and surgery, and preoperative radiotherapy. Treatment algorithms have been proposed based on the magnitude of the injury [16]. Small injuries such as avulsion of a small branch can be effectively controlled with bipolar electrocautery. Larger injuries require focal packing or sacrifice of the vessel. Direct suturing is very difficult to perform. A muscle patch appears to be superior to other materials for covering the defect. The vessel may be partially or completely occluded with an aneurysm clip. Intraoperative neurophysiologic monitoring (SSEP) is critical to determine impact on intracranial perfusion. Once the intraoperative bleeding is controlled, the patient is transferred immediately to the endovascular suite for endovascular evaluation and/or control (with continued monitoring). Angiography identifies the site and extent of the injury (occlusion, stenosis, pseudoaneurysm, etc.) and assesses collateral circulation. Treatment options include observation, stenting, or permanent occlusion. Close follow-up is warranted due to the high risk of pseudoaneurysm formation.

Visual Loss

Visual loss may occur as a result of direct trauma to the optic nerve or loss of blood supply. With tumor erosion of the optic canal, the ophthalmic artery is at increased risk inferior to the optic nerve and distal perfusion via the ethmoidal arteries may already be compromised. Excessive cauterization or careless dissection in this region can injure the nerve and its blood supply.

Cranial Nerve Injury

Other than the optic nerve, the nerves at greatest risk are the branches of the second division of the trigeminal nerve. The infraorbital nerve may be injured as tumor is dissected from the floor of the orbit and foramen rotundum. It can be helpful to find the nerve peripherally or at Meckel's cave and follow it through the tumor. The descending palatine nerve is often displaced or engulfed by large tumors and can be very difficult to identify in the pterygopalatine space. It is helpful to identify it in the palatal canal where its position is fixed. Injury of the third division of the trigeminal nerve is also possible if the tumor extends to foramen ovale or there is a large component in the masticator space. It is helpful to first locate Meckel's cave and the lateral pterygoid plate. The foramen ovale is directly inferior to the trigeminal ganglion at the posterior edge of the lateral pterygoid plate.

Injury to the oculomotor nerves (III, IV, VI) is rare, as lateral cavernous sinus invasion is very unusual. These nerves are more likely to be injured if there is tumor invasion of the superior orbital fissure. As a result, this may be a site of small residual in the interest of preservation of function.

CSF Leak

Dural injuries typically occur along the floor of the middle cranial fossa when tumor extends lateral to the orbital apex. Although true dural invasion is rare, the dura may be adherent, especially if prior surgical dissection in this area has been performed or past embolization resulted in local inflammation. If a small dural defect results, this can be repaired with inlay and onlay fascial grafts and coverage with an adipose tissue graft. Nasal packing is placed for 5–7 days. A vascularized nasoseptal flap is not usually a realistic option, as the ipsilateral pedicle is often involved and the contralateral flap unlikely to reach.

Blood Transfusion

The surgeon must not lose sight of the goals of surgery and stick to the surgical plan. Excessive blood loss results in a coagulopathy, which further compounds the blood loss. Excessive blood loss requiring multiple transfusions has its own morbidity. Hypovolemia and hypotension can also precipitate visual loss when the optic nerve is already compromised by tumor compression. In addition, transfusion reactions become more likely; transfusion-related lung injury may result with large transfusion volumes.

Residual Tumor/Recurrence

The risk of leaving tumor behind is much greater with large tumors with residual vascularity. The multinodular growth pattern of the tumor, extensive bone infiltration, and poor visualization all contribute. The most common sites for residual tumor are in the base of pterygoid where it infiltrates the cancellous bone, in the masticator space behind the hard palate, and surrounding the cavernous ICA. When there is brisk bleeding from vascular contributions from the ICA, residual tumor may be intentionally left in proximity to it (Fig. 12.10). It is also easy to miss a small nodule within the inferior orbital fissure at the orbital apex. Not all residual tumors will grow during follow-up. If residual tumor is detected on a postoperative radiologic study, it is reasonable to follow it with serial scans to establish a growth pattern, especially if it is adjacent to the ICA or difficult to dissect. Younger patients are more likely to experience regrowth of their residual tumor. Radiation for residual is never recommended as a first option and small residual tumors can usually be allowed to grow prior to attempts at repeat resection, which may be facilitated by tumor growth.

Outcomes

The outcomes of surgery for advanced JA depend on multiple factors as previously discussed. In our own experience with endoscopic and endoscopic-assisted surgery, a complete removal of tumor can be achieved in most patients without significant morbidity and without the need for radiation therapy (Fig. 12.11).

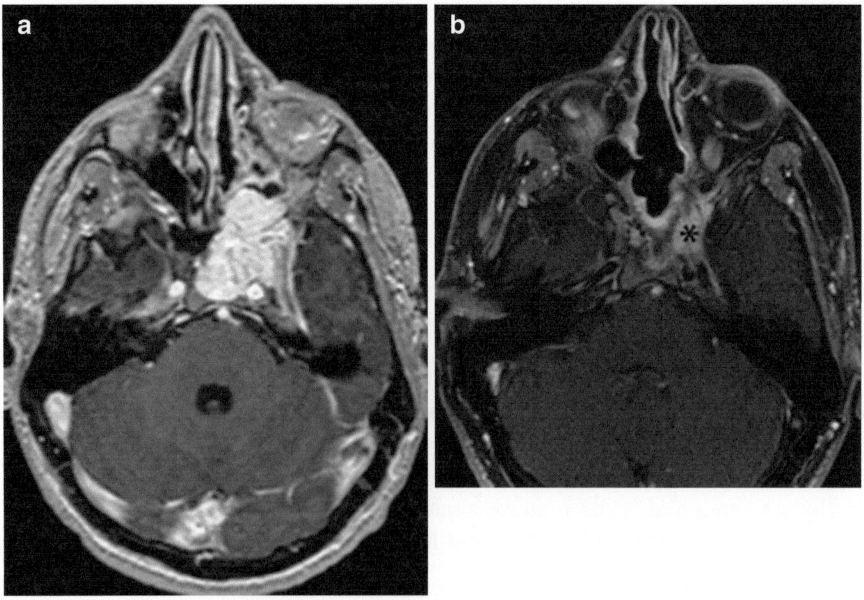

Fig. 12.10 Following excision of this UPMC stage 5 tumor (**a**), residual tumor (*asterisk*) was left in proximity to the internal carotid artery (**b**). This was observed without the need for surgical intervention

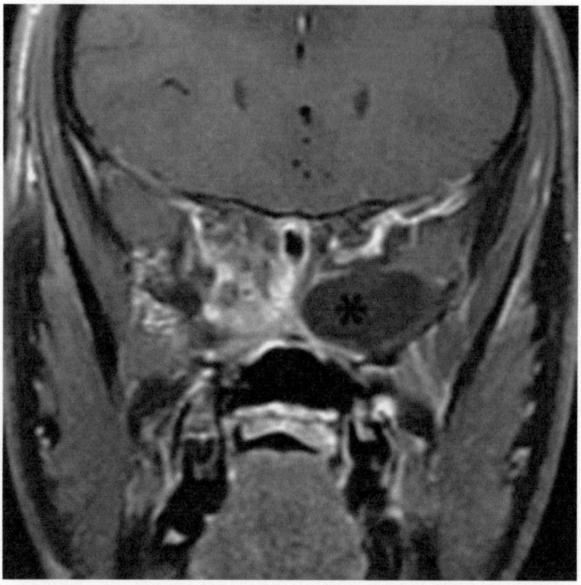

Fig. 12.11 A complete resection of the tumor in Fig. 12.2 was achieved. There is a small meningocele (*asterisk*) at the site of the middle fossa component of the tumor

In a recent review of our own experience (unpublished data), 12/34 patients were found on preoperative imaging to have intracranial extension. The average age was 13 years (range 7–16 years). Six patients (50 %) had prior surgical treatment; none had prior radiation treatment. Six of the 12 cases underwent staged surgery and a total of 20 surgeries were performed. All patients underwent preoperative embolization of the ECA contribution to their tumor. All patients had persistent blood supply to the tumor from small branches of the cavernous and petrous segments of the ICA (UPMC stage 4 or 5). Radiographic gross total resections were seen in seven patients (58 %). In the remaining patients, there was a greater than 90 % resection of the tumor. The most common sites for residual tumor were the cavernous ICA, Meckel's cave, or the middle cranial fossa. The average length of stay in the hospital was 6.8 days (range 1–22 days), usually related to staged procedures. Postoperative complications were seen in six patients, the most common being transient cranial nerve VI palsy in four patients, all with complete resolution. One patient suffered unilateral blindness secondary to central retinal artery occlusion 2 days after surgery, possibly related to vasospasm. Another patient suffered a carotid injury requiring carotid sacrifice without postoperative neurological sequelae. There were no postoperative cerebrospinal fluid leaks, meningitis, infections, or mortalities. With an average follow-up of 29 months, two patients with growth of their residual tumor (17 %) required further endoscopic endonasal surgery. No patient required radiation therapy.

Conclusions

With proper planning, even large JA with intracranial extension can be managed using endoscopic techniques. The biggest challenges are bleeding from tumor vessels derived from the intracranial circulation. The UPMC staging system is useful in devising a surgical strategy based on the degree of residual vascularity and the route of intracranial extension. A staged approach with excision of vascular territories of the tumor allows safe resection with minimal morbidity. There is a higher risk of residual tumor with advanced JA with skull base involvement, but not all patients require further surgery. Radiation therapy can be avoided with a comprehensive surgical strategy.

References

1. Thakar A, Hota A, Bhalla AS, Gupta SD, Sarkar C, Kumar R. Overt and occult vidian canal involvement in juvenile angiofibroma and its possible impact on recurrence. Head Neck. 2016;38:E421–5.
2. Vescan AD, Snyderman CH, Carrau RL, Mintz A, Gardner P, Branstetter 4th B, et al. Vidian canal: analysis and relationship to the internal carotid artery. Laryngoscope. 2007;117:1338–42.
3. Boghani Z, Husain Q, Kanumuri VV, Khan MN, Sanghvi S, Liu JK, et al. Juvenile nasopharyngeal angiofibroma: a systematic review and comparison of endoscopic, endoscopic-assisted, and open resection in 1047 cases. Laryngoscope. 2013;123:859–69.
4. Khoueir N, Nicolas N, Rohayem Z, Haddad A, Abou Hamad W. Exclusive endoscopic resection of juvenile nasopharyngeal angiofibroma: a systematic review of the literature. Otolaryngol Head Neck Surg. 2014;150:350–8.
5. Leong SC. A systematic review of surgical outcomes for advanced juvenile nasopharyngeal angiofibroma with intracranial involvement. Laryngoscope. 2013;123:1125–31.
6. Snyderman C, Kassam A, Carrau R, Mintz A, Gardner P, Prevedello DM. Acquisition of surgical skills for endonasal skull base surgery: a training program. Laryngoscope. 2007;117:699–705.
7. Liu J, Pinheiro-Neto CD, Fernandez-Miranda JC, Snyderman CH, Gardner PA, Hirsch BE, et al. Eustachian tube and internal carotid artery in skull base surgery: an anatomical study. Laryngoscope. 2014;124:2655–64.
8. Snyderman CH, Pant H. Endoscopic management of vascular sinonasal tumors including angiofibroma. Otolaryngol Clin North Am 2016;49:791–807.
9. Snyderman CH, Pant H, Carrau RL, Gardner P. A new endoscopic staging system for angiofibromas. Arch Otolaryngol Head Neck Surg. 2010;136:588–94.
10. Rowan NR, Zwagerman NT, Heft-Neal ME, Gardner PA, Snyderman CH. Juvenile nasal angiofibromas: a comparison of modern staging systems in an endoscopic era. J Neurol Surg B (Accepted for publication, May 2016).
11. Alshaikh NA, Eleftheriadou A. Juvenile nasopharyngeal angiofibroma staging: an overview. Ear Nose Throat J. 2015;94:E12–22.
12. Lutz J, Holtmannspotter M, Flatz W, Meier-Bender A, Berghaus A, Brückmann H, et al. Preoperative embolization to improve the surgical management and outcome of juvenile nasopharyngeal angiofibroma (JNA) in a single center: 10-year experience. Clin Neuroradiol. 2015 Jan 29:1–9. [Epub ahead of print].
13. Ballah D, Rabinowitz D, Vossough A, Rickert S, Dunham B, Kazahaya K, et al. Preoperative angiography and external carotid artery embolization of juvenile nasopharyngeal angiofibromas in a tertiary referral paediatric centre. Clin Radiol. 2013;68:1097–106.
14. Grandhi R, Hunnicutt CT, Harrison G, Zwagerman NT, Snyderman CH, Gardner PA, Hartman DJ, Horowitz M. Comparing angiographic devascularization with histologic penetration after preoperative tumor embolization with Onyx: what indicates an effective procedure. J Neurol Surg A Cent Eur Neurosurg. 2015;76:309–17.

15. Godoy MD, Bezerra TF, Pinna FD, Voegels RL. Complications in the endoscopic and endoscopic-assisted treatment of juvenile nasopharyngeal angiofibroma with intracranial extension. Braz J Otorhinolaryngol. 2014;80:120–5.
16. Carrau RL, Fernandez-Miranda JC, Prevedello DM, Gardner PA, Snyderman CH, Kassam AB. Management of vascular complications during endoscopic skull base surgery. In: Stamm AC, editor. Transnasal endoscopic skull base and brain surgery. New York: Thieme; 2011. p. 386–91.

Chapter 13
Excision by Midfacial Degloving Approach

José Luis Llorente and C. Suarez

Abstract Complete removal of juvenile angiofibroma is essential to prevent recurrence, and most, if not all, recurrences could be reflecting incomplete resection of the tumor. The use of a midfacial degloving approach allows a good uni- or bilateral exposure of maxillary area and avoids several adverse functional and aesthetic sequelae associated to open approaches. Because of the modular design of the facial translocation approach, it accommodates the surgical needs for different procedures at the skull base and sinonasal area. Juvenile angiofibromas with extensive nasopharyngeal and sinonasal involvement, moderate to large extension into the infratemporal fossa, and upper displacement of the inferior part of the cavernous sinus is managed with a unilateral medial facial translocation. In MFD, circumvestibular release is performed by joining full transfixation, intercartilaginous and sublabial incisions. Sublabial incision is extended between maxillary first molars and beyond and round the maxillary tuberosity in the pathological side. Subsequently, soft tissue over the nasomaxillary skeleton is elevated in subperiosteal plane. Infraorbital nerve and lacrimal sac are sectioned. With the help of osteotomies, the anterolateral wall of the maxilla, lateral bony nasal wall, and part of medial wall of maxillary antrum are removed as single block of bone, and it is preserved. Posterior maxillary wall is removed for clamping and/or ligation of sphenopalatine and maxillary artery. The tumor is separated from the surrounding tissues and removed. The block of bone is replaced and fixed with microplates and screws and the wound is closed. The patients should be followed up to 5 years to detect recurrence.

Osteomyelitis of the bone subunits is a major complication after a facial translocation approach. The interference of osteotomies with the facial growth is still controversial. Other complications include vestibular stenoses, nasal crusting and associated foul nasal smell, and anesthesia of the cheek.

J.L. Llorente, MD, PhD (✉)
Depto. Otorrinolaringología, Hospital Universitario Central de Asturias, Avenida de Roma s/n, 33011 Oviedo, Spain
e-mail: llorentependas@telefonica.net

C. Suarez, MD, PhD
University of Oviedo, Oviedo, Spain
e-mail: csuareznieto@gmail.com

S.P. Dubey, B. Schick (eds.), *Juvenile Angiofibroma*,
DOI 10.1007/978-3-319-45343-9_13

In spite each case must be individualized, midfacial degloving approach offers an excellent exposure in tumors with extensive involvement of the nasopharynx, infratemporal fossa, nasal cavity, and maxillary sinus with very few sequelae. It is an interesting alternative to other approaches.

Keywords Juvenile angiofibroma • Nasopharyngeal angiofibroma • Midfacial degloving • Facial translocation approach • Complications • Sequelae

Introduction

A number of anterior and lateral approaches to neoplasms within the nasopharynx and the infratemporal fossa have been described. These are transantral or transmaxillary, transpalatal, subtemporal-infratemporal, subfrontal, Le Fort I access, maxillary swing, facial translocation, endoscopic, etc. Transfacial-transmaxillary open approaches with removal of structures of the middle third of the face offer wide access to the median structures of the skull base but may produce severe adverse sequelae, such as a notable paranasal depression originated by the removal of part of the maxilla, and visible facial scars.

Indication

The use of a midfacial degloving (MFD) allows a good bilateral exposure of maxillary area and avoids several adverse functional and aesthetic sequelae. In juvenile angiofibroma (JA) occupying nasal cavity, paranasal sinuses, nasopharynx, sphenoid sinus, infratemporal fossa, extracranial clivus, and middle cranial fossa, the facial translocation by MFD approach, can be the simplest and most direct way to expose these areas and to facilitate extensive tumor removal. It provides the surgeon a better exposure than that obtained by other infratemporal procedures.

Surgical Technique

A full standard transfixion incision is carried out extending from the roof of the nose onto the nasal floor. This incision is continued by a full-thickness incision down through the periosteum of the pyriform margin and nasal floor. Intercartilaginous incisions are joined to the superior end of the transfixion incision medially, extending beyond the lateral margin of the upper lateral cartilages and completing the circumvestibular release. Nevertheless, a circular incision is more prone to produce a stenosis in the nasal vestibule. To avoid this, it seems preferable to not complete the circular incision in the roof of the nose. Dissection through the intercartilaginous

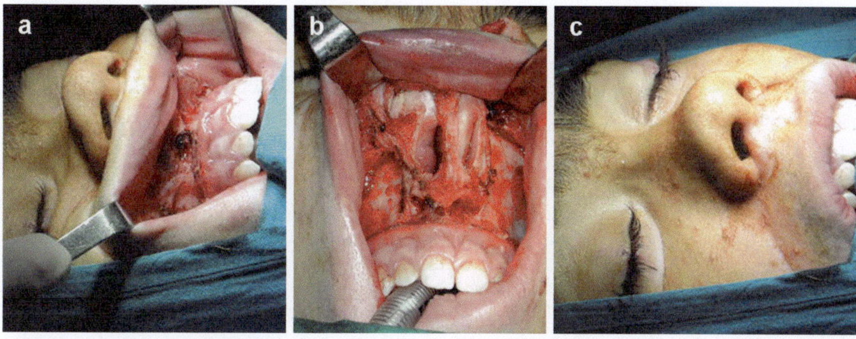

Fig. 13.1 Midfacial degloving technique. (**a**) Sublabial incision. (**b**) Intranasal circular incision interrupted at the tip of the nose and exposure of the anterior wall of the maxillary sinus. (**c**) Final aspect after closure of the wound

incision exposed the dorsum of the upper lateral cartilage that led to the nasal bones. The periosteum is incised, and soft tissues are widely elevated. Elevation extends laterally to the nasomaxillary sutures and superiorly to the glabella. All adhesions between the nasal skeleton and soft tissue are released to allow full elevation. The sublabial incision is made with electrocautery. The incision is carried down through the periosteum of the canine fossa. The standard incision is made from one first molar to the contralateral first molar; it is extended around the maxillary tuberosity on the pathological side. Soft tissue over the anterior maxilla is elevated in the subperiosteal plane, extending laterally to the zygoma and up to the infraorbital rim. Superiorly, the neurovascular bundle of the infraorbital nerve is visualized and sectioned. The nasal floor and sublabial incisions are connected. Full retraction of the facial soft tissues, including the upper lip, intact columella, and nasal tip, is performed up to the level of the medial canthus (Fig. 13.1).

Once the MFD has been carried out, we proceed to perform a transmaxillary approach which is performed according to the author's technique of minifacial translocation, central, and minifacial translocation, lateral [1–5].

The orbital content is then reflected posteriorly to expose the lacrimal sac. The lacrimal sac is sectioned horizontally at the entrance in its bony canal and divided vertically, the orbital content is retracted, and the soft tissues lining the inner aspect of the piriform aperture are elevated. The inferior orbital nerve is electively sectioned along the floor of the orbit, tagged, and repaired at the end of the procedure. Titanium miniplates are molded and screwed to the bones of the nasomaxillary and orbital regions. This guaranteed that the mobilized bones would return to their exactly original position at the end of the surgical procedure. The plates are then removed and preserved for its later use. Osteotomies of the orbitomaxillary skeleton are then performed using an electric oscillating saw to free the anterior face of the maxilla, malar eminence, and inferior orbital rim, as well as the orbital floor.

At first, an osteotomy through the anterior part of the floor of the orbit is made with a right-angled saw. A second osteotomy across the frontal process of the maxilla and through the lacrimal bone connects the superior piriform aperture with the osteotomy in the medial part of the floor of the orbit. Next step consists of dividing the lateral wall of the nose/medial wall of the antrum along the floor of the nasal cavity up to the posterior wall of the antrum. The dissection is halted when the osteotome hits up against the solid pterygoid bone. This osteotomy is continued laterally in the plane of the floor of the nasal cavity across the anterior wall of the maxillary sinus. Finally, a vertical osteotomy through the anterolateral wall of the maxilla at the level of the junction with the malar eminence is performed, joining the osteotomy in the lateral part of the floor of the orbit. This en bloc segment is preserved for later reconstruction (Fig. 13.2).

The bone of the posterolateral maxillary wall is removed, and the sphenopalatine and/or internal maxillary artery is clamped and divided. The pterygoid plates can be removed with a high-speed pneumatic drill. We proceeded with the resection using blunt and bipolar dissection; suction bipolar electrocautery is first used to ablate feeding vessels along the surface of the tumor; a suction elevator or knife is used to release adhesions and dissect tumor off adjacent structures.

JA occupying nasal cavity, maxillary sinus, nasopharynx, and sphenoid sinus, with moderate to large extension into the infratemporal fossa and upper displacement of the inferior part of the cavernous sinus, is dissected and resected en bloc through this approach. Endoscopes are also valuable adjunct in MFD approach and are used to assess the extent of the tumor and the adequacy of the resection, especially in the sphenoid sinus.

Once the tumor has been removed (Fig. 13.3), the lacrimal sac is marsupialized into the nasal cavity and the bone is repositioned with the help of the preserved microplates (Fig. 13.4).

Closure of the nasal incision began with transfixion stitches. The precise placement of this suture is critical in determining the final position of the nasal tip, if the

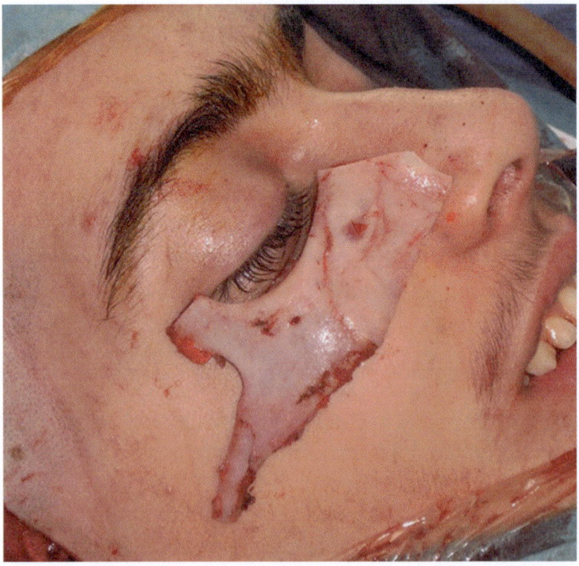

Fig. 13.2 Detail of maxillary osteotomies over the patient´s face in an extended midfacial degloving approach

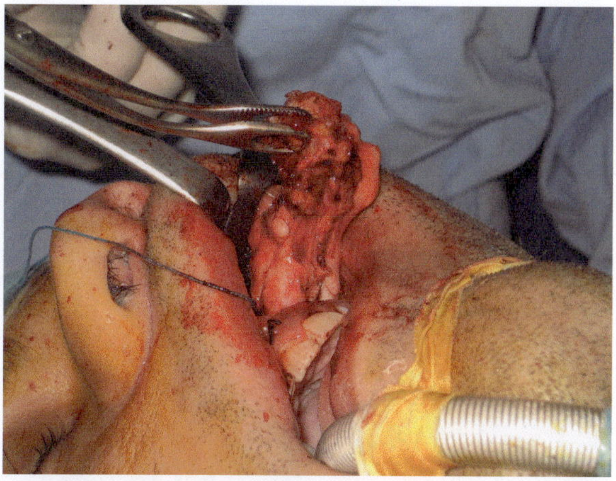

Fig. 13.3 Removal of a juvenile angiofibroma via midfacial degloving approach

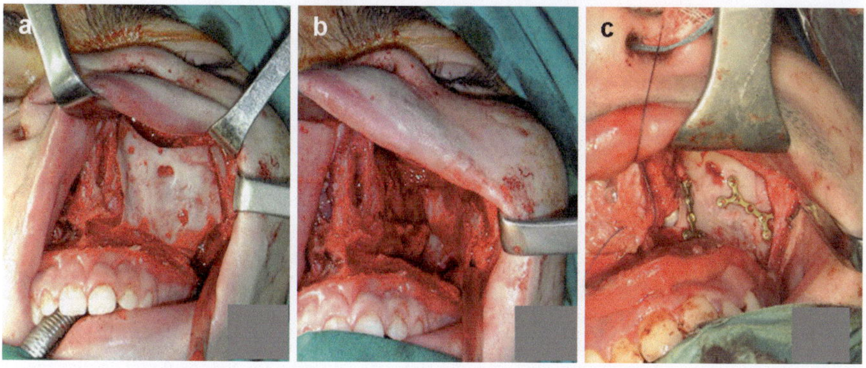

Fig. 13.4 Medial translocation technique. (**a**) Osteotomies across the anterior wall of the maxilla. (**b**) Operative cavity after resection of the posterolateral maxillary wall and the tumor. (**c**) Replacement of the anterior wall of the maxilla with microplates

nasal incision had been circumferential. The circumvestibular incisions are carefully reapproximated with three or more stitches placed at the intercartilaginous, pyriform, and nasal floor areas. Hemostasis is achieved by packing of the nasal cavity bilaterally using Netcell® (*Network Medical Prod., England*) to be removed after 48 h. Closure of the sublabial incision is done through reapproximation at the frenulum using polyglycologic acid material [6].

JA with massive involvement of the infratemporal fossa or even the temporal fossa and moderate to large middle fossa involvement and extending laterally to the cavernous sinus is unsuitable for excision by endoscopic approach or by medial facial translocation. These cases are the best candidates for a standard facial translocation (Fig. 13.5). Because the high likelihood of producing significant morbidity and due to JA are benign lesions, tumor fragments located near the orbital apex, into the cavernous sinus or attached to the internal carotid artery are better not removed avoiding the mobilization of critical neurovascular structures. This approach could be useful in

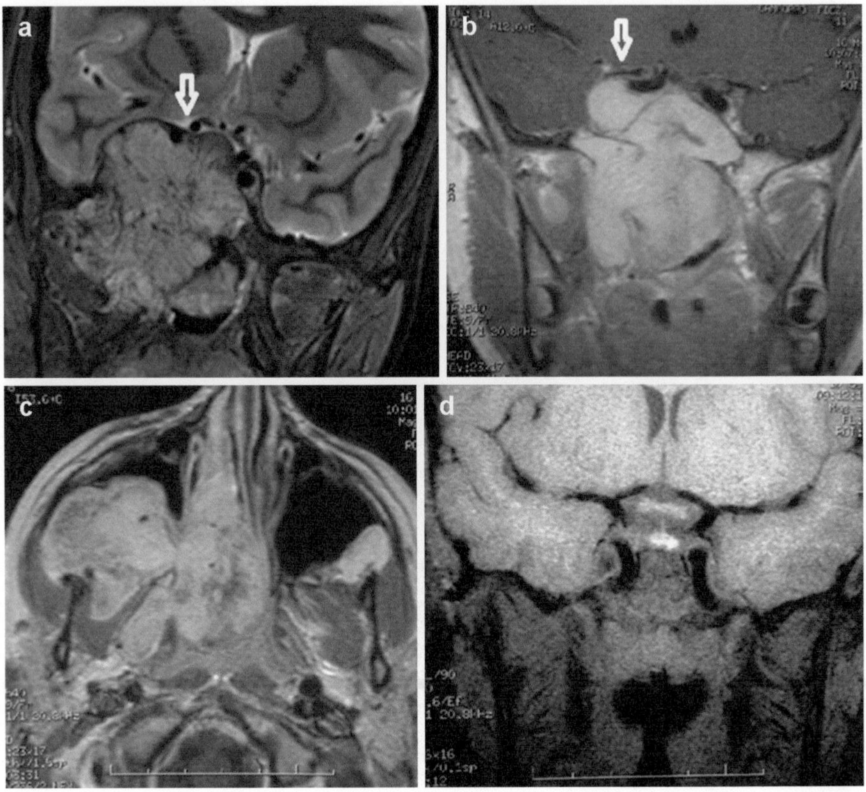

Fig. 13.5 Indications for a standard facial translocation. (**a**, **b**) Coronal MRI of two different patients with juvenile angiofibroma showing an extensive parasellar involvement and displacement of the internal carotid artery, cavernous sinus (*white arrow*), and middle fossa. (**c**) Axial MRI in a patient with moderate parasellar invasion and extension into the infratemporal fossa. (**d**) Postoperative MRI showing the total resection of the tumor (case b)

order to control the middle fossa if necessary or when we have planned a reconstruction with the anterior part or the total temporalis muscle filling any dead space in the infratemporal fossa. It is important to note that the blood supply to the temporalis muscle, which may be used for reconstruction, could be compromised by embolization.

MFD can be combined with lateral preauricular approach which is described in Chap. 16.

Complications

1. *Related to incision*: Incidence of vestibular stenosis is markedly reduced by avoiding incision at the roof of the nasal vestibule. Epiphora, lower lid ectropion, and scarring can also happen postoperatively; they become more marked when external incision are used [1–7].

2. *Osteomyelitis*: Osteomyelitis of the bone subunit is a major postoperative complication of facial translocation approach [6, 8]. This complication is more pronounced when the patient undergoes repeated operations or receives postoperative irradiation. These situations are rare with JA patients. Different modifications have been proposed to avoid this complication [9–11].
3. *Facial growth*: The growth of male craniofacial skeleton continues until at least 18 years. The practice of craniofacial surgery in the pediatric patients has been limited by the apprehension that facial growth would be disrupted by osteotomies. Nevertheless this concern has not been substantiated [12]. The use of absorbable microplates may overcome problems associated with metal plates and growth restriction.
4. *Others*: Nasal crusting and foul nasal smell are encountered in the postoperative period [8]. Some degree of anesthesia of the cheek usually remains as the infraorbital nerve is transected during flap elevation. Much less frequent is the occurrence of mild to moderate trismus. Abducens nerve palsy and temporary ophthalmoplegia can rarely be seen following removal of large tumors, as it happened in one patient of our series.

Follow-Up

Complete removal of juvenile angiofibroma is essential to prevent recurrence, and most, if not all, recurrences could be reflecting incomplete resection of the tumor. Performing a postoperative MRI (better after removing the nasal packing), we can detect residual tumor and is especially useful in big tumors. Follow-up clinical examinations (including nasal endoscope) usually take place in the first month, every 6 months for the first year and annually thereafter up to 5 years, if there is no evidence of recurrence. An MRI is obtained once a year if there is any suspicion of tumor remnant or in years 3 and 5 after surgery if we have a low chance of recurrence. A CT is helpful if MRI is not available. Sometimes additional explorations or tests (CT or MRI) are indicated if the patient has recurrent symptoms or signs suggestive of tumor regrowth.

In the case of recurrent or residual tumor, a second surgery is considered as the best option if the tumor can be removed completely. Depending of the extension tumor, salvage surgery can be performed by MFD or better by another open or endoscopic approach. In case of using the same MFD, more fibrosis during surgery and a higher incidence of osteonecrosis can be expected.

However, each case must be individualized, and they should not be routinely operated because complete removal of the tumor from areas such as the cavernous sinus, carotid artery, or orbit apex would cause a significant morbidity that is hardly justified during excision of a benign tumor. The use of radiotherapy is still a matter of debate if radiation can be considered a safe therapeutic option in young patients. In our department, taking into account the new and more precise modalities of radiotherapy (radiosurgery, intensity-modulated radiotherapy) [13], we agree that the risk of complications from radiation is less than the morbidity and possible mortality associated with surgical resection especially if there is a transdural extension of angiofibroma [14]. However, the role of the "wait and see" strategy and radiosurgery in residual tumors will require further prospective studies.

The role of radiotherapy in JA is described in Chap. 18.

References

1. Janecka IP, Sen C, Sekhar LN, Arriaga M. Facial translocation: a new approach to the cranial base. Otolaryngol Head Neck Surg. 1990;103:413–9.
2. Janecka IP. Classification of facial translocation approach to the skull base. Otolaryngol Head Neck Surg. 1995;112:579–85.
3. Llorente JL, López F, Suárez V, Costales M, Suárez C. Evolution in the treatment of juvenile nasopharyngeal angiofibroma. Acta Otorrinolaringol Esp. 2011;62:279–86.
4. Suárez C, Llorente JL, Muñoz C, García LA, Rodrigo JP. Facial translocation approach in the management of central skull base and infratemporal tumors. Laryngoscope. 2004;114:1047–51.
5. Arriaga MA, Janecka IP. Facial translocation approach to the cranial base: the anatomic basis. Skull Base Surg. 1991;1:26–33.
6. Fagan JJ, Snyderman CH, Carrau RL, Janecka IP. Nasopharyngeal angiofibromas: selecting a surgical approach. Head Neck. 1997;19:391–9.
7. Kekatpure VD, Rajan GP, Patel D, Trivedi NP, Arun P, Iyer S, Kuriakose MA. Morbidity profile and functional outcome of modified facial translocation approaches for skull base tumors. Skull Base. 2011;21:255–60.
8. Hao SP, Pan WL, Chang CN, Hsu YS. The use of the facial translocation technique in the management of tumors of the paranasal sinuses and skull base. Otolaryngol Head Neck Surg. 2003;128:571–5.
9. Hao SP. Facial translocation approach to the skull base: the viability of translocated facial bone graft. Otolaryngol Head Neck Surg. 2001;124:292–6.
10. Hao SP. Modified facial translocation to prevent necrosis of bone graft. Laryngoscope. 2002;112:1691–5.
11. Chen CW, Hao SP, Pan WL. Bone graft necrosis of facial translocation: comparison of 3 different techniques. Otolaryngol Head Neck Surg. 2006;135:719–23.
12. Lang DA, Neil-Dwyer G, Evans BT, Honeybul S. Craniofacial access in children. Acta Neurochir (Wien). 1998;140:33–40.
13. Gutiontov SI, Shin EJ, Lok B, Lee NY, Cabanillas R. Intensity-modulated radiotherapy for head and neck surgeons. Head Neck. 2016;38:E2368–73.
14. López F, Suárez V, Costales M, Suárez C, Llorente JL. Treatment of juvenile angiofibromas: 18-year experience of a single tertiary centre in Spain. Rhinology. 2012;50:95–103.

Chapter 14
Modified Transpalatal Approach and Total Maxillary Swing Approach

Siba P. Dubey and Charles P. Molumi

Abstract Many surgical techniques have been described for resection of juvenile angiofibroma (JA). There is a high tendency for incomplete removal of the tumor within the confines of the anterior and middle skull base. Repeat surgical procedure to remove regrowth from residual tumor is difficult and it results in high morbidity. The ease and complete onetime removal depends on perfect exposure. Excellent visualization and unhindered surgical manipulation result in successful postoperative results. The authors designed surgical technique of "modified transpalatal" and "total maxillary swing" to approach the anterior, middle, and lateral skull base for onetime complete removal of limited and advanced juvenile angiofibroma, respectively. Tumor localized to the nasopharynx, oropharynx, and sphenoid sinus without lateral extension is removed by modified transpalatal with palatal osteomucoperiosteal (POMP) flap approach. During the procedure the hard palate and, if necessary, the soft palate are reflected like a "lid," thereby opening up the nasal cavity and nasopharynx. This provides excellent view of the tumor and helps to coagulate the feeding vessels. In contrast to the conventional procedure, no part of the bony palate is removed and discarded. Consequently, patient did not develop scarred smaller palate and palatal insufficiency in postoperative period. Total maxillary swing (TMS) approach completely opens up the origin and most extensions of extensive juvenile angiofibroma. TMS allowed removal of the tumor from the pterygoid base, basisphenoid, clivus, pterygoid canal, and other extensions. Tumor with intracranial extensions is also dealt with. Despite the extensiveness of TMS, no maxillofacial bone is lost, and the growth of the adolescent facial skeleton is not disturbed. The facial scar gradually became indistinct over time.

Keywords Juvenile angiofibroma • Total maxillary swing • Transpalatal • Advanced juvenile angiofibroma • Complete excision

---

S.P. Dubey, MS (✉) • C.P. Molumi, MMed
Department of Otolaryngology – Head and Neck Surgery, Port Moresby General Hospital, Boroko, NCD, Papua New Guinea
e-mail: dr_sp_dubey@yahoo.com; pmolumi@gmail.com

S.P. Dubey, B. Schick (eds.), *Juvenile Angiofibroma*,
DOI 10.1007/978-3-319-45343-9_14

Introduction

The main objective of open surgical approaches to the skull base in the excision of JA is to have maximum exposure for complete tumor removal. Adequate surgical access allows complete tumor removal to avoid regrowth of residual tumor and reduce surgical complications from injury to important structures. JA has various routes of extension and is located in the confines of the nose, nasopharynx, paranasal sinus, skull base, and intracranial cavity [1]. The surgical approach depends on the extensions and location of the tumor. In our institution, we perform transpalatal approach by palatal osteomucoperiosteal (POMP) flap for excision of JAs without lateral extensions [2] and the total maxillary swing (TMS) approach for large JAs with lateral and intracranial extensions [3].

Palatal Osteomucoperiosteal (POMP) Flap

The conventional way of performing transpalatal approach involves elevation of the palatal mucoperiosteum and permanent removal of the bony hard palate [4, 5]. But this technique leads to temporary and permanent complications in the immediate and late postoperative period, namely, palatal fistula, palatal insufficiency, hypernasility, and nasal synechiae [6]. Removing and discarding the major part of the bony hard palate and scarring of the soft palate are responsible for these complications. The authors modified this technique to preserve the entire hard palate bone to avoid the complications. This procedure is suitable for JA extensions medially from the site of origin (vide Fig. 5.1 in Chap. 5) and minimal lateral extension confined to the pterygopalatine fossa.

Surgical Technique

The patient is anesthetized with orotracheal intubation and placed in supine tonsillar position. The surgical steps are described below.

Reflection of Nasal Floor Mucoperiosteum

Through a midline sublabial incision, the nasal floor mucoperiosteum is elevated from the pyriform aperture to the posterior end of the hard palate and side to side as much as possible. With a heavy scissors, the junction of the maxillary crest and nasal septum is cut all the way from its anterior to the posterior ends. In this way, a space is created between the bony and soft tissues of the nasal floor where a malleable copper retractor is placed. It prevents injury to the nasal floor mucoperiosteum during subsequent osteotomy of the ipsilateral hard palate.

Osteotomy of Ipsilateral Hard Palate Margin

The tags of hard palate mucosa joining the gingivolabial mucosa in between the teeth are incised, and the palatal mucoperiosteum is elevated from the last molar tooth of the pathological side to the junction between the contralateral canine and first premolar teeth. The palatal mucoperiosteum is elevated just medial to the greater palatine canal posteriorly and just posterior to the incisive foramen anteriorly to expose sufficient hard palate for osteotomy. The ipsilateral greater and lesser palatine arteries are coagulated. Using a mastoid drill and a small cutting burr, the hard palate bone is cut just medial to the greater palatine canal and carried posteriorly to the end of the hard palate. The osteotomy is continued anteriorly and stopped just posterior to the incisive foramen (Fig. 14.1).

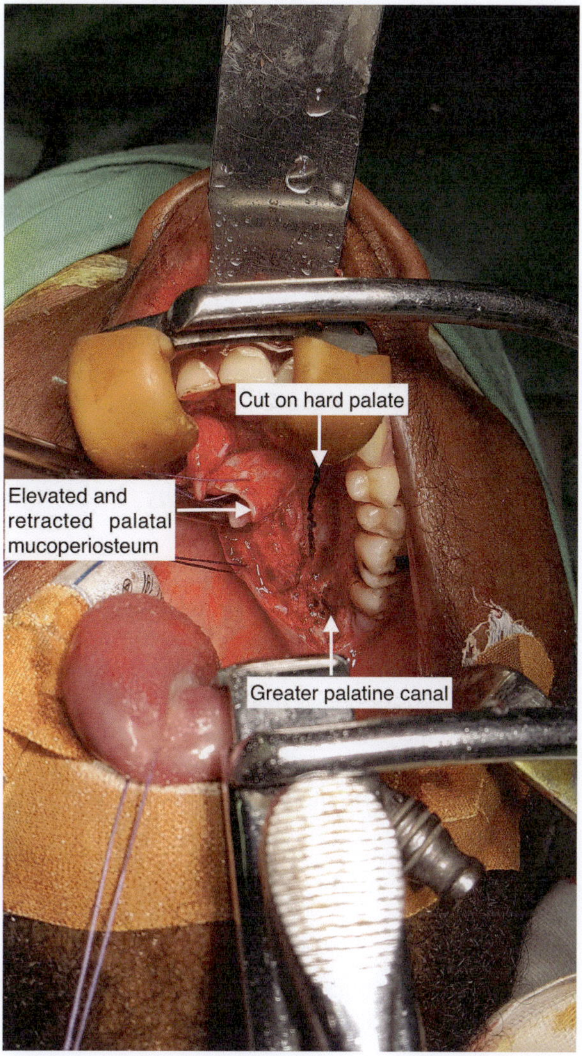

Fig. 14.1 The palatal mucoperiosteum on the pathological side is elevated, and a hard palate cut is made medial to the greater palatine canal. The greater palatine artery is coagulated

Osteotomy of Contralateral Hard Palate

The contralateral hard palatal cut is made through the midline sublabial incision. A through and through osteotomy is done without injuring the palatal mucoperiosteum with the help of Joseph lateral osteotome which is used in rhinoplasty; the right one is for the left palatal half and vice versa. The knob at the tip of the osteotome is felt through the palatal mucoperiosteum which in turn prevents the accidental injury or buttonhole of the palatal mucoperiosteum. The osteotomy has begun just posterior to the incisive foramen where the ipsilateral osteotomy was ended and continued along the contralateral hard palate margin to the end.

Exposure of Surgical Field and Removal of Tumor

Pressure with a periosteum elevator from the nasal side toward the oral side opens up the palatal osteomucoperiosteal (POMP) flap (like the "lid" of a box) in the oral cavity. The flap is pedicled on the mucoperiosteum from the first premolar to the last molar tooth of the normal side where the greater and lesser palatine arteries are intact. This exposes the nasal floor mucoperiosteum of both sides. The POMP flap is either reflected with a retractor or sutured and anchored with a weight at the non-pathological side. The nasal floor mucoperiosteum of the pathological side is cut open to expose the tumor (Fig. 14.2). The tumor is then removed. Any residual tumor in pterygoid base, basisphenoid, and pterygoid canal is drilled and removed by focusing the operating microscope through the oral cavity with 300 mm lens. Control of bleeding is discussed later in this chapter.

Variations of Soft Palate Incisions

The posterior part of this incision varies according to the size of tumor and extent of surgery. In the case of limited lesion, the incision extends from the last molar tooth transversely along the junction of the hard and soft palate and falls just short of the contralateral last molar tooth. In the case of a bigger pathology which needed wider exposure, the posterior end of the incision is carried past the last molar tooth and extends up to the junction of the soft palate and upper end of the anterior tonsillar pillar of the pathological side. By this way the soft palate is reflected together with the hard palate to the contralateral side.

Closure

At the completion of the procedure, the medial and the lateral incised halves of the nasal mucoperiosteal floor are stitched together. Subsequently, the POMP flap is

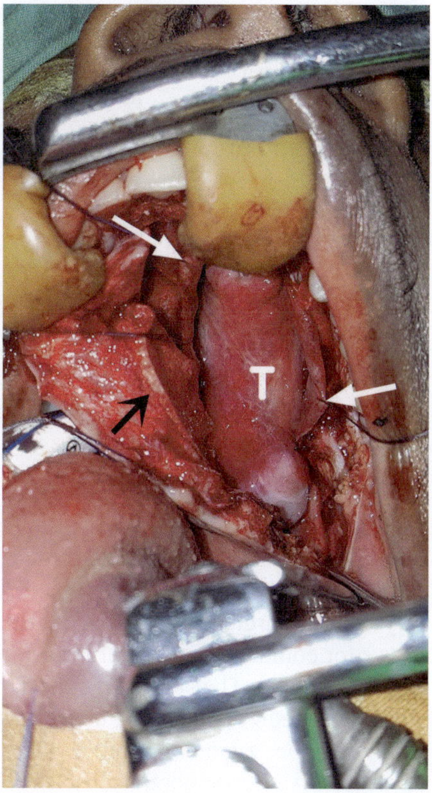

Fig. 14.2 The intact hard palate bone within the reflected POMP flap (*black arrow*), the cut and reflected nasal mucoperiosteal floor (*white arrows*), and exposed tumor in the nasal cavity and nasopharynx (*T*)

placed back. Three to four sutures are placed between the elevated palatal mucoperiosteum with the mucoperiosteum of the gingivolabial sulcus across the spaces between the teeth. The sublabial incision is closed in two layers. A light nasal packing is done to be removed in 2–3 days. When soft palate incision is made, it is closed using 3/0 Vicryl sutures in three layers as the nasopharyngeal surface mucosa, the muscle layer, and the oral surface mucosa. Very rarely, patient may develop small fistula at the lateral end of the extended incision in the immediate postoperative period, and it heals with minimal scarring (Fig. 14.3).

Total Maxillary Swing

The approach is called TMS as the entire maxilla is cut from all its bony attachments and swinged laterally with attached soft tissues of the cheek [3]. It is total in contrast to subtotal maxillary swing where the inferior orbital wall is kept in place [7]. TMS approach completely exposes the nasal cavity, nasopharynx, sphenopalatine foramen, pterygopalatine and infratemporal fossae, orbital apex, and adjoining skull base regions [3]. The pterygoid base, basisphenoid, and pterygoid canal are the sites where the tumor is thought to be attached [8]. Residual tumor in these areas leads to regrowth. TMS allows complete removal of the tumor from these areas [9].

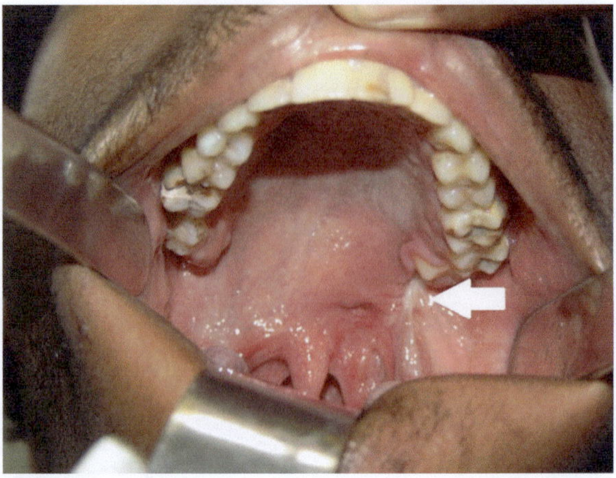

Fig. 14.3 Postoperative picture after 6 weeks showing the hard and soft palate. In the immediate postoperative period, there was a small fistula at the lateral end which healed with minimal scarring (*white arrow*)

Maximum exposure of TMS is also advantageous in managing sphenoid sinus and cavernous sinus involvement and bleeding from the latter [9].

Given the well-circumscribed character of JA and its "pushing" growth pattern, very careful surgical dissection, especially in the area of the skull base, often allows for complete removal of intracranial extension from below without formal craniotomy [10]. The surgical field can be expanded more laterally to the temporal and infratemporal fossa by converting TMS to extended TMS by making osteotomy at the zygomatic process instead of maxillozygomatic suture [9]. Subsequently, the temporalis muscle is elevated from its fossa for craniotomy [9]. The entire clivus can be exposed from the sella turcica down to the level of the foramen magnum [9].

Surgical Techniques

The patient is intubated with endotracheal tube and placed in supine tonsillectomy position. The surgical steps are described below.

Reflection of Ipsilateral Palatal Mucoperiosteum

The ipsilateral hard palate mucoperiosteum is marked out and infiltrated with lignocaine and adrenaline. The tags of hard palate mucosa joining the gingivolabial mucosa in between the teeth are incised, and the palatal mucoperiosteum is elevated. Reflection of the palatal mucoperiosteum is continued till the greater palatine artery in the greater palatine canal is encountered. The artery is coagulated and the palatal mucoperiosteum is reflected up to the midline (the contralateral hard palate mucoperiosteum is kept intact). The posterior retraction is continued till the end of the hard palate is reached.

Exposure of Osteotomy Site

A Weber-Ferguson incision (without the gingivolabial component) is marked out on the face. The infraciliary incision is marked out 3–5 mm from the ciliary line. The incision is deepened to the bone from the upper lip to the medial canthal region. Bleeding encountered in the medial canthal region is controlled with diathermy. The incision is carried into the nasal cavity along the nasal bone taking care not to injure the tumor, and the nasal ala is reflected medially and anchored with suture (Fig. 14.4). This exposes the frontal process of the maxilla. The infraciliary incision is carried above the orbital fat till the level of the infraorbital margin is reached. By this way the infraorbital edema, which happens after standard Weber-Ferguson incision, is avoided. The infraorbital margin periosteum is elevated till the zygoma is reached. The periosteum from the nasal side is elevated laterally to the level of the infraorbital foramen.

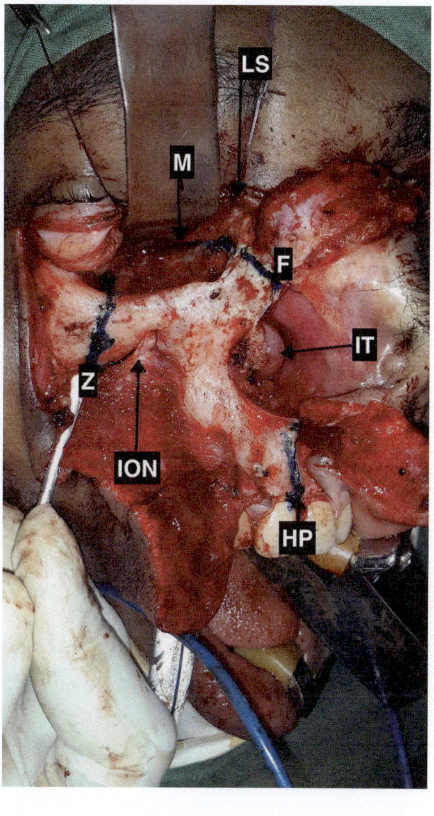

Fig. 14.4 After Weber-Ferguson incision, the nasal ala is reflected medially, the lacrimal sac (*LS*) is transected and reflected and anchored with sutures, the orbital floor periosteum is elevated, and the sites of osteotomies (*Z* zygomaticomaxillary suture, *F* frontal process of the maxilla, *M* maxilloethmoidal suture, *HP* the hard palate in the midline) are marked out with methylene blue (Note the inferior turbinate (*IT*) to be reflected attached to the maxilla and infraorbital nerve (*ION*) which is preserved)

The "V"-shaped notch of the anterior nasal process of the maxilla is exposed (Fig. 14.4). The bone anterior to the inferior part of the lacrimal sac is drilled till the lower end of the sac is exposed. The lacrimal sac is transected at its lowest end and anchored with a 4/0 Vicryl suture to be placed back during closure (Fig. 14.4). The orbital floor periosteum is reflected, and the entire orbital floor periosteum is elevated to the level of the orbital apex. The infraorbital nerve is preserved as it comes out of the foramen. The osteotomy sites, namely, frontal process of the maxilla, maxillozygomatic suture, the hard palate in the midline, and maxilloethmoidal suture, are exposed (Fig. 14.4).

Osteotomies and Outward Reflection of the Maxilla

A curved artery forceps is placed in the inferior orbital fissure from the orbital side and passed to the infratemporal fossa till it is visible under the zygoma. A micro-oscillating saw is used to cut the zygomaticomaxillary suture till the artery forceps is reached. The saw is also used to cut the frontal process of the maxilla to the remaining bone behind the lacrimal sac.

The maxilloethmoidal suture is disarticulated using a fine osteotome (with measuring scale) which is hammered gently till the orbital apex is reached (approximately 6 cm from the anterior lacrimal crest). The palatal halves are separated in the midline by placing an osteotome in between the "V"-shaped anterior nasal process of the maxilla and hammered gently. The osteotome is directed along the exposed hard palate in the midline and observing from the oral cavity. The palatal halves open up in the line of fusion. The final osteotomy is done to disarticulate the pterygoid process from the maxilla by placing a curved osteotome behind the last molar tooth and gently hammered till the pterygoid plates are disarticulated. In patients with nonerupted third molar tooth, the third molar tooth is removed, and through this space, the maxilla is separated from the pterygoid process. This osteotomy is performed carefully in patients with partial destruction of the pterygoid process by the tumor. After completion of all osteotomies, the nasal floor mucoperiosteum is incised, and the entire maxilla (with the attached cheek tissues and most of the inferior turbinate) is reflected laterally like opening a swing door, thereby exposing the entire surgical field (Fig. 14.5).

Removal of Tumor

The feeding vessel to the tumor, if identified, is coagulated to reduce bleeding (Fig. 14.5). The JA is grasped and pulled caudally and medially, and all attachments of the tumor are dissected out meticulously. The intracranial portion of the tumor through the orbital apex is removed by gentle traction. Residual tumor in the

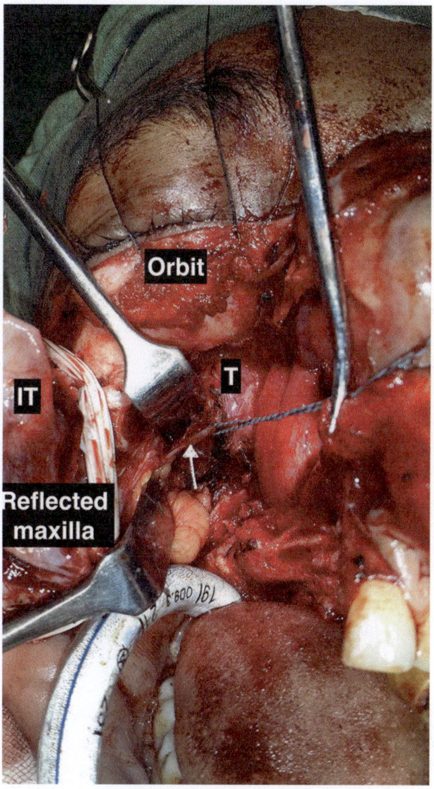

Fig. 14.5 Reflection of the maxilla laterally with the attached inferior turbinate (*IT*) and cheek skin exposing the nasal and lateral extension of the tumor (*T*). In this case the sphenopalatine artery (*arrow*) feeding the tumor (*T*) is exposed and anchored with a suture

cancellous bone at the base of the pterygoid process and pterygoid canal is looked for and removed. Tumor removal from these areas leaves a bony excavated area (Fig. 14.6). The bony surface of the basisphenoid and clivus is drilled to remove any tumor remnant.

Repositioning of the Maxilla

The orbit is lifted by placing a malleable retractor at its inferior aspect, the reflected palatal mucoperiosteum is retracted laterally, the lacrimal sac is repositioned, and the maxilla is placed back like the "closing of a swing door." The maxilla is first held together by placing interdental wires around the upper central incisors, and the osteotomy sites are fixed with miniplates and screws at the frontal process of the maxilla, maxillozygomatic suture, and intermaxillary suture at the inferior margin of the pyriform aperture. In patients below the age of 15 years, absorbable miniplates and screws are used. The palatal mucoperiosteum is reflected back and sutured across the upper teeth. The facial incision is closed in layers.

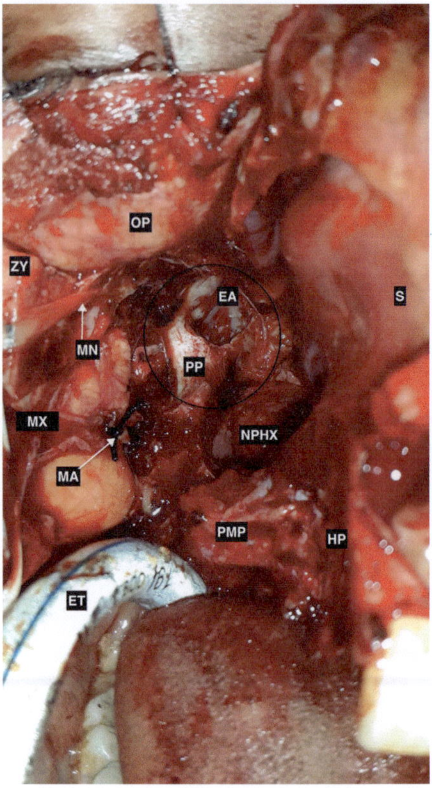

Fig. 14.6 Photograph of the operative field after removal of tumor. The maxilla (*MX*) with attached inferior turbinate is reflected laterally. Residual tumor was removed from the excavated area (*EA*) within the *circle* located at the junction of pterygoid processes (*PP*) with the body of the sphenoid including pterygoid canal. Other visible structures are the orbital periosteum (*OP*), nasal septum (*S*), nasopharynx (*NPHX*), reflected palatal mucoperiosteum (*PMP*), hard palate (*HP*), ligated maxillary artery (*MA*), maxillary nerve (*MN*) coming out of foramen rotundam, endotracheal tube (*ET*), and zygoma (*ZY*)

The nasal pack is removed after 3 days and interdental wiring after 4 weeks. The wounds heal satisfactorily after 6 weeks, and the facial incision scars disappear with time [9].

Complications

Swelling below the lower eyelid due to collection of serous fluid may be encountered on the third postoperative day. It is drained by aspiration with a wide bore needle. Between the fourth and sixth postoperative day, edema subsides, and nasal encrustations and hyperlacrimation due to injury to the lacrimal sac may become apparent. A dilated pupil may be seen on the side of the tumor due to ciliary ganglion injury in cases with orbital apex and intracranial extension. Complications depend on the extension of the tumor, and complete improvement occurs within 6 months [9]. Dry eyes due to lacrimal hyposecretion have been observed after tumor removal from the pterygopalatine fossa due to injury to the pterygopalatine ganglion [11].

Most authors are reluctant to excise extensive JA due to incomplete resection, high rate of complications, and death [12, 13]. The authors made every attempt to remove the tumor completely with the wide exposure presented by TMS. Complications encountered in 16 consecutive advanced JAs operated by TMS are described by authors [9]. Complications such as neuralgia due to the sectioning of the V nerve, hearing loss, or trismus due to sectioning of the pterygoid muscles and mandible condyle displacement can occur after any lateral approach to the skull base [14]. These complications were not encountered in of the patients who underwent TMS [3, 9]. The occlusion was perfect at the end of the procedure; hence no trismus was encountered [3, 9]. The vascularity of the maxilla is maintained by keeping the soft tissues of the cheek attached with it in TMS [3]. Otherwise, free reinsertion of the bone with or without irradiation has the possibility of the grafted bone undergoing avascular necrosis leading to sequestrum formation [1]. Avascular necrosis of the maxilla, osteomyelitis, and facial asymmetry have been reported when facial bone grafts are used [15–17]. Postoperative encrustation of the nasal cavity is reduced by keeping the inferior turbinate mucosa attached with the maxilla [3, 9].

Reduction of Intraoperative Bleeding in the Absence of Embolization

The use of preoperative embolization to reduce intraoperative blood loss during excision of JA is discussed in Chap. 9. In nonembolized patients, intraoperative strategies to reduce blood loss include head-end elevation, infiltration of lignocaine and adrenaline to the site of incision, subperiosteal dissection, cauterization of the overlying mucosa [18], the use of surgical aids like laser [19], cryotherapy, and selective ligation of feeding vessels [20]. Anesthesia and management of intraoperative bleeding are described in Chap. 10.

During the POMP flap approach, after reflecting the POMP flap to the nonpathological side, the operating microscope with 300 mm lens is fixed at the operating field. Subsequently, the mucoperiosteum of the lateral nasal and nasopharyngeal wall is elevated in continuity with the nasal floor. The greater palatine artery in its canal is exposed by drilling it in the caudocranial direction. By following this artery cranially, the third part of the maxillary artery and its sphenopalatine branch is also reached. Bleeding is reduced considerably by coagulating all these arteries (Fig. 14.7).

In the TMS approach, the authors identified the external carotid artery through a neck incision and placed vascular clamps on both external carotid arteries before making facial incisions. The vascular clamps were placed very close to the bifurcation of the common carotid artery to include the ascending pharyngeal artery within the clamp. By this way, the bleeding from the facial incisions and tumor was significantly reduced. In patients with intracranial extension, vascular clamp is placed in the ipsilateral internal carotid artery (ICA) also. In few cases, the feeding vessels to the tumor are identified and ligated (Fig. 14.5). During the surgical incisions and osteotomies, accidental injury to the tumor is avoided as it causes bleeding before removal. Dissection along the pseudocapsular plane with fine surgical hemostatic instruments significantly reduces bleeding [21].

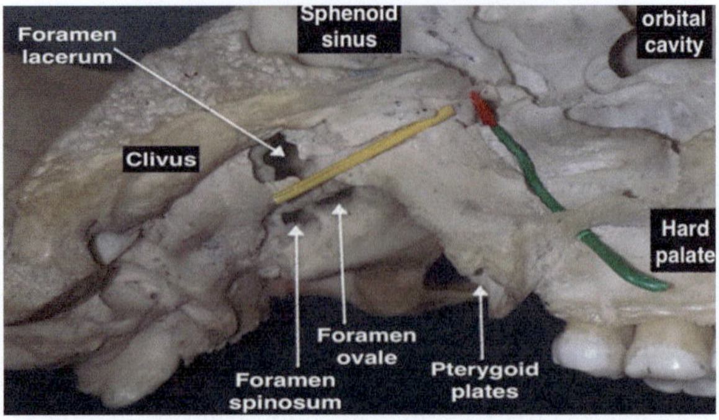

Fig. 14.7 Medial view of the sagitally sectioned skull showing the greater palatine artery (*green marker*) leading to the sphenopalatine and the third part of the maxillary artery (*red marker*). The pterygoid canal is opened and demonstrated with *yellow marker*

During tumor removal excessive bleeding is experienced. Quick removal of the tumor bulk significantly reduces blood loss. Subsequently, the surgical cavity is packed with surgical sponge which is removed slowly while coagulating the bleeding vessels. Despite these measures, bleeding may continue to come from residual tumor in the vidian canal, base of the pterygoid process, basisphenoid, and clivus. Removal of residual tumor and drilling these areas reduce bleeding considerably. Small bleeding from the spongy bone in this area is controlled by application of bone wax. Surgicel is placed and held with neuropatty in case of bleeding after removal of tumor at the orbital apex. The thin-walled pterygoid venous plexus continues to bleed despite the use of bipolar diathermy; in this situation Surgicel is placed and pressure is applied for sometime. The application of fibrin glue to the pterygoid plexus also controls pterygoid venous plexus bleeding [22]. Cell saver replaces large volumes of blood loss from the cavernous sinus [19]. Surgicel supported by roughly oval or circular bone wax is placed within the sphenoid sinus in case of suspected bleeding from the cavernous sinus following tumor removal [9].

After tumor removal and hemostasis, the vascular clamps over carotids are released to identify and ligate any additional bleeding vessels which were not already coagulated or ligated. Continuous intraoperative bleeding follows after tumor removal in a patient with large intracranial extension; the internal carotid artery (ICA) was clamped when the bleeding is reduced markedly, and then the ICA was ligated (patient in Fig. 7.19 in Chap. 7). Ligation or clamping the internal carotid artery at this young age usually does not produce any neurological deficit as in adults [20]. Last but not the least, light nasal packing is done for 3 days to prevent oozing from raw mucosal area. Wide surgical exposure by TMS allowed us to achieve hemostasis with ease.

References

1. Sennes LU, Butugan O, Sanchez TG, et al. Juvenile angiofibroma: the routes of invasion. Rhinology. 2003;41:235–40.
2. Dubey SP, Molumi CP. Transpalatal approach with pedicled palatal osteo-mucoperiosteal flap. ANZ J Surg. 2012;82:439–42.

3. Dubey SP, Molumi CP. Critical look at the surgical approaches of nasopharyngeal angiofibroma excision and "total maxillary swing" as a possible alternative. Ann Otol Rhinol Laryngol. 2007;116:723–30.
4. Hsu M, Ko J, Sheen T, et al. Salvage surgery for recurrent nasopharyngeal carcinoma. Arch Otolaryngol Head Neck Surg. 1997;123:305–9.
5. Crumley RL, Gutin PH. Surgical access for clivus chordoma: University of California, San Francisco, experience. Arch Otolaryngol Head Neck Surg. 1989;115:295–300.
6. Waldman SR, Levine HL, Astor F, Wood BG, Weinstein M, Tucker HM. Surgical experience with nasopharyngeal angiofibroma. Arch Otolaryngol. 1981;107:677–82.
7. Wei WI, Lam KH, Sham JST. New approach to the nasopharyngeal: the maxillary swing approach. Head Neck. 1991;13:200–7.
8. Liu Z, Wang D, Sun X, Wang J, Hu L, Li H, Dai P. The site of origin and expansive routes of juvenile nasopharyngeal angiofibroma (JNA). Int J Pediatr Otorhinolaryngol. 2011;75:1088–92.
9. Dubey SP, Molumi CP, Apaio LM. Total maxillary swing approach to the skull base for advanced intracranial and extracranial nasopharyngeal angiofibroma. J Craniofac Surg. 2011;22:1671–6.
10. Radkowski D, McGill T, Healy GB, Ohlms L, Jones DT. Angiofibroma changes in staging and treatment. Arch Otolaryngol Head Neck Surg. 1996;122:122–9.
11. Rong Z, Zixiang Y, Chang L, et al. Lacrimal hyposecretion: a surgical complication of juvenile nasopharyngeal angiofibroma. Am J Otolaryngol Head Neck Med Surg. 2008;29:367–71.
12. Jafek BW, Krekorian EA, Kirsch WM, Wood RP. Juvenile nasopharyngeal angiofibroma: management of intracranial extension. Head Neck Surg. 1979;2:119–28.
13. Donald PJ, Enepikedes D, Boggan J. Giant juvenile nasopharyngeal angiofibroma: management by skull-base surgery. Arch Otolaryngol Head Neck Surg. 2004;130:882–6.
14. Herman P, Lot G, Chapot R, Salvan D, Tran Ba Huy P. Long-term follow-up of juvenile nasaopharyngeal angiofibromas: analysis of recurrence. Laryngoscope. 1999;109:140–7.
15. Hao S. Facial translocation approach to the skull base: the viability of translocated facial bone graft. Otolaryngol Head Neck Surg. 2001;124:292–6.
16. Suarez C, Llorente JL, Munoz C, et al. Facial translocation approach in the management of central skull base and infratemporal tumors. Laryngoscope. 2004;114:1047–51.
17. Sharma PK, Schuller DE, Goodman JH, et al. Maxillary removal and reinsertion for anterior cranial base tumors: long-term result. Arch Otolaryngol Head Neck Surg. 1998;124:149–52.
18. Fonseca AS, Vinhaes E, Boaventura V, et al. Surgical treatment of non-embolized patients with nasoangiofibroma. Rev Bras Otorrinolaringol. 2008;74:583–7.
19. Mair EA, Battiata A, Casler JD. Endoscopic laser-assisted excision juvenile nasopharyngeal angiofibromas. Arch Otolaryngol Head Neck Surg. 2003;129:454–9.
20. Spector JG. Management of juvenile angiofibroma. Laryngoscope. 1988;98:1016–26.
21. Romani R, Touminen H, Hernesniemi J. Reducing intraoperative bleeding of juvenile nasopharyngeal angiofibroma. World Neurosurg. 2010;74:497–500.
22. Chang L, Xixiang Y, Zmeing F, et al. Managgement of pterygoid plexus hemorrhage during resection of a large juvenile angiofibroma: a review of 27 cases. Ear Nose Throat J. 2013;92:204–8.

Chapter 15
Excision by Le Fort I Osteotomy Approach

S. Girish Rao

Abstract The treatment of juvenile angiofibroma is a challenge for the operating surgeon as getting access to this deeply seated midface tumor is difficult and complete excision of the lesion is even a bigger challenge. Many approaches are available to excise this lesion, the usual ones being the lateral rhinotomy, Weber-Ferguson, transpalatal, facial translocation, midface degloving, and endoscopic approaches. Each of these has their own merits and demerits, while very extensive lesions and recurrent lesions are extremely difficult to manage.

The Le Fort osteotomy gives an excellent access to excise the tumor in toto under direct vision and leaves behind no facial scars. This approach is from an intraoral maxillary vestibular incision; the plates are preadapted once the osteotomy is marked on the anterolateral surface of the maxilla. The plates are removed; the maxilla is down fractured which gives direct access to the juvenile angiofibroma in the nasopharyngeal region. The lesion is excised, and the maxilla is fixed back to its original position using the preadapted plates without affecting the occlusion.

A simple technique, with a bit of training, helps the operating surgeon to get total clearance of the tumor leaving behind no facial scars and no functional deficits.

Keywords Juvenile angiofibroma • Le Fort osteotomy • Access osteotomy • Maxillary osteotomy • Skull base tumors • Midfacial approach

Introduction

The concept of access surgery involves dismantling of the facial skeleton based on the pedicled blood supply, getting access to deeper structures, excision of pathology, and putting the hard and soft tissues back to its original position. This novel procedure was first carried out by Langenbeck in 1859 where a horizontal osteotomy was carried out in the maxilla to excise tumor in the nasopharyngeal area. Le

S.G. Rao, MDS, FDSRCS(Eng), FFDRCSI(Ire)
Department of Oral & Maxillofacial Surgery, RV Dental College & Hospital,
JP Nagar 1st Phase, Bangalore 560078, India
e-mail: girishrao66@gmail.com

S.P. Dubey, B. Schick (eds.), *Juvenile Angiofibroma*,
DOI 10.1007/978-3-319-45343-9_15

Fort in 1901 described the fracture pattern in the facial skeleton and showed the fractures of the middle third of the face that usually follows three levels. The low-level fracture called Le Fort I is a horizontal fracture separating the entire dental alveolar component from the midface. Le Fort II fracture is a pyramidal fracture which involves the nasomaxillary dysjunction from the facial skeleton. The Le Fort III fracture is a high-level fracture which separates the orbito-naso-ethmoid-maxillary components from the skull base.

The access surgery most often used to reach the nasopharyngeal area is the conventional Le Fort I level or in the younger age group a modification of this osteotomy called the high Le Fort I osteotomy where the bone cuts are made at a slightly higher level in order to avoid damage to the erupting permanent teeth buds (Fig. 15.1). The bone cuts (osteotomy) are made with either a reciprocating saw or a fine drill. Prior to down fracturing of the maxilla, low-profile titanium or resorbable plates are adapted and fixed to the maxilla (Fig. 15.2). These plates and screws are then removed, the osteotomy is completed with osteotomes, and the maxilla is down fractured. This access provides an increased and more direct exposure to both vital normal structures and the pathology. Once the pathology is fully removed and hemostasis is achieved, the facial skeleton is put back into its original position and secured in place with the preadapted plates and screws.

Being an intraoral approach, there are no facial scars. Uninvolved normal structures are not removed. With the maxilla down fractured, the central skull base area extending from the cribriform plate of the ethmoid to the craniocervical junction can be easily accessed by this approach (Fig. 15.3). The exposure may be further increased inferiorly to C1/C2 levels by a midline split of the maxilla and division of the hard and soft palate.

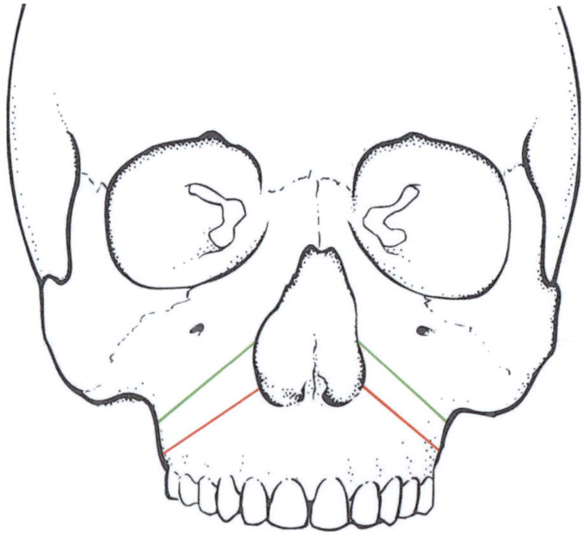

Fig. 15.1 Illustration showing conventional Le Fort I osteotomy (*red line*) and high Le Fort I osteotomy (*green line*)

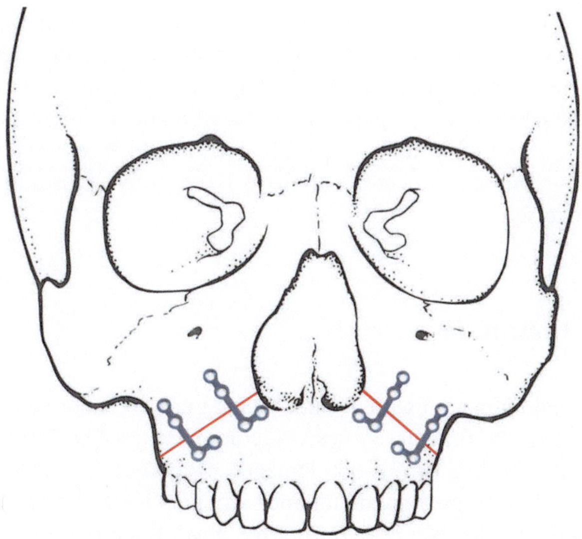

Fig. 15.2 Illustration showing preadaptation of *L-shaped* plates prior to maxillary down fracture

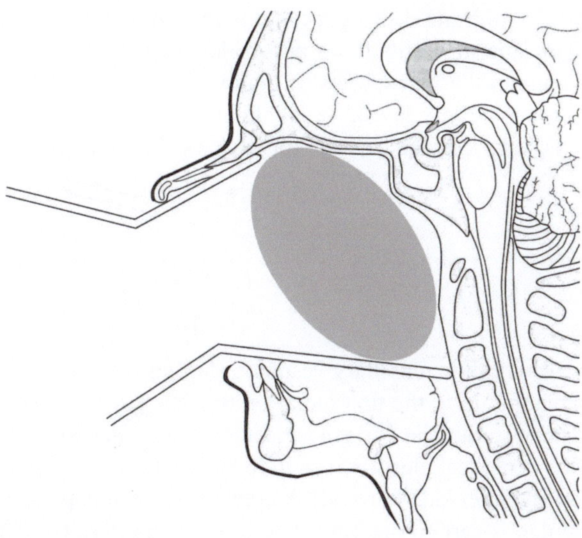

Fig. 15.3 Illustration showing Le Fort I access from the cribriform plate of the ethmoid to C1–C2 junction

Surgical Procedure

Preoperative Work-Up

CT scan or MRI, MR angiogram, or conventional angiogram should be done preoperatively to identify the extent of the lesion.

Preoperative embolization of the lesion either through direct puncture intralesional embolization or through a conventional trans-arterial embolization should be carried out to reduce the bleeding during the surgical excision. The patient should be taken up for surgery within 24–48 h after embolization.

Two to four units of packed cells and FFP should be kept reserved for use during surgical procedure if there is excessive bleeding while the tumor is being excised.

Anesthesia

Oral intubation with a south-facing guarded endotracheal tube is employed so that, when the maxilla is down fractured and pushed further down using the gag, the endotracheal tube is not damaged. Hypotensive anesthesia is beneficial, and a systolic blood pressure maintained around 90–100 mmHg will greatly benefit in reducing the bleeding both during the down fracturing of the maxilla and excising this vascular lesion.

Local anesthetic infiltration of lignocaine with 1 in 80,000 adrenaline injected into the maxillary buccal vestibule on both sides helps in reducing the bleeding while the incision and the mucoperiosteal flap is being raised. Usually 5–6 ml of infiltration into the maxillary buccal vestibule of the local anesthetic agent should suffice, and it is very crucial to wait for at least 3–5 min before making the incision.

Incision

The incision is made in the maxillary vestibule starting from the first molar region on one side extending up to the first molar on the opposite side. The blade should directly hit the bone so that the flap raised would be a full thickness mucoperiosteal flap. A sharp fine periosteal elevator is used to elevate the flap (Fig. 15.4). Austen's retractor is used on either side to retract the mucoperiosteal flap. The subperiosteal elevation of the flap is carried out both superiorly and posteriorly. The infraorbital nerves are identified and protected throughout the procedure.

Anteriorly, the anterior nasal spine is exposed, and the subperiosteal dissection is carried on in the pyriform fossa to elevate the nasal mucosa from the nasal floor. Two periosteal elevators are then placed in the pyriform fossa between the nasal mucosa and the floor of the nose. This helps in reducing the amount of bleeding from the nasal cavity if the nasal mucosa is damaged during the osteotomy procedure. A copper malleable retractor is inserted into the pterygomaxillary fissure to retract the flap posteriorly. Care should be taken not to put too much of traction; otherwise the buccal pad of fat tends to herniate into the operating site.

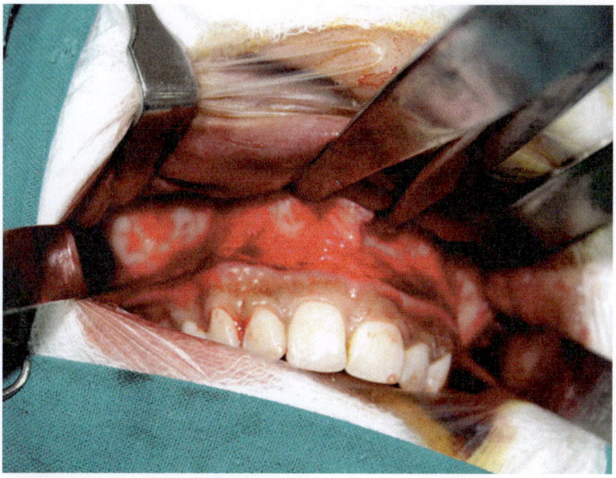

Fig. 15.4 Intraoperative photograph showing Le Fort I incision from the right upper first molar to the left upper first molar along with mucoperiosteal flap elevation

Osteotomy

In conventional Le Fort I osteotomy, bone marking starts from the lateral aspect of the pyriform fossa going at least 5 mm above the apices of all the teeth and extending up to the tuberosity or to the pterygomaxillary fissure. A high Le Fort I osteotomy is used when multiple unerupted teeth are there in the maxilla. The bone marking would start about a centimeter above the base of the pyriform fossa extending on the anteriolateral wall of maxillary sinus up to the tuberosity.

The bone cuts are usually made with a fine reciprocating saw or using a drill and 1 mm fine straight fissure bur. The osteotomy created using a reciprocating saw is a very fine cut, and in the younger age group where the anterolateral wall of the maxilla is very thin, the use of the saw will be like hot knife going through butter. Extreme care has to be taken while using the saw; otherwise the soft tissues of the cheek and lips can be damaged. The use of the drill with a fine fissure bur is much easier for the novice operator; a postage stamp method can be used to initially mark the osteotomy from the pyriform fossa to the tuberosity, and subsequently all of them could be joined to complete the osteotomy (Fig. 15.5).

Adaptation and Fixation of Plates

Prior to down fracturing of the maxilla, four "L"-shaped titanium plates or resorbable polylactic plates are passively adapted onto the anterior wall of the maxilla and fixed using miniscrews. The final tightening of the screws is not carried out at this stage. This positioning of the plates prior to the down fracture is necessary so that when the maxilla is fixed back after the excision of the tumor, it is repositioned to its original position and there is no change in occlusion (Fig. 15.6).

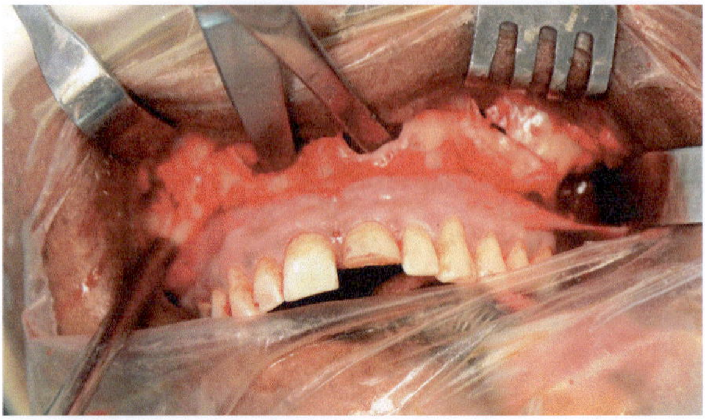

Fig. 15.5 Intraoperative photograph showing Le Fort I osteotomy cut made from the pyriform fossa to the tuberosity

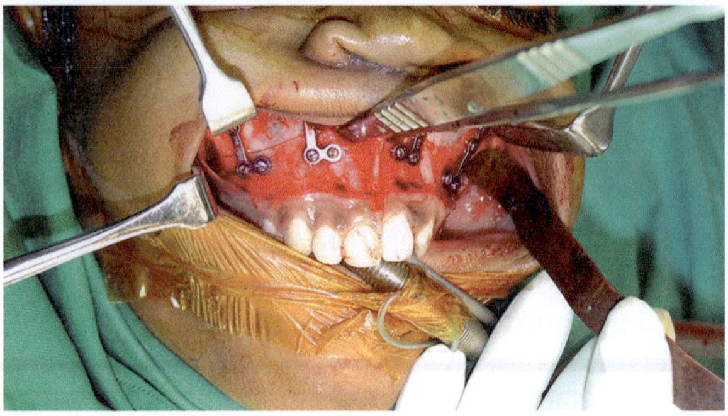

Fig. 15.6 Intraoperative photograph showing the preadaptation of four low-profile or resorbable plates

Removal of the Preadapted Plates

These preadapted plates are removed and placed in specifically marked four gallipots so that the corresponding plates and screws are fixed back into their preadapted and drilled position at the end of the surgery.

Down Fracture of the Maxilla

The osteotomy is now completed using fine osteotomes, all along the length of the bone cuts (Fig. 15.7). A guarded nasal chisel is used to separate the nasal septum from the maxilla, and a curved pterygoid osteotome is used in the pterygomaxillary fissure or at the tuberosity level itself to separate the anterior maxilla from the pterygoid plates. A Smith's spreader is employed to down fracture the maxilla (Fig. 15.8). Care has to be taken to place the Smith's spreader in the zygomatic buttress region and at the lateral wall of the nose. In these areas the bone is much more stronger. Once the maxilla is down fractured, a heavy-duty bone hook can be used to pull the maxilla down. The vascularity to the down-fractured maxilla is maintained throughout, with the intact palatal mucoperiosteal flap hinged on the greater palatine

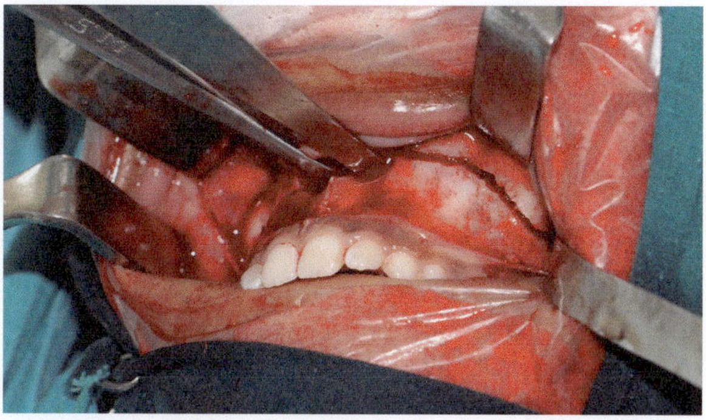

Fig. 15.7 Intraoperative photograph showing removal of the preadapted plates and completion of the osteotomy

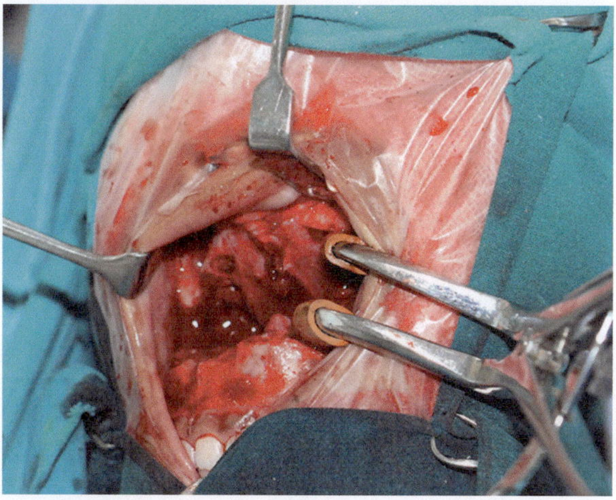

Fig. 15.8 Intraoperative photograph showing down fracture of the maxilla

vessels. A mouth gag can then be applied between the osteotomy cuts to facilitate further distraction of the osteotomy, and this facilitates direct access to the maxillary sinus, nasopharyngeal area, infratemporal fossa, and anterior and middle cranial fossa (Fig. 15.9).

The tumor is excised under direct vision (Fig. 15.10). An operating microscope can also be used at this stage to get better direct access and clear vision into the inaccessible areas. An endoscope can also be used directly through this osteotomy, which will facilitate further excision of tumor in areas, which could be challenging.

Once the tumor has been excised, hemostasis is achieved with bipolar cautery, and a ribbon gauze pack soaked in white head varnish or an antibiotic ointment can be packed into the operated area. The maxilla is repositioned into its original position, and the previously adapted plates and screws are fixed into the corresponding predrilled holes (Fig. 15.11). This ensures that the maxillary plane and occlusion are not altered following the down fracture and excision of the tumor.

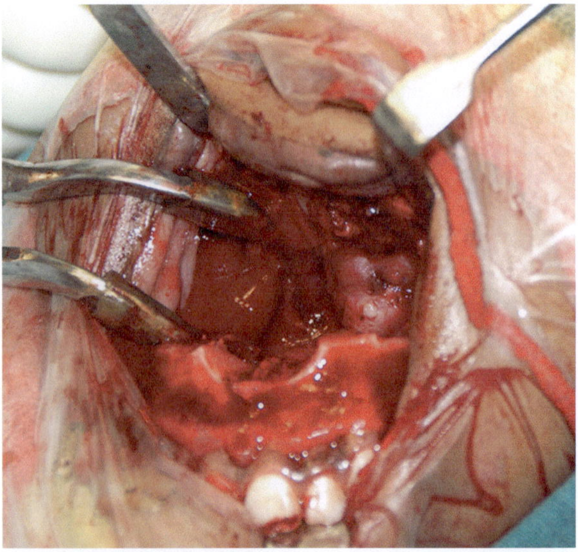

Fig. 15.9 Intraoperative photograph showing the direct exposure of the tumor following down fracture of the maxilla

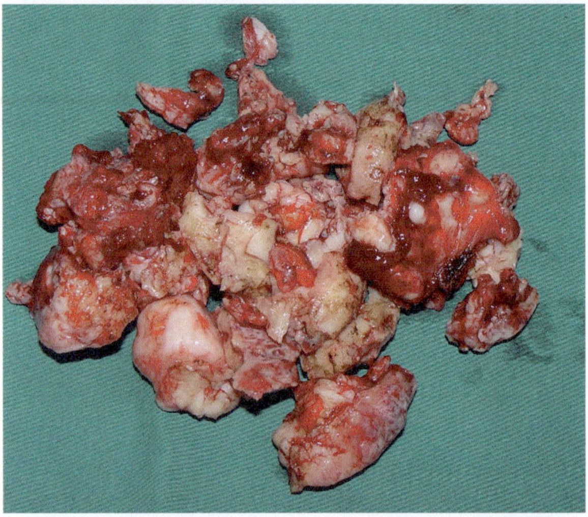

Fig. 15.10 Intraoperative photograph showing excision of the tumor

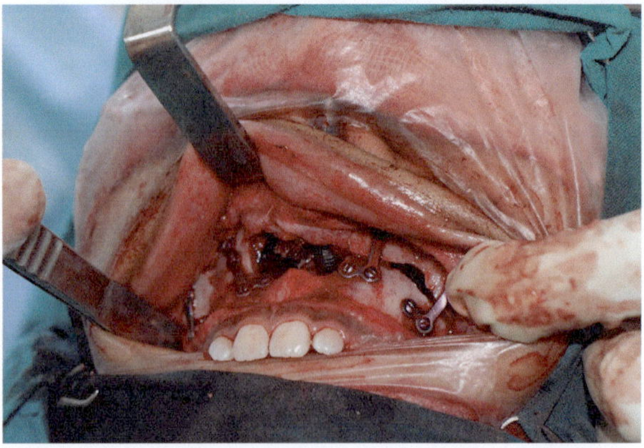

Fig. 15.11 Intraoperative photograph showing the final fixation of the preadapted plates and screws

Closure of the Incision

The mucosal closure is carried out with a fine resorbable suture either Vicryl or Dexon (Fig. 15.12). Care should be taken to ensure small bites of the mucosa so that the vestibule is not obliterated.

Postoperative Care

Cold packs are advised for first 24–48 h. The nasal pack is usually removed after 48 h.

Complications

Bleeding

Bleeding can happen, as the tumor is very vascular. Preoperative embolization carried out prior to the surgery largely facilitates the reduction in bleeding. Hypotensive anesthesia also helps in reducing the intraoperative bleeding. The most common bleeding in a Le Fort osteotomy is from pterygoid plexus of veins, the maxillary artery, greater palatine vessels, and the posterior superior alveolar artery. The broad exposure of the central skull base and the direct line of vision through the Le Fort access osteotomy provide easy identification of the bleeder and ligation of the vessel.

Infection of the Plate

Dehiscence of the incision site can lead to exposure of the plates and subsequent infection. Care should be taken to get watertight closure with good approximation of the mucosal edges.

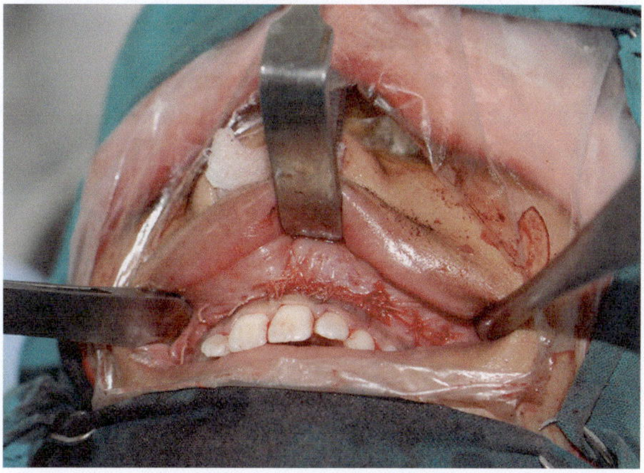

Fig. 15.12 Intraoperative photograph showing mucosal closure with resorbable sutures

Malocclusion

Preadaptation of the plates and fixation of the screws prior to down fracture of the maxilla largely prevent a change in the position of the maxilla. In the younger age group, where the anteriolateral wall of the maxilla is very thin, this bone can easily shatter during the process of down fracture. In such circumstances it becomes difficult to refix the maxilla in its original position. This may lead to slight alteration in the position of the maxilla and can lead to malocclusion. In the mixed dentition phase where the permanent teeth are not fully erupted, doing a conventional Le Fort osteotomy, where in the bone cuts area made from the lateral aspect of base of the pyriform fossa to the tuberosity. The reciprocating saw can damage the tooth buds of the erupting canines and premolars. This can be avoided by making the cuts from the middle of the pyriform fossa going over to the tuberosity, which is termed as a high Le Fort osteotomy [1].

CSF Rhinorrhea

When the tumor is very extensive and extending into the intracranial region, sometimes the dura can be torn leading to CSF rhinorrhea. In such circumstances there is a high risk of meningitis. The dura can be repaired, and antibiotic cover should be employed to minimize the risk of meningitis [2].

Concerns with growth discrepancy following Le Fort osteotomy in the younger age group have been raised; however, the disruption of facial growth is unlikely as the osteotomy does not pass through growth centers [1, 3].

Recurrence is common following excision of juvenile angiofibroma. Most recurrences develop as a consequence of invasion of the basisphenoid; the tumor is very extensive or has not been fully excised [4, 5]. The Le Fort access provides a more meticulous exploration of this area at the time of primary surgery and has a dramatic effect on the reduction of the rate of recurrence [3, 6–8].

Other reported rare complications with this procedure include subcutaneous emphysema, unilateral abducens nerve palsy, upper lip hypesthesia [9–11], aseptic necrosis of the maxilla [12, 13], fatal arteriovenous fistula, and blindness [14, 15].

Conclusion

There has been a paradigm shift in all branches of surgical practice with the introduction of minimal invasive and endoscopic surgery. With better instrumentation, excellent training of surgeons, and the introduction of robotic surgery, tumors in inaccessible areas have been easily removed with least amount of morbidity to patients. Small- to medium-sized juvenile angiofibroma can be easily managed with an endoscopic approach. However, very extensive lesions, recurrent JAs, and the ones with intracranial extensions pose the greatest challenge. The Le Fort osteotomy is a versatile procedure, which in the authors experience is of immense value in extensive juvenile angiofibromas or in recurrent lesions.

The key advantages of the Le Fort access osteotomy are (i) being an intraoral approach, there is no facial scar, (ii) there is no need to resect uninvolved normal structures, (iii) it provides an increased and more direct access to both vital normal structures and pathology, (iv) it has excellent access to the central skull base from the cribriform plate of the ethmoid to craniocervical junction and with a midline split of the maxilla and division of the hard and soft palate, exposure may be increased inferiorly to C1/C2, (v) it better controls hemostasis, (vi) it has less operating time, (vii) its preadaptation and fixation of the plates and screws help in maintaining the original anatomy and function of the facial skeleton, and (viii) there is no change in the dental occlusion and hence patients can get back to early normal mastication.

References

1. Lowlicht RA, Jassin B, Kim M, Sasaki CT. Long term effect of Le Fort I osteotomy for resection of Juvenile nasopharyngeal angiofibroma on maxillary growth and dental sensation. Arch Otolaryngol Head Neck Surg. 2002;128:923–7.
2. Singh R, Hazarika P, Nayak DR, Balakrishnan R, Pillai S, Hazarika M. Role of Le Fort Type I osteotomy approach in Juvenile nasopharyngeal angiofibroma. Int J Oral Maxillofac Surg. 2011;40:1271–4.
3. Rao SG, Reddy SK, Sampath S. Le Fort I access for juvenile nasopharyngeal angiofibroma (JNA): a prospective series of 22 cases. J Craniomaxillofac Surg. 2012;40:e54–8.
4. Lin Y, Qiu J-H, Qiao L. Le Fort I osteotomy for extensive juvenile nasopharyngeal angiofibroma: a retrospective study. Adv Ther. 2008;25:1057–64.
5. Marshall AH, Bradley PJ. Management dilemmas in the treatment and follow-up of advanced juvenile nasopharyngeal angiofibroma. ORL. 2006;68:273–8.
6. Moorthy PNS, Reddy BR, Quiyum HA, Madhira S, Kolloju S. Management of juvenile nasopharyngeal angiofibroma. A 5 year retrospective study. Indian J Otolaryngol Head Neck Surg. 2010;62:390–4.
7. Amin AAW. Maxillary swing approach for surgical resection of recurrent nasopharyngeal tumours. J Egypt Natl Cancer Inst. 2007;19:219–23.
8. Eisig SB, Joseph F, Hall C, Goodrich JT. The 2-piece Le Fort I osteotomy for cranial base access: an evaluation of 9 patients. J Oral Maxillofac Surg. 2000;58:482–6.
9. Mello-Filho FV, Freitas LCCD, Dos Santos AC, Rui Celso Mamede M. Resection of juvenile angiofibroma using the Le Fort I approach. Am J Otolaryngol. 2004;25:157–61.
10. Avelar RL, Santos TS, Antunes AA, Dourado E, Filho JRL. Horizontal maxillary osteotomy approach for resection of juvenile nasopharyngeal angiofibroma. J Craniofac Surg. 2011;22:1027Y1030.
11. Belmont JR. The Le Fort I osteotomy approach for nasopharyngeal and nasal fossa tumors. Arch Otolaryngol Head Neck Surg. 1988;114:751–4.
12. Naraghi M, Bayat M, Yahyavi S, Kashfi A, Yazdi ARK, Khorsandi MT. Le Fort I osteotomy approach for advanced nasopharyngeal angiofibroma with intracranial extension: report of a case. Acta Med Iran. 2002;40:256–60.
13. Roy S, Patel PK, Tomita T. The Le Fort I transmaxillary approach to skull base tumors. Clin Plastic Surg. 2007;34:575–83.
14. Lo LJ, Hung KF, Chen YR. Blindness as a complication of Le Fort I osteotomy for maxillary distraction. Plast Reconstr Surg. 2002;109:688.
15. Filho FVM, Netto PBM, Filho RCT, Araujo FCF, Filho FJFP, Faria AC. Resection of a juvenile nasoangiofibroma by Le Fort I osteotomy: experience with 40 cases. J Craniomaxillofac Surg. 2015;43:1501–4.

Chapter 16
Excision by Lateral Skull Base Approach

J. Dale Browne and Eric R. Oliver

Abstract The lateral approach is a preauricular, subcranial technique that traverses the infratemporal fossa (ITF) for surgical resection of juvenile angiofibroma (JA). Although these lesions originate medially relative to the ITF within the nasal cavity, it is not necessary to visualize the point of origin directly to achieve safe removal with this technique. Thus, the angle of approach for removal can be superior, medial, and smaller than a more extensive classically described posterior infratemporal fossa approach that compromises the overall structure of the middle ear. The lateral approach is ideal for JAs that extend lateral to the foramen rotundum and abut the cavernous sinus. The effectiveness of this technique relies on both successful preoperative endovascular embolization and the fibrous nature of the tumor. These fibrous characteristics allow initial mobilization and subsequent extraction by lateral traction of the tumor from its medial point of origin, obviating the need to further compromise sinonasal structures associated with other approaches. This chapter presents the lateral approach features, indications, patient selection considerations, techniques, modifications, and potential complications with illustrative figures.

Keywords Subcranial • Subtemporal • Infratemporal fossa • Juvenile • Angiofibroma • Preauricular • Rotundum

Introduction

The lateral approach evolved from modifications of the infratemporal fossa approaches to the jugular foramen, apical petrous temporal bone, clivus, parasellar region, and nasopharynx developed and refined by Professor Ugo Fisch at the University of Zurich over three decades ago. These approaches, designated types A, B, and C, represent a generally more anterior and medial surgical exposure [1–4]. Each of the classic techniques includes both a postauricular incisional approach that

J.D. Browne, MD (✉) • E.R. Oliver, MD
Department of Otolaryngology, Wake Forest University, Baptist Medical Center, Medical Center BLVD, Winston-Salem, NC 27157-1034, USA
e-mail: jdbrowne@wakehealth.edu

S.P. Dubey, B. Schick (eds.), *Juvenile Angiofibroma*,
DOI 10.1007/978-3-319-45343-9_16

transects the external auditory canal and a subtotal petrousectomy, thus compromising the conductive hearing mechanism. For more anteriorly located lesions, inclusion of the middle ear within the surgical field is not necessary. Thus, preauricular incisional modifications were created, designated as type D approach [5–9]. However, the more anterior incision with this modification alters the angle of approach and may limit the ability to directly access more medial pathology that extends to the posterior nasopharynx and parasellar region. Nevertheless, the less invasive exposure decreases morbidity and allows for excellent exposure of the lateral and superior margins of a JA.

Chapter 8 reviews JA staging schemes. Generally, these schemes describe ascending degrees of involvement of adjacent structures relative to tumor origin vicinity of the sphenopalatine foramen within the posterior nasal cavity. The advancing stages correspond to a spectrum of tumor extension ranging from confinement within the posterior nasal cavity and nasopharynx to infiltration and invasion of the cavernous sinus and pituitary fossa. Intracranial extension of the tumor is present in approximately 10–20 % of cases [10, 11]. Tumors which are confined to the nasal cavity, nasopharynx, paranasal sinuses, and pterygomaxillary fossa region are candidates for a transnasal endoscopic approach for resection, and multiple series have demonstrated tumor control with this approach [12–17]. Extensive tumors that border the cavernous sinus, invade the orbit, or extend intracranially generally mandate an open approach for optimization of both safety and probability of a complete resection.

The knowledge and understanding of a modified lateral infratemporal fossa (ITF) approach continues to secure a position within the armamentarium of the multidisciplinary JA treatment team. The ITF refers to the anatomic area located inferior to the temporal fossa, located deep to the masseter muscle and its superior attachment, the zygomatic arch (Fig. 16.1). The detailed surgical anatomy of this region is described in Chap. 2.

The successful application of the lateral approach for excision of JA highly depends on careful and effective preoperative endovascular embolization of external carotid system feeders. Endovascular embolization for treatment of JA is described in Chap. 9. A critical principle for embolization in conjunction with the lateral technique is the complete obstruction of the major vessels well lateral to the tumor itself. As illustrated in Fig. 16.2, robust feeding branches from the external carotid artery are visualized, most prominently from the internal maxillary artery and middle meningeal artery. Given the relative narrow field of operative exposure with this technique, direct visualization of the larger vessels is impaired. As the surgeon pulls the tumor from the surgical wound, he or she is dependent on successful vessel occlusion lateral to the tumor to prevent significant bleeding that can only be easily managed by intraoperative packing.

Surgical Technique

Intraoperatively, the patient is under general anesthesia and positioned supine on the surgical bed, 180° rotated from the anesthesiology team. This allows room for the operating surgeon and assistants; the scrub nurse is positioned opposite the surgeon.

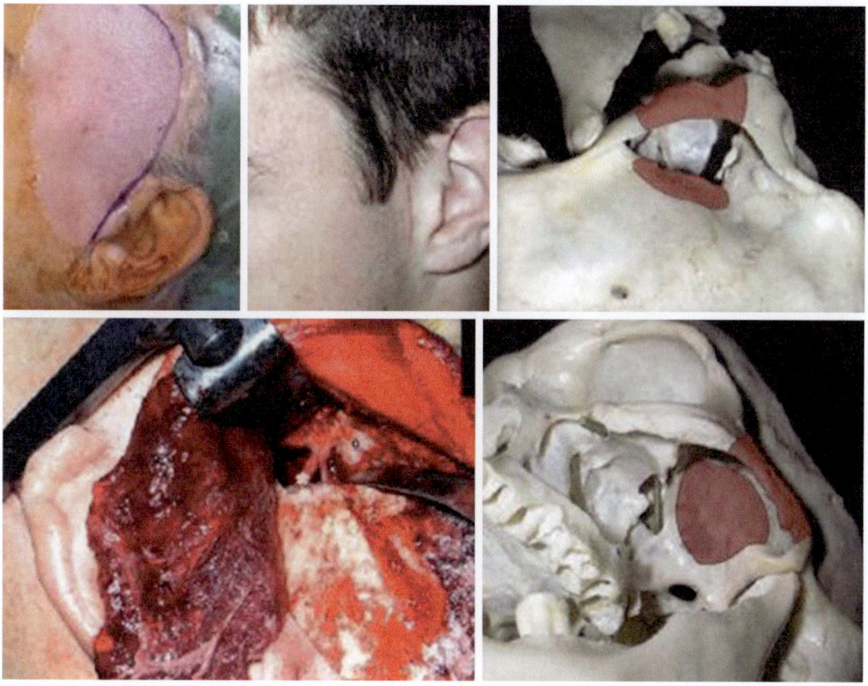

Fig. 16.1 (*Upper left*) A typical preauricular incision is made in the pretragal region and curved along the periphery of the temporal fossa. (*Center left*) Once hair growth returns, the incision is almost hidden. (*Upper* and *lower right*) On a skull, the area of bone removal is demonstrated in *red*. The zygomatic arch is replaced at the conclusion of the procedure, with part of the floor of the middle cranial fossa drilled away to expose the tumor and foramen rotundum. The path of the second division of the trigeminal nerve is shown in *gold*. (*Lower left*) An intraoperative view showing the temporalis muscle reflected posteriorly. The second division of the trigeminal nerve (*) and lateral orbit (0) are shown as a retractor elevates the dura of the temporal lobe

The patient is positioned supine on the surgical bed with 15° of head of bed elevation to decrease cerebral venous pressure and limit bleeding. The neck is slightly extended and rotated contralaterally approximately 45°. A soft headrest is utilized.

The temporal scalp is generally shaved if necessary just beyond the temporal fossa. Cotton pledgets soaked in 0.05 % oxymetazoline solution are placed intranasal to the anterior border of the tumor. Following surgical preparation and draping, 1 % lidocaine with epinephrine 1/100,000 is injected along the proposed temporal fossa incision line (Fig. 16.1). The incision begins in the pretragal area, and extends 1 cm inferior to the level of the zygomatic arch, and then extends superiorly and medially in a curvilinear fashion along the superior border of the temporal fossa just anterior to the hair-bearing scalp. This will maximize concealment of the incision once the hair has grown back (Fig. 16.1). The medial extent of the planned incision reaches the same vertical plane as the lateral brow.

The initial incision is made with a scalpel or needle-tipped monopolar pencil with low current to the level of the deep temporal fascia, and the scalp flap is elevated anteriorly to the level of the deep temporal fat pad. The deep temporal fascia is incised diagonally from the posterior zygomatic arch toward the superior lateral

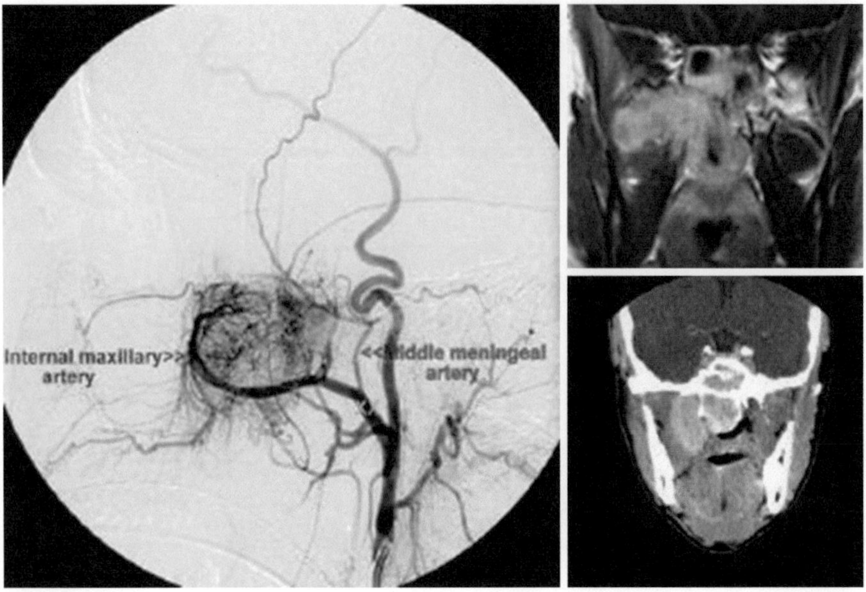

Fig. 16.2 Preoperative endovascular embolization is key to the approach, taking care to not only distantly occlude feeding vascular supply, but obstructing the larger proximal vessels well lateral to the tumor to allow for dissection of lateral extensions, demonstrated in the images on the *right*

orbital rim. At this point, the periosteum of the posterior zygomatic arch is incised and the periosteum and deep temporal fascia are elevated *as a unit* off the zygomatic arch to the level of the lateral orbital rim anteriorly. A key point in elevation is the preservation of the zygomatic arch periosteum. Similarly, incision of the lateral orbital rim periosteum allows complete skeletonization of the zygoma, zygomatic arch, and lateral orbital rim without damage to the frontal branches of the facial nerve as the temporal scalp flap is elevated anteriorly.

Next, the now exposed zygomatic arch is temporarily removed with a drill from its posterior root to the lateral zygoma; it is stored in saline. The scalp is back elevated to expose the entire periphery of the temporalis muscle. A curvilinear incision through the temporalis muscle is created to the skull at the border of the temporal fossa. The muscle is elevated from the skull and lateral orbital wall in a subperiosteal fashion. Bone wax is applied for venous perforators through the bone. The visible bone in this dissection includes the parietal, frontal, greater wing of sphenoid, and squamous portion of temporal bones. The temporalis muscle attachments to the coronoid process are preserved. The elevation concludes at the roof of the ITF where either the tumor is visualized or the root of the lateral pterygoid plate is palpable in the depths of the dissection.

Cutting and diamond burs are used to thin the bone at the lateral orbit and adjacent greater sphenoid wing so as to outline the shape of the temporal horn of the middle cranial fossa dura (Fig. 16.3b, c). This maneuver will provide maximal exposure in the operative regions. In most instances, removal of a small (3 × 3 cm)

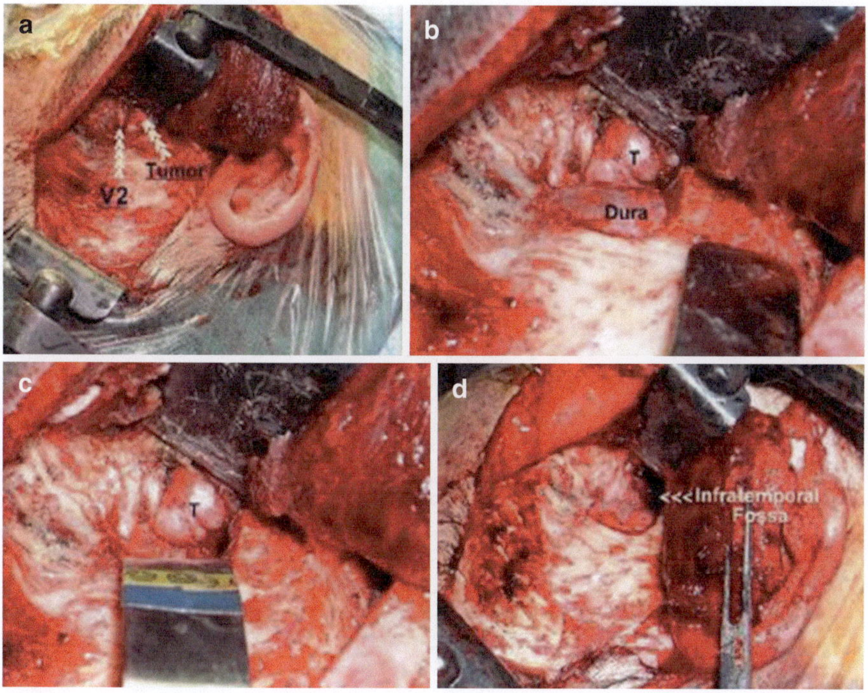

Fig. 16.3 Intraoperative view of a right-sided tumor resection. (**a**) The temporalis muscle has been exposed and reflected posteriorly. The tumor can be seen under the second division of the trigeminal nerve, V2. (**b, c**) To expose the tumor, a small craniectomy is performed of the greater sphenoid wing bone over the temporal horn, allowing dural retraction above the tumor. (**d**) The defect created after the removal of the tumor

section of the bone overlying the temporal lobe dura can allow gentle dural retraction. This can afford complete exposure of the superior and lateral extent of the tumor, especially its relationship to the second trigeminal nerve division (V2). If necessary, the bone along the floor of the middle fossa can be removed to include the foramen rotundum for superior exposure and protection of V2. As shown in Fig. 16.1, lower left, the normal pathway of V2 as it exits the foramen rotundum is approximately a 30° angle relative to lateral orbit. This relationship is altered in tumors that extend far laterally and usually displace the nerve laterally, as shown in Fig. 16.2a, upper left. Knowledge of such anatomical variations due to tumor displacement of the nerve allows for gentle separation of the nerve from the angiofibroma during the dissection.

It is the fibrous and somewhat compressible nature of the tumor that allows for manipulation and mobilization of its periphery with blunt dissectors and ultimately the removal of the angiofibroma. Frequently, the exposure defect is slightly smaller than the tumor, which can be removed with traction as it and the surrounding soft tissue deform enough to allow extraction. The first layer of dissection clears the temporalis muscle from the superior extent of the tumor and moves V2 away from

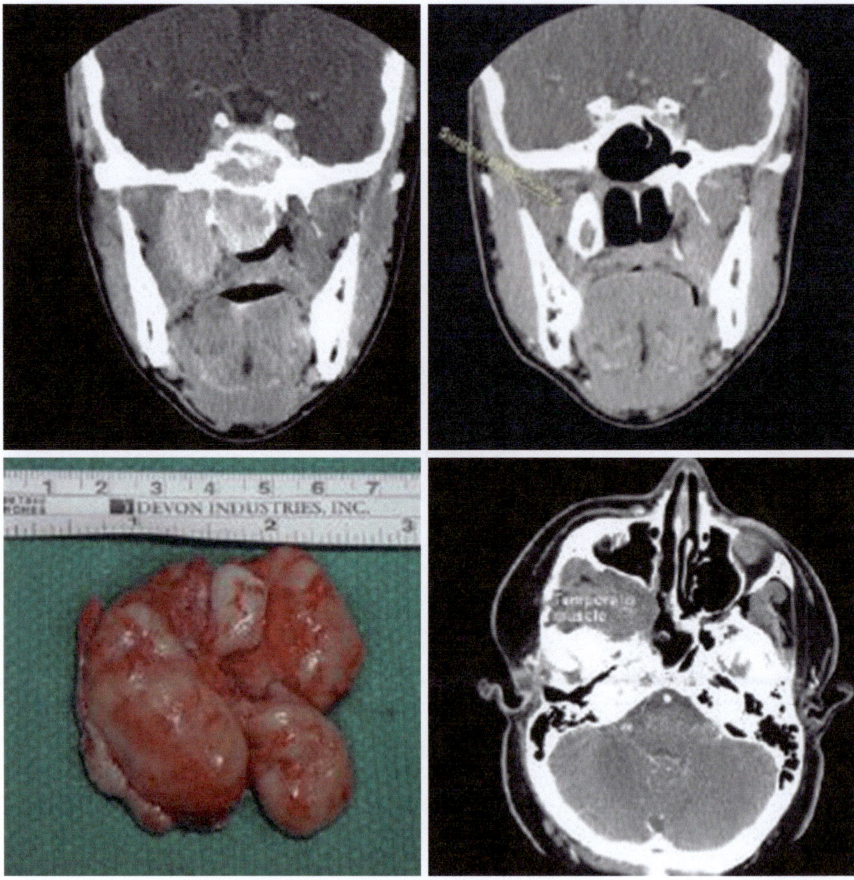

Fig. 16.4 (*Upper left*) A coronal view of a juvenile angiofibroma with a lateral extension ideal for removal for the lateral technique. (*Upper right*) A postoperative scan demonstrating the pathway of dissection. (*Lower right*) A transverse, postoperative view highlighting the positioning of the temporalis muscle as it obliterates the defect created by tumor removal. (*Lower left*) The resected tumor

the mass, usually in a posterior direction. Working from lateral to medial, the angiofibroma is then separated from the floor of the middle fossa, lateral inferior orbit, and lateral sphenoid sinus. Much of the medial dissection is blind; the blunt dissector is used to palpate the bone from the tumor until the most medial extent is reached. Critical for safety in the dissection is knowledge of each bony dehiscence, especially those due to the tumor. Once the tumor is freed 360° from the surrounding soft tissue and bone in its lateral extent, the body of the angiofibroma is grasped with a toothed tenaculum or Allis forcep and pulled laterally out of the operative defect. The blunt dissector, placed medially, can act as a cantilever in the maneuver that provides additional force in the removal. The nasal cavity mucosa will tear to some extent with removal (Figs. 16.4 and 16.5).

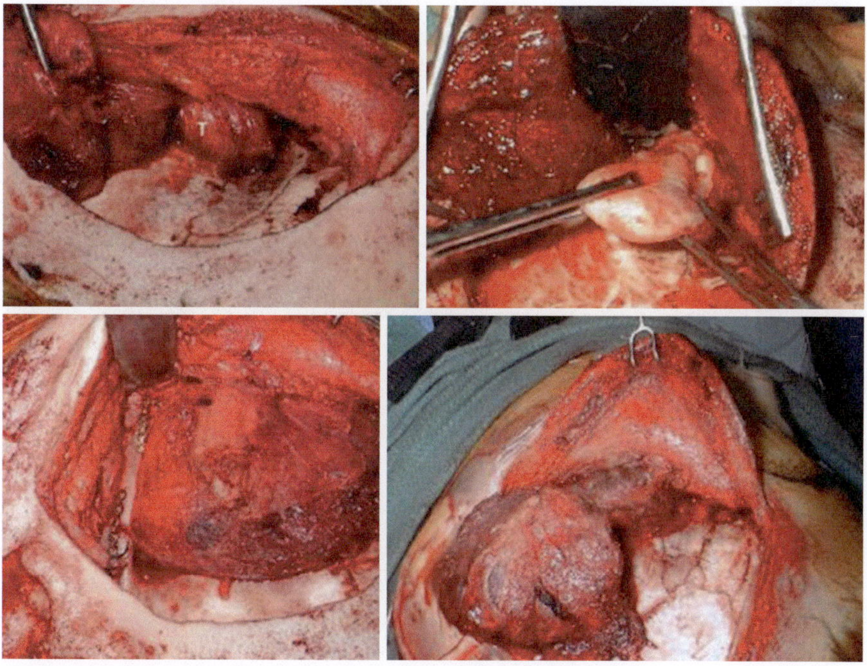

Fig. 16.5 (*Upper left*) The tumor (T) is visualized under some remnants of the temporalis muscle. (*Upper right*) The fibrous nature of the juvenile angiofibromas allows it to be firmly grasped and pulled out of the defect once critical attachments along the skull base are freed. (*Lower right*) After tumor removal, the temporalis muscle is split radially with a portion used to fill the defect. (*Lower left*) The remainder of the temporalis muscle is returned to fill the temporal fossa, and the zygomatic arch is replaced and secured

Modifications of this exposure chiefly involve bone removal of the greater sphenoid wing at the lateral orbit to allow for greater dural elevation in order to remove the tumor extending to the inferior cavernous sinus extradurally. For more extensive involvement, this exposure can be increased to a more traditional pterional craniotomy to allow for more significant dural elevation and, if necessary, intradural dissection (Fig. 16.6). Critical to the success of removal of more extensive lesions that may require such modifications is high-resolution CT preoperative imaging that allows the surgeon to recognize bone loss that signals involvement of the foramen rotundum, orbital floor and lateral wall, dural dehiscence from bone destruction, cavernous sinus extension, and carotid exposure in the lateral sphenoid wall.

Once the tumor is removed, visual inspection of the mass is important and centers on recognition of any disruptions that may signal residual disease left in the field. The most common areas of unremoved disease are (1) laterally for tumors with an extreme lateral extension to the level of the mandibular ramus, (2) medially within the sphenoid sinus, and (3) the soft tissue of the lateral nasopharynx. After copious irrigation, a nasal cavity and nasopharyngeal endoscopic examination with removal of any residual disease can be accomplished in a complementary fashion.

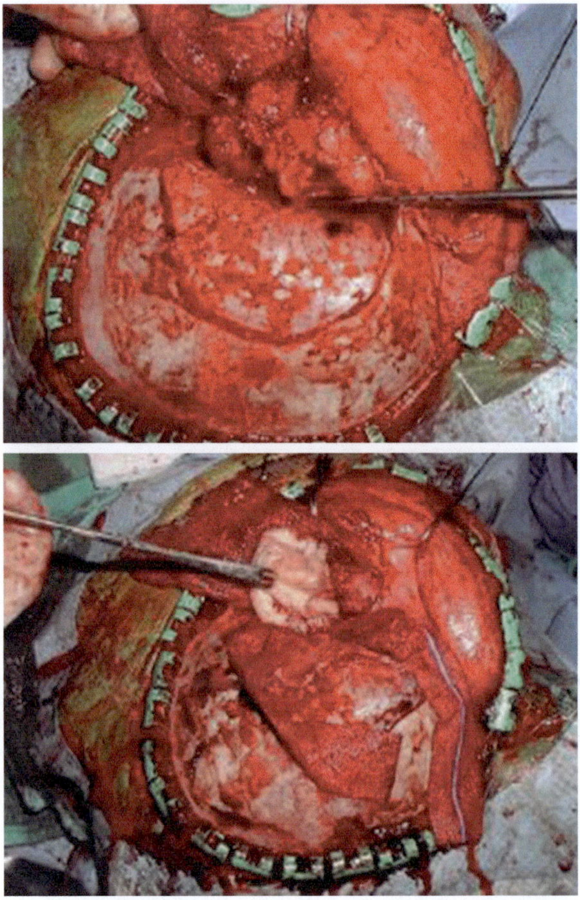

Fig. 16.6 (*Upper*) For larger tumors that involve the cavernous sinus more extensively, a wider craniotomy can be performed to provide operative access. (*Lower*) Once freed from skull base attachments, the tumor can be pulled from the wound in similar fashion used with smaller lesions

The space created by removal of the tumor provides wide endoscopic exposure without the need for further bone removal. Furthermore, the previous exposure of critical structures achieved by the lateral approach enhances the safety and orientation of the endoscopic examination.

Closure is preceded by copious saline irrigation and placement of collagen pledgets as a layer in the wound bed. An absorbent expandable tampon sponge is placed in the ipsilateral nasal vault. The zygomatic arch and craniectomy bone are replaced with titanium plating. The anterior one-third to one-half of the temporalis muscle is left pedicled on the bulk of the muscle and inserted into the operative defect. The remainder of the muscle is sutured to the soft tissue in and around the temporal fossa. If no dural disruption occurred, a suction drain is placed and the wound closed in layers. Except for extremely large tumors (Fig. 16.7), operative time averages less than 4 h with blood loss less than 500 cc; only two patients over 20 years have required transfusion (following removal of extremely large lesions with extensive cavernous sinus involvement).

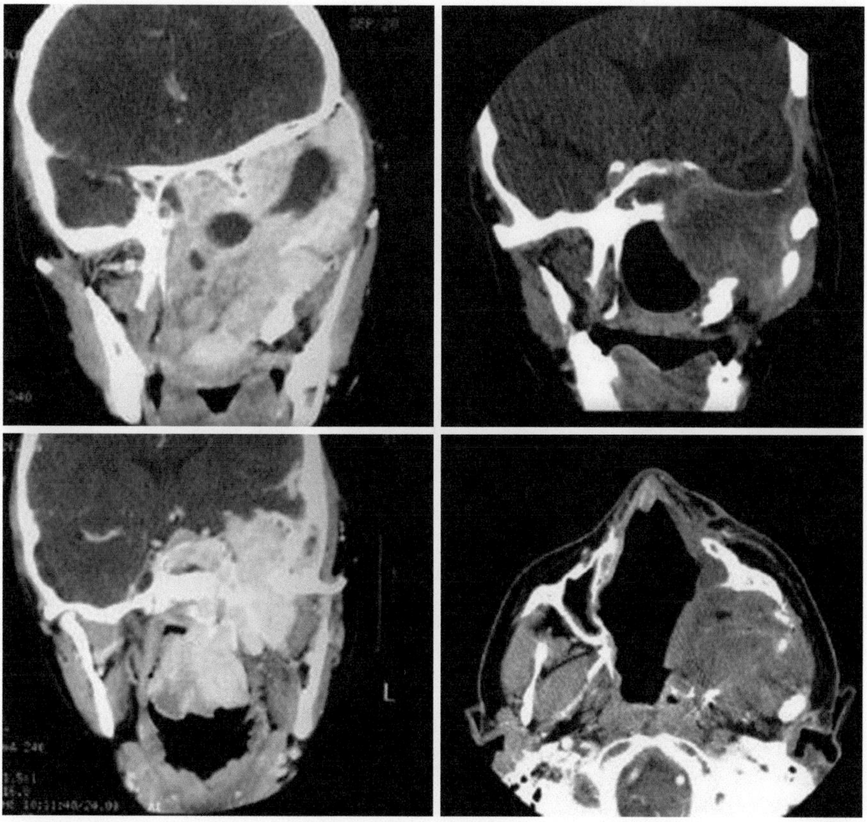

Fig. 16.7 (*Upper* and *lower left*) Coronal scans demonstrating massive juvenile angiofibroma approached with lateral technique as seen in Fig. 16.6. (*Upper and lower right*). Postoperative imaging showing tumor removal and utilization of the temporalis muscle to obliterate the defect and cover the exposed dura of the skull base

Nasal packing placed at the conclusion of the procedure is removed the following day. The drain is generally removed in 2 days; hospital discharge generally occurs on postoperative day 2–3 (except for the largest of tumors that have involved the cavernous sinus, indicative of more extensive dissection). Patients are started on an oral diet that evening (Fig. 16.8).

Advantages Over Other Open Procedures

Open surgical approaches for resection of JA include transpalatal, transmaxillary/maxillectomy by way of midfacial degloving or lateral rhinotomy, facial translocation, and subtemporal preauricular infratemporal fossa techniques. Transmaxillary approaches provide direct medial exposure of the tumor, and generally require either lateral rhinotomy or midfacial degloving incisional approaches, which include

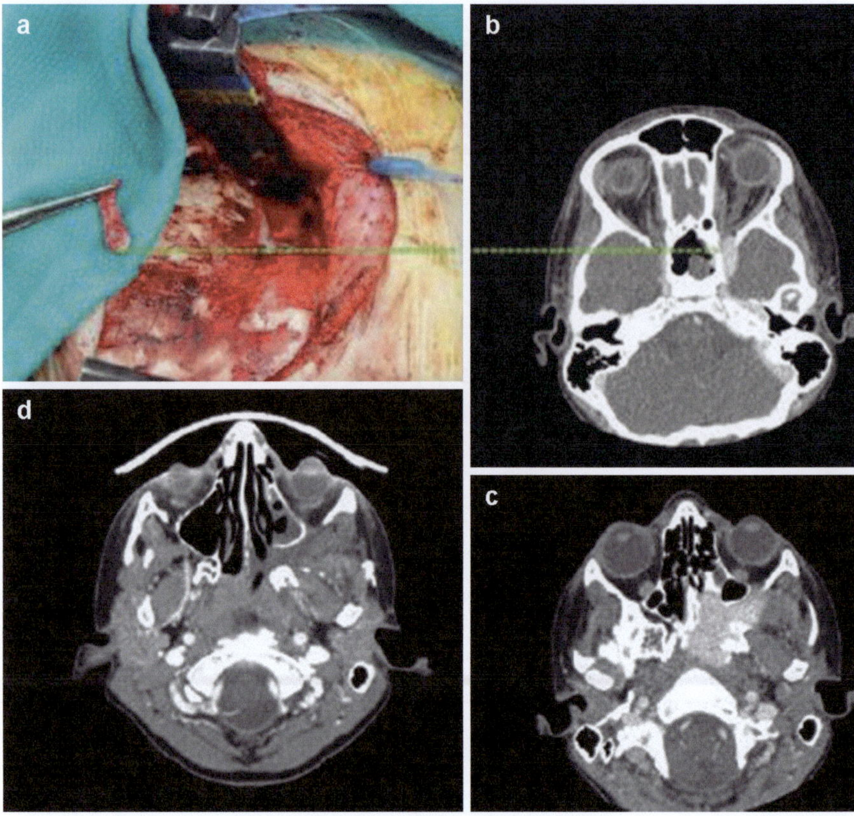

Fig. 16.8 (*Upper left* and *right*) The lateral technique can be used to remove smaller cavernous sinus extensions. (*Lower right*) Transverse CT imaging of the bulk of the tumor. (*Lower left*) Postoperative transverse view showing pathway of dissection and obliteration of defect with the temporalis muscle

facial and rhinoplasty incisions, respectively. These approaches independently may not provide optimal lateral and superior tumor exposure and traverse medial paranasal sinus and maxillofacial structure. In contrast, the lateral approach offers excellent lateral and superior tumor exposure at the expense of decreasing medial exposure.

The lateral approach is subcranial; all but the most extreme tumors require only minimal dural exposure and elevation. The subcranial approaches employed for removal of skull base lesions from the jugular foramen to the more medial nasopharynx resulted in obliteration of the middle ear space and ossicular chain for exposure. For these classic approaches, the more medial a lesion was located, there existed a greater need for sacrifice of the glenoid fossa and third division of the trigeminal nerve for direct exposure. In contrast, the lateral approach utilized for removal of JAs, which is a modification of the type C approach, is anterior to the glenoid fossa and foramen ovale and preserves otologic structures, the glenoid fossa, and divisions of the trigeminal nerve.

Although JAs arise medially, it is not necessary to visualize the point of origin directly to allow safe removal with the lateral technique. Thus, the angle of approach for removal can be superior, medial, and smaller than a more extensive posterior infratemporal fossa procedure that involves the middle ear. As mentioned earlier, the effectiveness of this technique relies on the success of preoperative embolization and the fibrous nature of the tumor to allow initial mobilization and then extraction by pulling the tumor from its point of origin. This angle of dissection also allows the second division of the trigeminal nerve to be visualized directly and then swept aside and preserved prior to tumor removal. Prior to tumor removal, the orbital floor can be directly assessed and protected if there is bony erosion. Similarly, loss of bone causing a dural dehiscence can be directly visualized and protected during removal. Should a dural disruption occur, direct access for repair with vascularized temporalis muscle is readily available.

The lateral approach technique as detailed in this chapter is ideal for tumors that extend *lateral* to the foramen rotundum and abut the cavernous sinus. Larger lesions that involve the petrous and cavernous carotid artery are most safely removed with direct visualization/access of that structure, either via a more extensive infratemporal approach or pterional craniotomy that permits direct exposure and the ability to control the internal carotid artery if necessary, especially if preoperative permanent occlusion of this artery was not performed. Another consideration in patient selection is the level of pneumatization of the sphenoid sinus and adjacent pterygoid plates. The more lateral the tumor or well pneumatized the lateral skull base, the more appropriate the lateral approach is. Patients with poorly pneumatized paranasal sinuses and medially based tumors can probably be removed more readily by an anterior open or endoscopic transnasal approach.

Postoperative Sequelae and Complications

Common postoperative sequelae from the lateral technique include mild transitory trismus and initial mild painful mastication and temporary infraorbital nerve hypesthesia. Given the lack of removal of nasal cavity/paranasal sinus structures to access the tumor, there is little postoperative nasal cavity crusting or need for postoperative care of the sinonasal cavity. There is little cosmetic impact, as the posterior temporalis muscle fills the temporal fossa, and the incision is predominantly within the hairline (Fig. 16.1). The risk of complications correlates with the nature of the tumor and the extent of surgery required to excise the pathology. Regardless of pathology, approximately 75 % who undergo this approach experience no complications. Minor complications occur in approximately 20 % and include hematoma, trigeminal paresthesia, minor cosmetic disfigurement, wound breakdown, and infection. Major complications occur in approximately 5 % and include cerebrospinal fluid leak, ocular damage, orbital hematoma, and development of an intracranial mucocele.

Conclusion

The lateral technique is an efficient method to remove JAs, especially those that extend lateral to the foramen rotundum. Common to most procedures aimed at total removal, effective preoperative vascular embolization is critical to minimize intraoperative blood loss; it is important that obstruction of larger feeding vessels be accomplished well lateral to the tumor. The fibrous but compressible nature of the tumor allows for extraction from an exposure cavity that is somewhat smaller than the tumor itself; normal sinonasal anatomy is preserved and postoperative care is minimized. Like any skull base surgical procedure, intimate knowledge of salient anatomy is critical to the safety and ultimate success in removal of these lesions.

References

1. Fisch U. Infratemporal fossa approach to tumours of the temporal bone and base of the skull. J Laryngol Otol. 1978;92:949–67.
2. Fisch U, Pillsbury HC. Infratemporal fossa approach to lesions in the temporal bone and base of the skull. Arch Otolaryngol. 1979;105:99–107.
3. Fisch U. The infratemporal fossa approach for nasopharyngeal tumors. Laryngoscope. 1983;93:36–44.
4. Fisch U. Infratemporal fossa approach for lesions in the temporal bone and base of the skull. Adv Otorhinolaryngol. 1984;34:254–66.
5. Browne JD, Jacob SL. Temporal approach for resection of juvenile nasopharyngeal angiofibromas. Laryngoscope. 2000;110:1287–93.
6. Mansour OI, Carrau RL, Snyderman CH, Kassam AB. Preauricular infratemporal fossa surgical approach: modifications of the technique and surgical indications. Skull Base. 2004;14:143–51.
7. Gates GA. The lateral facial approach to the nasopharynx and infratemporal fossa. Otolaryngol Head Neck Surg. 1988;99:321–5.
8. Zhang M, Garvis W, Linder T, Fisch U. Update on the infratemporal fossa approaches to nasopharyngeal angiofibroma. Laryngoscope. 1998;108(11 Pt1):1717–23.
9. Wetmore SJ, Suen JY, Snyderman NL. Preauricular approach to infratemporal fossa. Head Neck Surg. 1986;9:93–103.
10. Standefer J, Holt GR, Brown WE, Gates GA. Combined intracranial and extracranial excision of nasopharyngeal angiofibroma. Laryngoscope. 1983;93:772–9.
11. Leong SC. A systematic review of surgical outcomes for advanced juvenile nasopharyngeal angiofibroma with intracranial involvement. Laryngoscope. 2013;123:1125–31.
12. Garofalo P, Pia F, Policarpo M, Tunesi S, Valletti PA. Juvenile nasopharyngeal angiofibroma: comparison between endoscopic and open operative approaches. J Craniofac Surg. 2015;26:918–21.
13. Khoueir N, Nicolas N, Rohayem Z, Haddad A, Abou Hamad W. Exclusive endoscopic resection of juvenile nasopharyngeal angiofibroma: a systematic review of the literature. Otolaryngol Head Neck Surg. 2014;150:350–8.
14. Boghani Z, Husain Q, Kanumuri VV, Khan MN, Sangvhi S, Liu JK, Eloy JA. Juvenile nasopharyngeal angiofibroma: a systematic review and comparison of endoscopic, endoscopic-assisted, and open resection in 1047 cases. Laryngoscope. 2013;123:859–69.

15. Cloutier T, Pons Y, Blancal JP, Sauvaget E, Kania R, Bresson D, Herman P. Juvenile nasopharyngeal angiofibroma: does the external approach still make sense? Otolaryngol Head Neck Surg. 2012;147:958–63.
16. Midilli R, Karci B, Akyildiz S. Juvenile nasopharyngeal angiofibroma: analysis of 42 cases and important aspects of endoscopic approach. Int J Pediatr Otorhinolaryngol. 2009;73:401–8.
17. Hofmann T, Bernal-Sprekelsen M, Koele W, Reittner P, Klein E, Stammberger H. Endoscopic resection of juvenile angiofibromas – long term results. Rhinology. 2005;43:282–9.

Chapter 17
Combined Neurosurgical and Craniofacial Approach for Large Intracranial Tumor

M. Yashar S. Kalani, Nikolay L. Martirosyan, and Randall W. Porter

Abstract Craniofacial approaches may still be necessary, especially in those cases with significant intracranial tumor burden, those with intimate tumor association with the internal carotid artery (ICA), and those where the tumor has a significant extension laterally to the carotid artery. Complications including cerebrospinal fluid (CSF) leakage may necessitate reoperation or cerebrospinal fluid diversion. Meticulous closure using vascularized flaps minimizes the incidence of such complications. Given the proximity of the pathology to the intracranial circulation, the surgical team must be prepared for and able to perform standard revascularization procedures in the setting of inadvertent injury to these vessels. In this chapter, the craniofacial approach to juvenile angiofibromas is discussed along with outcomes in a cohort of patients treated using this strategy.

Keywords Craniofacial approach • Juvenile angiofibroma • Microsurgery

Introduction

A dramatic evolution in surgical techniques has occurred over the past two decades; the microsurgical removal of juvenile angiofibromas (JAs) has shifted from transfacial approaches to combined craniofacial approaches and ultimately to a pure endoscopic technique. The trend in most centers is that the majority of patients with JAs are now treated endoscopically [1], although those with intracranial extension remain in the domain of craniofacial surgery [2–4].

M.Y.S. Kalani, MD, PhD • N.L. Martirosyan, MD
Department of Neurosurgery, Barrow Neurological Institute, St. Joseph's Hospital and Medical Center, Phoenix, AZ, USA

R.W. Porter, MD (✉)
Department of Neurosurgery, Barrow Neurological Institute, St. Joseph's Hospital and Medical Center, Phoenix, AZ, USA

c/o Neuroscience Publications, Barrow Neurological Institute, St. Joseph's Hospital and Medical Center, 350 W. Thomas Road, Phoenix, AZ 85013, USA
e-mail: Neuropub@dignityhealth.org

S.P. Dubey, B. Schick (eds.), *Juvenile Angiofibroma*,
DOI 10.1007/978-3-319-45343-9_17

Factors limiting a pure endoscopic approach are tumors with significant intracranial extension, intimate association with the internal carotid artery (ICA), and lateral extension beyond the ICA. In these cases, preoperative embolization combined with craniofacial approaches can be used to safely remove these lesions. Craniofacial approaches allow the surgeon to osteotomize the orbits, retract the globes, and remove facial bones to provide a wide exposure to the anterior and middle cranial fossae. Here we review our experience with anterior craniofacial approaches to these lesions.

Surgical Technique of Craniofacial Approaches to Juvenile Angiofibromas

Patients should be treated only after their cases are extensively discussed among a multidisciplinary team comprising neurosurgeons; ear, nose, and throat surgeons; plastic surgeons; and radiation experts. In patients deemed inappropriate for endoscopic resection, craniofacial approaches are recommended.

The most commonly used craniofacial approaches for JAs include a modified transbasal approach with transmaxillary procedures with a sublabial incision where appropriate (Fig. 17.1). The osteotomies for these approaches have been described elsewhere and are summarized below [5, 6].

All patients at our center who cannot have endoscopic resections undergo anterior craniofacial approaches. We do not routinely use lumbar drains for our procedures, but do so when the degree of tumor extension and likelihood of not being able to reconstruct the skull base necessitates its use. A bicoronal incision is performed and a frontogaleal flap for reconstruction of the skull base is harvested. The flap is reflected anteriorly to expose the nasal bones and nasal process of the maxilla and to strip the periorbita. The nasolacrimal duct is exposed and preserved and the canthal ligaments are detached from the nasal bones. Next, a bifrontal craniotomy is performed and the orbital bandeau is osteomized and removed. It is important for the osteotomy to extend to the lateral orbital wall at the level of the infraorbital fissure to allow for retraction of the globes. This allows for enhanced working angles as one begins dissection (Fig. 17.1).

When necessary, in those cases with extensive maxillary extension, a transmaxillary procedure can be added to the surgical approach described above to enhance exposure. This is accomplished by performing a Le Fort I osteotomy with or without palatal splitting. An upper buccal sulcus incision is sufficient to expose the anterior maxilla. For more extensive lesions that require palatal splitting, the midline is incised through the oral mucosa and the soft palate on one side of the uvula. Once the Le Fort I osteotomy is performed, the maxillary fragments are rotated laterally to expose the clivus and provide enhanced working angles.

The dura is mobilized and opened to allow for complete lesion removal. Once the resection is complete, the osteotomies are fixed with rigid fixation. The skull base is reconstructed, and flaps are used to obtain a watertight closure and prevent leakage of cerebrospinal fluid. In cases where a transmaxillary approach was necessary, reassembly is performed with prepared interdental splints and fixation plates. In rare cases where a complete closure is not obtained, a lumbar drain is left in situ for

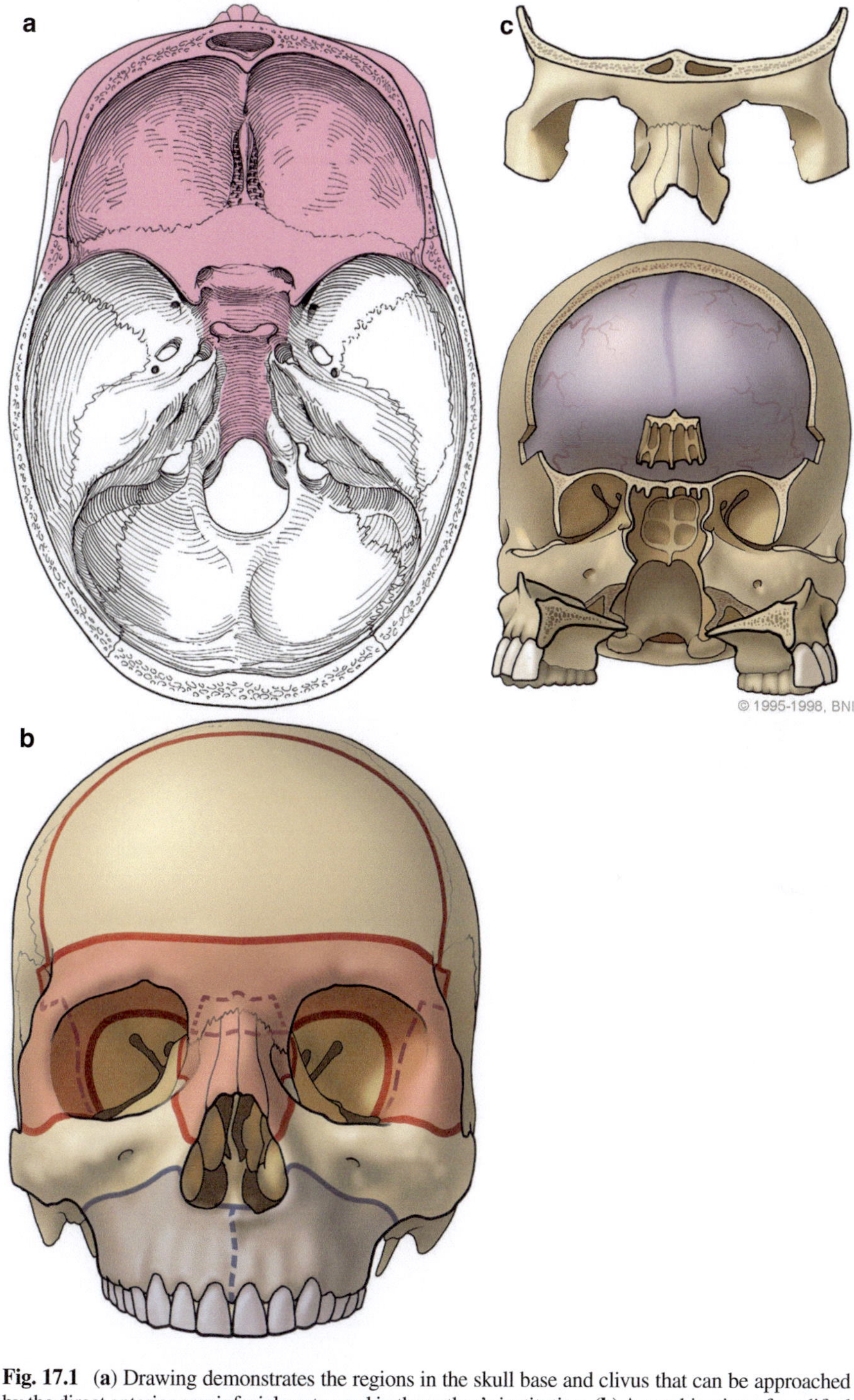

Fig. 17.1 (**a**) Drawing demonstrates the regions in the skull base and clivus that can be approached by the direct anterior craniofacial route used in the author's institution. (**b**) A combination of modified transbasal (*red* region) and transmaxillary (*blue* region) approaches to the midline skull base is shown. Two variations for performing the transmaxillary approach are indicated by the *dotted* and *solid lines*. (**c**) Illustration shows the combined approaches; the cribriform plate is preserved, and depth of exposure is depicted (Used with permission from Barrow Neurological Institute, Phoenix, Arizona)

Table 17.1 Clinical summary of 22 patients with JAs

Case no.	Age (years)	Stage[a]	Presenting symptoms	EBL	LOS (days)	Complication	EOR	Recurrence	Other treatment	FU (months)
1	11	IIIB	Epistaxis, facial swelling, diplopia	800	11	Musculoskeletal defect	GTR	No		12
2	18	IIIB	Nasal obstruction	2,500	10	Central frontal defect	GTR	No	Multiple revisions	38
				NR		Infection		No		
						Chronic drainage		No		
						CSF leak		No		
3	13	IIIB	Nasal obstruction	1,500			STR	No	Residual treated by Peacock XRT; 45 GY in 25 fractions	11
4	11	IIIB	Epistaxis	400			GTR	No		2
5	14	IIIB	Headache, facial swelling	4,900	8		GTR	No		20
6	13	IIIB	Facial swelling, epistaxis	2,500		Nasal voice	STR	No	Residual treated by surgery	144
	13			1,200			STR	No	Residual treated by Peacock XRT; 54 GY in 25 fractions	
7	18	IIIB	Nasal obstruction, epistaxis	1,100	8	CSF leak	GTR	No		8

8	13	IIIB	Nasal obstruction	700	4		GTR	Yes; 26 months	Recurrence treated by surgery	32
			Headache, severe epistaxis	NR			STR	No	Residual treated by CyberKnife	
9	13	IIIB	Nasal obstruction	400	9		GTR	No		1
10	13	IIIB	Epistaxis	1,800	4		GTR	Yes; 24 months	Recurrence treated by surgery	28
	15	IIIB		800	5			No		
11	26	IIIB	Epistaxis	1,000	3	Sinusitis	GTR	No		10
12	14	IIIB	Epistaxis	1,400	6	CSF leak	GTR	No		19
				NR		Wound infection; abscess				
13	14	IIIB	Epistaxis	2,250	20	Meningitis; CSF leak	GTR	No		36
14	9	IIIB	Sinusitis, facial swelling	1,200	6		STR	No	Residual treated by Peacock XRT; 45 GY in 25 fractions and endoscopic removal	54
15	26	IIIB		700			GTR	Yes; 23 months		24
	27	IIIB		2,000				No		

(continued)

Table 17.1 (continued)

Case no.	Age (years)	Stage[a]	Presenting symptoms	EBL	LOS (days)	Complication	EOR	Recurrence	Other treatment	FU (months)
16	11	IIIB	Nasal obstruction, epistaxis	400	10		STR	Yes; 11 months	Recurrence treated by CyberKnife; 40 Gy in five fractions	12
17	16	IIIB	Airway obstruction	NR	10	Headache, nasal stuffiness	GTR	No		29
18	14	IIIB	Difficulty breathing	2,800	10	CSF leak, epistaxis	GTR	No		12
19	15	IIIB	Nasal bleeding	NR	10		GTR	No		25
20	16	IIIB	Nasal obstruction	NR	7		GTR	No		38
21	14	IIIB	Nasal obstruction, epistaxis, loss of hearing	1,500	6		GTR	No		2
22	14	IIIB	Nasal obstruction, epistaxis	NR	8		GTR	No		22

Modified from Kalani et al. [3] Used with permission from *Journal of Neurosurgery: Pediatrics*

CSF cerebrospinal fluid, *EBL* estimated blood loss, *EOR* extent of resection, *FU* follow-up, *GTR* gross total resection, *LOS* length of hospital stay, *NR* not recorded, *STR* subtotal resection, *XRT* radiation therapy

[a]Staging based on Radkowski et al. [7]

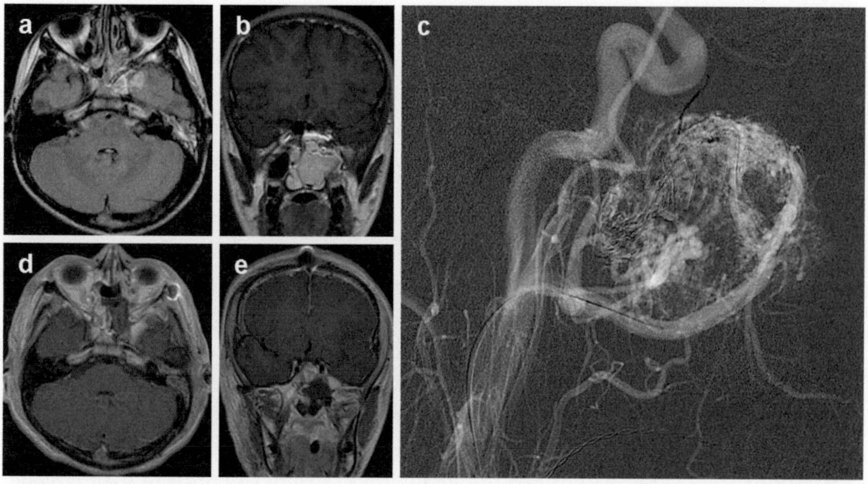

Fig. 17.2 Preoperative axial (**a**) and coronal (**b**) magnetic resonance (MR) images demonstrate a JNA with intracranial involvement. Postembolization angiogram (**c**) after Onyx (ev3 Endovascular, Inc., Plymouth, MN) embolization demonstrates the highly vascular nature of the JA. (**d**) Postoperative axial and (**e**) coronal MR imaging demonstrates gross total resection of the tumor (Modified from Kalani et al. [3])

3–5 days. If the cerebrospinal fluid leak remains recalcitrant to lumbar drainage, the patient is taken back for surgical repair of the leak.

Patient Outcomes at the Barrow Neurological Institute

We have reported our experience with treating 22 patients with Radkowski stage IIIB [3, 7]. An example of a patient treated is presented in Fig. 17.2. All patients were male with a mean age at presentation of 15 years (range, 9–27 years). The majority of patients presented with epistaxis and nasal obstruction. All patients underwent preoperative embolization of extracranial carotid artery vascular pedicles irrigating the tumor. Preoperative embolization was performed using a liquid embolic agent and n-butyl cyanoacrylate glue.

The mean blood loss in these operations was 1,480 mL (range 400–4,900 mL). The mean hospital stay was 8.2 days (range, 3–20 days). Using the techniques described above, we obtained gross total resection in 17 cases and subtotal resection in 5 cases. In five cases of residual tumor, radiation therapy was used as an adjunct therapy.

There were no cases of procedure-related mortality, but there was a significant rate of morbidity. The rate of postoperative complications was 41 %, with cerebrospinal fluid leak being the most common (23 %). Other complications included superficial infection (14 %), aesthetic defect requiring reoperation (10 %), deep infection/meningitis (10 %), and other minor complications (4 %). Despite orbital osteotomies, no patient developed vision loss, cranial nerve deficits, or neurological decline.

At a mean follow-up of 27.7 months (range, 2–144 months), the mean Karnofsky Performance Scale score was 90. The overall recurrence or progression rate was 18 %, and the mean time to recurrence was 21 months (range, 11–26 months).

Prevention and Management of Intraoperative Complications

By far the most common complication associated with the use of extensive craniofacial approaches is postoperative cerebrospinal fluid (CSF) leakage. This complication was observed in 23 % of cases in our experience and often requires re-exploration and repair of the fistula. In a subset of cases, the patient may require placement of permanent means of CSF diversion, often a ventriculoperitoneal shunt. In some cases, lumbar drain placement may result in spontaneous closure of the CSF fistula. In general, a multilayered meticulous closure can prevent CSF leakage postoperatively.

Intracranial vascular injury is a rare but potentially disastrous complication of craniofacial approaches. Although we did not encounter this complication in our experience, surgical teams should be prepared for and have the facility to repair vascular injuries using standard microsurgical techniques [8]. In cases where direct repair is not possible, endovascular sacrifice or treatment of vasculature should be attempted.

Other less common complications associated with the use of craniofacial approaches include injury to the facial bones, poor cosmetic results as a result of reconstruction, or cranial neuropathies. In general these complications can be avoided by being meticulous during exposure and closure of wounds. In the case of anosmia after transbasal approaches, the inclusion of cribriform plate osteotomies can reduce the incidence of olfactory nerve dysfunction [9].

Craniofacial Approaches and Comparison with Other Techniques

Prior to the advent and improvement of neuroendoscopic techniques, craniofacial approaches were the workhorses for resection of deep-seated lesions involving the anterior and middle cranial fossae. Craniofacial approaches were an extension of the pioneering work performed by Tessier on reconstruction of facial birth defects [10, 11]. Tessier and Derome expanded these techniques for resection of anterior and middle fossa pathologies [12]. However, due to the growing craniofacial skeleton in children, the use of these approaches in the pediatric population has been performed with some reluctance, albeit with good results [13–15].

The extent of tumor resection is closely related to the approach used to resect JAs. In cases of tumors with significant intracranial or infratemporal fossa extension, radical resection may not be possible with simple transfacial approaches. Using a lateral rhinotomy approach, for example, the extent of residual tumor may range between 20 and 50 % [15–17], while midfacial degloving results a lower incidence of residual tumor (15–37 %) [18, 19]. In cases of tumors with involvement of the infratemporal fossa and cavernous sinus, the infratemporal fossa approach [20] can provide excellent results with complete resection in 87 % of patients [21]. More extensive lesions, especially those with a significant intracranial burden, may require the use of craniofacial approaches, as described above. However, caution must be exercised in drawing conclusions from the results of meta-analyses and systematic reviews that combine all JAs because more complex lesions may require more extensive approaches and may be associated with critical structures, limiting the surgeon's ability to obtain a gross total resection and, because of this, resulting in a higher residual rate.

Proponents of endoscopic techniques have challenged the utility of craniofacial approaches given the morbid nature of the operation, the high rates of postoperative complications, and the significant blood loss associated with these approaches [22, 23]. A report from the Pittsburgh group [4] noted good outcomes using a predominantly endoscopic/endoscopic-assisted technique in a group of 31 patients with Radkowski stage IIIA or greater JAs. This study reported five cases of recurrence and noted that association of the tumor with feeders from the internal carotid artery was not a contraindication for the use of endoscopy. A systematic review [23] of 1,047 cases demonstrated a recurrence rate of 4.7 % in patients undergoing endoscopic resection of JAs (as compared with the 22.6 % in those undergoing open surgery and 20.6 % in the endoscopic-assisted group) with a significant reduction in blood loss when compared with open surgery. However after controlling for extent of tumor, there was no difference in recurrence rates, which supports the notion that endoscopic approaches were likely used to treat predominantly smaller tumors in most centers.

Despite favorable results with endoscopy in experienced hands, the majority of patients with JAs with extensive intracranial involvement continue to undergo craniofacial approaches for resection, while pure endoscopy is used to treat all small and medium lesions and select large lesions [2, 24, 25]. As noted, the use of endoscopy is currently limited when treating tumors with significant lateral extension to the internal carotid artery and, for most surgeons, when treating tumors with significant vascular contribution from branches of the ICA. Although more effective embolization and better endoscopic techniques may nullify these limitations, current practice results in either incomplete endoscopic resection of the subset of tumors with lateral extension to the carotid (and, in most cases, subsequent treatment with radiation) or the use of craniofacial approaches to address these tumors.

Conclusions

In the subset of tumors with extension lateral to the ICA and the subset with supply from the ICA that are not amenable to embolization, craniofacial approaches remain a treatment option. This situation may arise where the diagnosis may be delayed, and these lesions may present at sizes where craniofacial resection is the only safe option.

Partial resection of these lesions and treatment with radiation should be avoided when possible given the long-term risk of radiation to this mostly pediatric population of patients. Surgical teams must be prepared for the rare possibility of injury to the internal carotid artery and have facility to revascularize the carotid circulation using standard revascularization techniques. In a subset of patients, cerebrospinal fluid leaks may require reoperation for repair or CSF diversion.

References

1. Rogers DJ, Bevans SE, Harsha WJ. Endoscopic resection of juvenile nasopharyngeal angiofibroma. Adv Otorhinolaryngol. 2012;73:132–6.
2. Leong SC. A systematic review of surgical outcomes for advanced juvenile nasopharyngeal angiofibroma with intracranial involvement. Laryngoscope. 2013;123:1125–31.
3. Kalani MY, Kalani MA, Kalb S, Albuquerque FC, McDougall CG, Nakaji P, et al. Craniofacial approaches to large juvenile angiofibromas. J Neurosurg Pediatr. 2011;8:71–8.
4. Hackman T, Snyderman CH, Carrau R, Vescan A, Kassam A. Juvenile nasopharyngeal angiofibroma: the expanded endonasal approach. Am J Rhinol Allergy. 2009;23:95–9.
5. Beals SP, Joganic EF, Hamilton MG, Spetzler RF. Posterior skull base transfacial approaches. Clin Plast Surg. 1995;22:491–511.
6. Feiz-Erfan I, Han PP, Spetzler RF, Horn EM, Klopfenstein JD, Porter RW, et al. The radical transbasal approach for resection of anterior and midline skull base lesions. J Neurosurg. 2005;103:485–90.
7. Radkowski D, McGill T, Healy GB, Ohlms L, Jones DT. Angiofibroma. Changes in staging and treatment. Arch Otolaryngol Head Neck Surg. 1996;122:122–9.
8. Kalani MY, Rangel-Castilla L, Ramey W, Nakaji P, Albuquerque FC, McDougall CG, et al. Indications and results of direct cerebral revascularization in the modern era. World Neurosurg. 2015;83:345–50.
9. Feiz-Erfan I, Han PP, Spetzler RF, Horn EM, Klopfenstein JD, Kim LJ, et al. Preserving olfactory function in anterior craniofacial surgery through cribriform plate osteotomy applied in selected patients. Neurosurgery. 2005;57(1 Suppl):86–93; discussion 86–93.
10. Tessier P. Complete and forme fruste vertical and oblique orbito-facial clefts (colobomas). Ann Chir Plast. 1969;14:301–11.
11. Tessier P. The definitive plastic surgical treatment of the severe facial deformities of craniofacial dysostosis. Crouzon's and Apert's diseases. Plast Reconstr Surg. 1971;48:419–42.
12. Derome P. The trans-bucco-pharyngeal approach and tumoral pathology of the clivus. Neuro-Chirurgie. 1977;23:298–306.
13. Teo C, Dornhoffer J, Hanna E, Bower C. Application of skull base techniques to pediatric neurosurgery. Childs Nerv Syst. 1999;15:103–9.
14. Posnick JC, Goldstein JA, Armstrong D, Rutka JT. Reconstruction of skull defects in children and adolescents by the use of fixed cranial bone grafts: long-term results. Neurosurgery. 1993;32:785–91; discussion 91.
15. Roche PH, Paris J, Regis J, Moulin G, Zanaret M, Thomassin JM, et al. Management of invasive juvenile nasopharyngeal angiofibromas: the role of a multimodality approach. Neurosurgery. 2007;61:768–77; discussion 77.
16. Danesi G, Panizza B, Mazzoni A, Calabrese V. Anterior approaches in juvenile nasopharyngeal angiofibromas with intracranial extension. Otolaryngol Head Neck Surg. 2000;122:277–83.
17. Jones GC, DeSanto LW, Bremer JW, Neel 3rd HB. Juvenile angiofibromas. Behavior and treatment of extensive and residual tumors. Arch Otolaryngol Head Neck Surg. 1986;112:1191–3.
18. Fagan JJ, Snyderman CH, Carrau RL, Janecka IP. Nasopharyngeal angiofibromas: selecting a surgical approach. Head Neck. 1997;19:391–9.

19. Close LG, Schaefer SD, Mickey BE, Manning SC. Surgical management of nasopharyngeal angiofibroma involving the cavernous sinus. Arch Otolaryngol Head Neck Surg. 1989; 115:1091–5.
20. Fisch U, Pillsbury HC. Infratemporal fossa approach to lesions in the temporal bone and base of the skull. Arch Otolaryngol. 1979;105:99–107.
21. Andrews JC, Fisch U, Valavanis A, Aeppli U, Makek MS. The surgical management of extensive nasopharyngeal angiofibromas with the infratemporal fossa approach. Laryngoscope. 1989;99:429–37.
22. Dahl JP, Zopf DA, Parikh SR. Do open and endoscopic resection approaches to juvenile nasopharyngeal angiofibroma result in similar blood loss and recurrence rates? Laryngoscope. 2015;125:2436–7.
23. Boghani Z, Husain Q, Kanumuri VV, Khan MN, Sangvhi S, Liu JK, et al. Juvenile nasopharyngeal angiofibroma: a systematic review and comparison of endoscopic, endoscopic-assisted, and open resection in 1047 cases. Laryngoscope. 2013;123:859–69.
24. Garofalo P, Pia F, Policarpo M, Tunesi S, Valletti PA. Juvenile nasopharyngeal angiofibroma: comparison between endoscopic and open operative approaches. J Craniofac Surg. 2015;26:918–821.
25. Huang Y, Liu Z, Wang J, Sun X, Yang L, Wang D. Surgical management of juvenile nasopharyngeal angiofibroma: analysis of 162 cases from 1995 to 2012. Laryngoscope. 2014; 124:1942–6.

Chapter 18
Radiation Therapy

Curtis Bryant and William M. Mendenhall

Abstract Juvenile angiofibroma (JA) is a benign vascular tumor that develops almost entirely in young males. JA originates at the superior margin of the spheno-ethmoidal suture which is located at the junction of the nasal cavity and nasopharynx, and JA is defined by its propensity for local invasion and bony destruction of the nasal cavity, nasopharynx, and skull base. No reports are available of nodal or distant metastasis. The preferred treatment for JA is selective embolization of the vascular supply of the tumor bed followed by surgical resection. For patients with extensive skull base invasion or intracranial extension, complete surgical resection may not be possible without accepting a high risk for severe acute and chronic complications. In these cases, we recommend definitive radiation therapy. Evidence supports the delivery of fractionated radiation therapy for JA tumors and reports suggest that the rate of local control ranges between 73 and 100 % following moderate doses of radiation therapy (36–45 Gy) (Amdur et al. Pract Radiat Oncol 1(4):271–278, 2011; Kuppersmith et al. Int J Pediatr Otorhinolaryngol 52(3):261–268, 2000; Lee et al. Laryngoscope 112(7 Pt 1):1213–1220, 2002; Mallick et al. Acta Otorhinolaryngol Ital 35(2):75–79, 2015; McGahan et al. Int J Radiat Oncol Biol Phys 17(5):1067–1072, 1989). Serious complications are uncommon; consequently, radiation therapy is an attractive alternative to surgery for patients with locally advanced disease.

Keywords Benign tumors • Radiotherapy • Head and neck cancer

Introduction

Juvenile angiofibroma (JA) is a benign vascular tumor that develops most commonly in adolescent and teenage males. These tumors originate at the junction of the sphenoidal process of the palatine bone and the pterygoid process of the sphenoid bone, which is located just superior to the sphenopalatine foramen [6]. JA does

C. Bryant, MD, MPH (✉) • W.M. Mendenhall, MD
Department of Radiation Oncology, University of Florida,
2015 North Jefferson St., Gainesville, Jacksonville, FL 32206, USA
e-mail: cbryant@floridaproton.org

S.P. Dubey, B. Schick (eds.), *Juvenile Angiofibroma*,
DOI 10.1007/978-3-319-45343-9_18

not metastasize but typically displays locally destructive behavior. As the tumor grows anteriorly, it extends further into the nasal cavity and from there can flatten the turbinates and push the septum into the opposite side of the nasal cavity. The tumor can erode into the maxillary sinus laterally and while filling the nasal cavity [7, 8]. Base-of-skull invasion exists in up to 74 % of patients at the time of presentation [1–5, 9]. A common access point to the base of the skull is laterally through the sphenopalatine foramen and into the pterygopalatine fossa. From the pterygopalatine fossa, the tumor can then extend to the infratemporal fossa through the pterygomaxillary fissure. Intracranial extension is present in 10–20 % of patients at the time of diagnosis [10, 11]. Although surgery is the preferred treatment, many patients require radiation therapy because of the size and extent of disease at the time of diagnosis [7]. The following chapter focuses on the role of radiation therapy in the management of locally advanced JA.

Diagnosis, Workup, and Imaging

For the treating radiation oncologist, the pretreatment evaluation should include a thorough medical history, physical examination, and advanced imaging since the diagnosis of JA is primarily made by clinical evaluation. Patients usually present with unilateral nasal obstruction and recurrent epistaxis. Less common symptoms can include nasal discharge or conductive hearing loss secondary to obstruction of the eustachian tube. Patients with locally aggressive tumors may present with facial pain and swelling of the cheek. Patients with orbital invasion may present with unilateral blindness, orbital pain, or proptosis. Patients with invasion of the base of the skull can present with cranial nerve deficits including trigeminal nerve palsies [7]. These patient characteristics, symptoms, imaging features, and growth pattern should be sufficient for diagnosis. Biopsy is discouraged because of the risk that instrumentation can cause serious bleeding. Additionally, a biopsy may lead to a false negative given the heterogeneous nature of these tumors [7, 12]. Before delivering radiation therapy, we recommend a biopsy only when clinical evaluation produces equivocal results and the diagnosis is still in doubt after a thorough workup [7].

Imaging should include multiplanar contrast-enhanced computed tomography (CT) and magnetic resonance imaging (MRI). Thin slices (1–2 mm) of both scans should be obtained through the nasal cavity, nasopharynx, sinuses, and base of the skull. CT imaging allows for demonstration of bony detail, in case bony erosion of the skull base is suspected, and should be performed with contrast enhancement to allow visualization of the primary tumor, which is vascular and should enhance with iodinated contrast. Obtaining T1- and T2-weighted multiplanar MRI is critical for diagnosis and for treatment planning. These images help define the tumor within the nasal cavity and nasopharynx and show the route of base-of-skull invasion and the extent of intracranial or orbital invasion. As Fig. 18.1 shows, JA usually demonstrates intense contrast enhancement on CT and T1-weighted MRI. T2-weighted MRI allows for the differentiation of tumor from obstructed sinuses. Flow voids are usually present and a vascular pedicle is often identifiable, which is characteristic of the diagnosis.

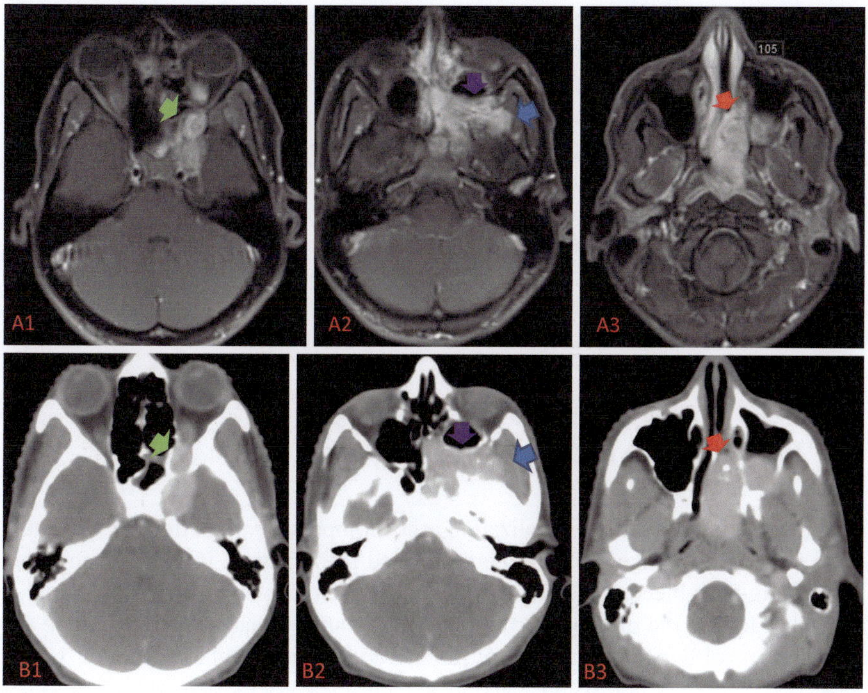

Fig. 18.1 Pre-radiation therapy imaging. A young male diagnosed with JA. He presented with headaches, blurry vision in the left eye, nosebleeds, and a mass in the left nasal cavity on exam. (A1–3) Contrast-enhanced T1-weighted image showing an enhancing mass involving the posterior orbit (*green arrow*) and left nasal cavity (*red arrow*) and entering the left sphenopalatine foramen to occupy the pterygopalatine fossa (*purple arrow*) and spreading to the infratemporal fossa (*blue arrow*). The images start superior to the tumor and each axial image is taken approximately 1.5 cm below the previous slice. (B1–3) Corresponding contrast-enhanced CT scan imaging showing the appearance of the mass and the erosion of the posterior wall of the maxillary sinus

Staging

Although several proposed staging systems exist, each was developed to predict tumor-related outcomes after surgery [13–16]. None of the available tumor-staging systems is known to correlate with the likelihood of local control after radiation therapy [1]. Consequently, radiation oncologists should stage patients primarily to help facilitate communication with surgical colleagues. The currently available staging systems do not guide radiation therapy decisions.

Indication for Radiation

Radiation therapy is the treatment of choice for patients with locally advanced disease for whom surgical resection would be incomplete or lead to unacceptable complications. Radiation therapy can be indicated for patients at the time of initial diagnosis or at the time of recurrence after surgery. In either case, we support radiation therapy for tumors that involve the cavernous sinus and optic nerve or display significant intracranial extension. We also recommend postoperative radiation therapy for patients initially managed with surgery, but with gross residual disease on postoperative examination or imaging. A positive microscopic margin is not an indication for adjuvant radiation therapy, though, and these patients should be managed with salvage therapy at the time of disease recurrence. The recommended dose of radiation therapy ranges between 36 and 45 Gy at 1.8 Gy per fraction and we prefer to deliver doses on the higher end of this range for large or recurrent tumors, particularly in patients 18 years old or older and patients for whom the dose constraints for the organs at risk (OAR) can be met.

The Role of Endovascular Embolization

Pretreatment endovascular embolization is not compulsory when treating with radiation therapy. Although it should be performed if the patient is experiencing life-threatening nose bleeds before therapy, no data exist showing that it aids in tumor control or lowers the risk for morbidity during or after radiation therapy. There are also theoretical concerns that embolization would lead to tumor hypoxia, which may contribute to radioresistance and local recurrence after radiation therapy [1].

Radiation Technique

Simulation

A summary of the technical details of fractionated radiation is included in Table 18.1. Patients require CT-based simulation with intravenous contrast and an Aquaplast mask to reduce motion and uncertainty. The patient's neck should be extended and an oral stent should be placed in the patient's mouth to push the tongue out of the treatment field. Multiplanar MRI should be obtained and fused to the CT planning scan. These images facilitate accurate contouring by defining the soft tissue extent of tumor within the nasal cavity, nasopharynx, and base of the skull and show the extent of intracranial invasion.

Target Delineation

The target volumes and OARs should be delineated on the planning CT scan according to the International Commission on Radiation Units and Measurements (ICRU) guidelines [17]. The gross tumor volume (GTV) should be contoured using the

Table 18.1 Technical details of fractionated radiation therapy

Indications for RT	Visible tumor on physical examination or imaging where surgical resection is not achievable without accepting significant morbidity
	Prior surgery with a grossly positive margin or gross disease present on examination or imaging after surgery
RT dose	36 Gy at 1.8 Gy per fraction
	Consider boosting areas of gross disease to 41.4–45 Gy at 1.8 Gy per fraction for patients 18 years old or greater and if doses to organs at risk are able to meet constraints
Radiation technique	Photon radiation delivered with IMRT. Radiation is delivered with 5–7 noncoplanar beams using a fixed beam approach. Alternatively, volumetric arc therapy may be applied
	Proton therapy delivered with 3–5 noncoplanar beams. Technique can include 3D conformal proton therapy or intensity-modulated proton therapy
RT simulation	Patient is supine in an Aquaplast mask with neck extended and arms by the side. An oral stent is placed in the mouth to push the tongue away from the treatment field
	CT simulation fused with an MRI scan
	CT: 1–2-mm contiguous slices from the skull vertex to the mid neck
	MRI: 1–2 mm contiguous slices with a T1-weighted sequence
Target definition	GTV = visible tumor on physical examination, CT, and MRI
	CTV = the entire pterygopalatine fossa and inferior orbital fissure on the ipsilateral side plus 1.0 cm expansion of the GTV in all directions where there is no barrier to tumor spread. The CTV is not expanded to cover the regional lymphatics. Include areas adjacent to presurgery tumor volume
	PTV = CTV plus 3–5 mm depending on availability of on treatment imaging
Target dose goal	95 % of the PTV receives 100 % of the prescription dose
	99 % of the PTV receives 93 % of the prescription dose
	No more than 20 % of the PTV receives 110 % of the prescription dose

Abbreviations: *3D* three-dimensional, *CT* computed tomography, *CTV* clinical target volume, *GTV* gross tumor volume, *IMRT* intensity-modulated radiation therapy, *MRI* magnetic resonance imaging, *PTV* planned target volume, *RT* radiation therapy

tumor extent visualized on CT and MRI as well as physical examination. If systemic therapy was delivered or surgery performed before radiation, the GTV should be outlined on the treatment planning CT according to its pretreatment extent. Although JA tumors are benign, we recommend providing generous margins to develop a clinical target volume (CTV) around the GTV. We recommend using a 1-cm margin around the GTV edited for anatomic boundaries to create the CTV. We also recommend including the entire pterygopalatine fossa and inferior orbital fissure on the ipsilateral side of the CTV. There is no role for elective nodal radiation; therefore, the CTV should not intentionally include any regional nodal stations [1]. The planning target volume (PTV) should be created by isocentrically expanding the CTV by 3–5 mm. The amount of expansion depends on the available image guidance technology and the reliability and accuracy of patient setup available at the treating institution. An example of contoured target volumes on a CT planning scan of a patient with JA is provided in Fig. 18.2.

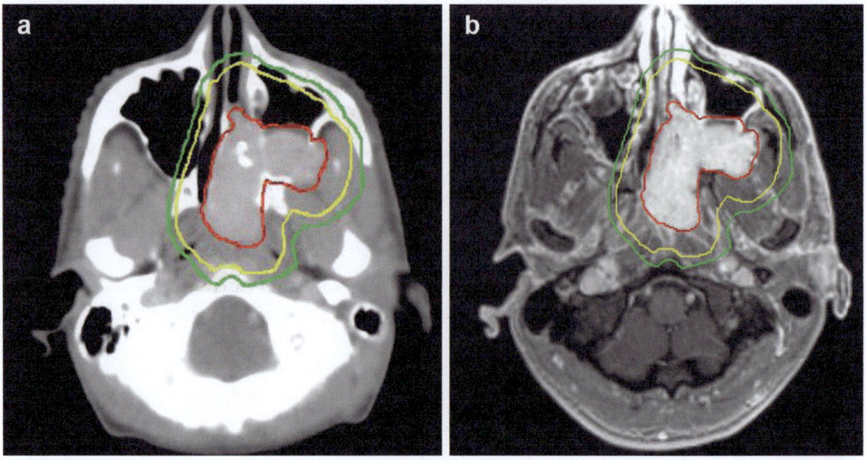

Fig. 18.2 Treatment planning target volumes. Young male with a locally advanced juvenile angiofibroma involving the left nasal cavity, left maxillary sinus, left pterygopalatine fossa, and infratemporal fossa. (**a**) CT planning scan. (**b**) Treatment planning MRI. In *red* the gross tumor volume (GTV) is contoured. In *yellow*, the clinical target volume is provided which is a 1-cm expansion of the GTV edited for anatomical boundaries for tumor spread. In *green* the planning target volume which was created by expanding the CTV by 3 mm

Treatment Planning

Treatment should be delivered with highly conformal radiation therapy and the treatment plan should be designed to provide the recommended dose to the target volume and to spare the organs at risk from any unnecessary radiation therapy. The location of JA tumors presents a technical problem for radiation therapy because of the proximity of these tumors to the normal tissues of the brain, facial structures, optic nerve, retina, lens, pituitary, hypothalamus, and hippocampus. It is critical to limit the doses to the organs at risk (OAR) as much as possible while maintaining adequate dose coverage of the PTV.

Photon-based radiation therapy can be delivered using three-dimensional (3D) conformal radiation. Normally, five to seven noncoplanar uniform beams are used to deliver the dose to the target using high-energy photon beams. This technology allows for conformal dose coverage around spherical targets. Intensity-modulated photon radiation therapy (IMRT) provides a stepwise improvement in dose conformality for tumors of the head and neck when compared to 3D conformal photon radiation therapy because it improves dose conformality for irregularly shaped targets [18]. IMRT is usually delivered using five to seven static noncoplanar beams. The intensity of each beam is modulated by delivering multiple beam segments per field designed to treat only portions of the target. By varying the number of beams, beam angles, beam segment size, location, shape, and the dose delivered by each, the prescribed radiation dose can be conformed around concave or horseshoe-shaped fields. Volumetric arc therapy is a type of IMRT that reduces treatment time and often improves conformality compared to static-beam IMRT by rotating the treatment gantry around the patient continuously with the beam on to provide a steady flow of radiation through various treatment angles [19]. The intensity of the beam can be modified continuously by changing the dose rate, gantry rotation speed, and shape of the multi-leaf collimators (MLCs) as the gantry rotates.

Proton therapy is an attractive alternative to photon-based radiation therapy. Photon radiation is characterized by a relatively high entrance dose along the beam path and a significant exit dose. Protons are subatomic particles with mass and charge. When a proton beam is used for radiation therapy, it delivers most of its energy at a single depth along the beam path called the Bragg peak. The beam delivers relatively little dose at the beam entrance and there is no exit dose. Consequently, compared with photon-based therapies, including IMRT, proton therapy delivers less radiation to surrounding OARs for head and neck tumors [20]. This dose reduction to the OARs can potentially reduce the risk for complications following radiation therapy, particularly complications that occur after exposure to low to moderate doses of radiation, like mucositis, dysgeusia, nausea, or second malignancies [21, 22]. Proton therapy might also make dose hypofractionation or escalation feasible, potentially shortening treatment schedules, reducing the cost of treatment, and improving local control [21]. An IMRT comparison plan for a patient with JA treated with proton therapy is provided in Fig. 18.3. The IMRT comparison plan delivers higher doses to the contralateral parotid gland, cochlea, and hippocampal head and a higher mean dose to the oral cavity which may increase the patients risk for acute and late side effects.

Skull base and intracranial stereotactic radiosurgery (SRS) has been proven to be safe and effective for carefully selected patients with benign and malignant tumors [23–25]. SRS involves the use of numerous beams of radiation aimed at a small immobilized target. The radiation dose is prescribed to deposit a large dose at the target with a very steep dose falloff outside the target. SRS is usually delivered in a single fraction at doses between 17 and 24 Gy making it more convenient than fractionated radiation therapy. It also has been shown to provide excellent local control for several benign and malignant tumors of the skull base and brain [24–26]. For JA, SRS should be considered as investigational given the paucity of supporting studies. To date, the results for a small number of patients have been reported detailing outcomes for JA treated with SRS. Each patient received prescribed doses of 17–23 Gy (with a 45 Gy maximum dose) using stereotactic techniques. Although results have been promising thus far [27–30], further investigation is warranted and we recommend careful consideration of the proximity of the primary tumor to the organs at risk before delivering SRS. The optic nerves, optic chiasm, retina, and brainstem are at significant risk with hypofractionated doses if this distance is less than 2–3 mm.

Target Coverage

The goals for target coverage for fractionated radiation should be explicit and followed closely. Our recommendation is to cover 95 % of the PTV with the target dose and to ensure that 99 % of the target gets at least 93 % of the target dose [1]. The

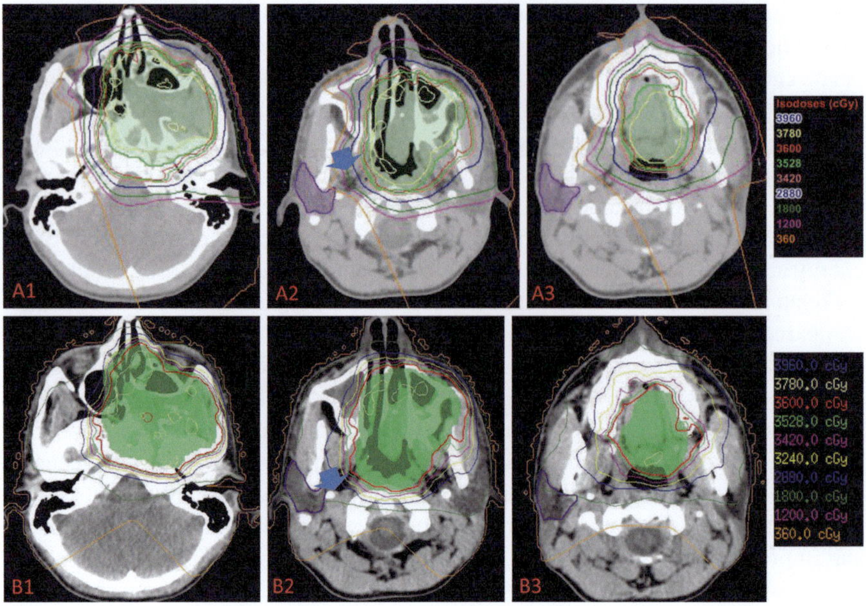

Fig. 18.3 Isodose distribution of a treatment plan for young male with juvenile angiofibroma of the left nasal cavity. The prescription dose was 36 Gy at 1.8 Gy per fraction. (A1–3) Treatment plan delivering proton therapy. (B1–3) Treatment plan delivering intensity-modulated photon radiation therapy (IMRT). The proton plan comparison plan shows lower doses delivered to the right parotid gland with (*blue arrow*) compared to IMRT which potentially lowers the risk for persistent xerostomia after radiation therapy. In general the volume of normal tissue receiving 2,880 cGy or lower is much lower with proton therapy than with IMRT. The DVH comparison table shows that proton therapy provides a lower mean dose to the contralateral organs at risk including the right cochlea and parotid gland and it provides a lower dose to the oral cavity

volume of tissue receiving more than 110 % of the target dose should be limited to 20 % of the PTV or less. We consider these rigid constraints as necessary to obtaining local disease control and preventing undue complications from excessive radiation dose due to radiation "hot spots," which are areas expected to receive significantly more radiation than intended [1].

Organs at Risk

The following normal structures should be contoured at the time of planning: parotids, larynx, submandibular glands, lacrimal glands, pharyngeal constrictors, lenses, retina, optic nerves, optic chiasm, pituitary, hypothalamus, cochlea, brainstem, hippocampi, and spinal cord. Example contours of the organs at risk are provided in Fig. 18.4. The radiation dose to these target structures should be calculated at the time of treatment planning and kept as low as possible. A recommended dose constraint guideline is listed in Table 18.2.

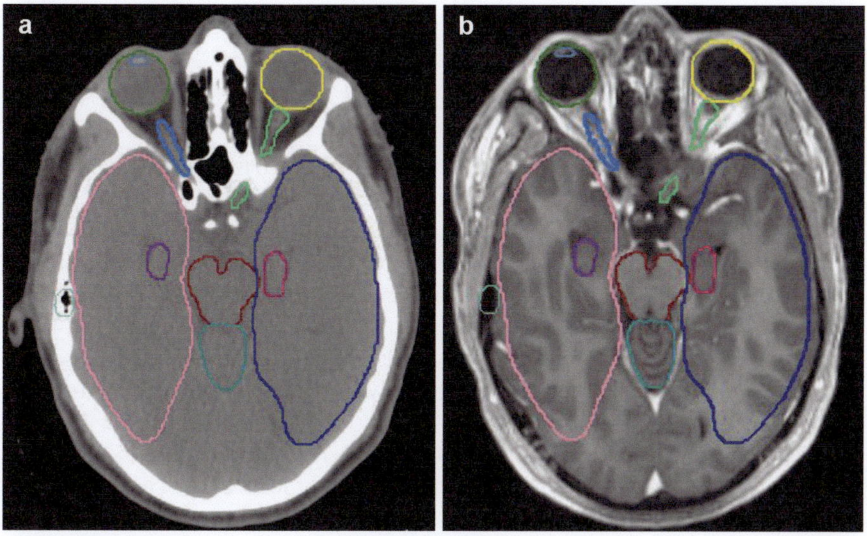

Fig. 18.4 Normal tissue contours (**a**) CT planning scan and (**b**) treatment planning MRI. *Pink* right temporal lobe. *Dark blue* left temporal lobe. *Green* left optic nerve. *Medium blue* right optic nerve. *Aqua* cerebellum. *Yellow* left retina. *Dark green* right retina. *Lightest blue* right lens. *Purple* right head of hippocampus head. *Fuchsia* left head of hippocampus

Table 18.2 Suggested radiation dose constraints for organs at risk for fractionated radiation therapy

Organ	Type	Goal
Brainstem	Dmax	<55 Gy
Cochlea	Mean dose	<36 Gy
Hippocampus head	Mean dose	<5 Gy
Hippocampus tail	Mean dose	<20 Gy
Lacrimal gland	Mean dose	<41 Gy
Lens	Mean dose	<10 Gy
Larynx	Mean dose	<36 Gy
	Dmax	<45 Gy
Mastoid	Mean dose	<30 Gy
Optic chiasm	Dmax	<55 Gy
Optic nerve	Dmax	<55 Gy
Retina	Dmax	<55 Gy
Oral cavity	Mean dose	<35 Gy
Parotid	Mean dose	<26 Gy
Spinal cord	Dmax	<50 Gy
Submandibular gland	Mean dose	<40 Gy
Temporal lobe	Volume receiving 20 Gy	<10 %
Pharyngeal constructor	Mean dose	<50 Gy

Radiation Therapy Results

Fractionated Radiation

Evidence supporting the use of radiation therapy is limited to retrospective reviews and case series, but in general the results are consistent and fairly promising (see Table 18.3). For the available data, three conclusions can be made about the effect of radiation therapy on JA: (1) The local control rate after moderate doses of radiation therapy (30–50 Gy) using conventional fractionation (1.8–2.0 Gy per fraction) is between 73 and 100 %. (2) Radiation therapy is generally well tolerated [1–4] but the presence of intracranial extension or the delivery of re-irradiation increases the risk for complications. (3) Doses above 36 Gy provided better local control than lower doses of fractionated RT [1, 5].

Cummings et al. [10], the largest published series documenting the effect of radiation therapy on JA, established the benchmark for local control and accurately describe the pattern of tumor regression after definitive radiation. In this series, 55 patients with JA were treated with conventional radiation therapy between 1946 and 1958. The median patient age was 15 years, and the series included two female patients thought to have JA. Most patients were treated with primary radiation (42 of 55) and the remaining patients were treated for a recurrence after surgery. Radiation was delivered with conventional two-dimensional planning and the prescription dose ranged from 30 to 35 Gy delivered over 14–16 fractions. Local control was achieved in 44 of 55 patients (80 %) and previous surgical resection had no effect on the potential for local control. Tumor regression was noted to be a slow process and at 12 months nearly 50 % of patients had an identifiable mass on examination. For patients with follow-up that included regular CT imaging, 6 of 22 had residual masses seen 3–15 years after radiation therapy. A biopsy of one of the masses 2 years after radiation showed only fibrous tissue. The most common acute side effect of radiation therapy was mucositis. Late complications included second tumor development in two patients. One patient developed a thyroid carcinoma and the other developed a basal cell carcinoma of the skin. Two patients developed cataracts after radiation therapy and one patient developed panhypopituitarism [10].

Two published reports suggest that radiation therapy doses of 36 Gy or higher improve expected local control of JA. Amdur and colleagues reported the outcomes of 24 patients treated for JA between 1975 and 2006 [1]. Patients were treated with radiation after incomplete resection (13 %) or for recurrence (55 %) with a median dose of 30 Gy. Most patients (88 %) had undergone an endovascular embolization procedure either before the initial surgery or to control bleeding before radiation therapy. The rate of local recurrence was 17 % and all of the recurrences occurred within the middle of the radiation field. There appeared to be a dose response for tumor control. The local control rate was 91 % for patients treated to 36 Gy, whereas it was 77 % for patients treated to 30 Gy or less. The four patients with local failure were successfully salvaged by surgical resection. Grade 3 complications occurred in two patients who developed ocular cataracts that required surgery. McGahan

Table 18.3 Fractionated radiation therapy results for juvenile angiofibroma

Study	No. of pts	Therapy	RT dose	Median F/U	Local recurrences	Late complications
Amdur et al. 2011 (University of Florida) [1]	24	3D conformal or IMRT or conventional	30–36 Gy at 1.8 Gy/fx	Median 18 years	4/22 (18 %)	Two patients had cataract formation
Kuppersmith et al. 2000 (Baylor University) [2]	3	IMRT	34–45 Gy at 1.8–2 Gy/fx	6–40 months	0/3	One patient experienced chronic rhinitis
Lee at al. 2002 (University of California, Los Angeles) [3]	27	3D conformal or conventional	30–55 Gy at 1.8 Gy/fx	6–17 years	4/27 (15 %)	One patient, growth retardation; one patient, panhypopituitarism; one patient, cataract formation; one patient, experienced brain necrosis, seizure, and keratopathy leading to orbital exenteration
Mallick et al. 2015 (AIIMS New Delhi) [4]	20	3D conformal or conventional	30–45 Gy at 1.8–2 Gy/f	Median 36 months	3/31 (9.7 %)	None
Chakraborty et al. 2012 (PGIMER Chandigarh, India) [37]	8	3D conformal or IMRT or conventional	30–46 Gy at 1.5–2 Gy per fraction	Median 17 months	1/8 (13 %)	One patient experienced chronic rhinitis
Fields et al. 1990 (Mallinckrodt Institute) [38]	13	3D conformal or conventional	36–52 Gy at 1.8–2 Gy/fx	Median 136 months	2/13 (15 %)	Xerostomia and dental caries
Cummings et al. 1984 (Princess Margaret) [10]	55	Conventional	30–35 Gy at 2–2.2 Gy/fx	3–26 years	11/55 (20 %)	Two patients developed second head and neck tumors

(continued)

Table 18.3 (continued)

Study	No. of pts	Therapy	RT dose	Median F/U	Local recurrences	Late complications
Wiatrak et al. 1993 (University of Michigan) [12]	3	Conventional	36.6–50.4 Gy at 1.8–2 Gy/fx	1.8–5 years	0/3	None
McGahan et al. 1981 (Baylor University) [5]	1	Conventional or 3D conformal	32–46 at 2 Gy per fraction	1.5–13 years	4/14 (27 %)	None

Abbreviations: *3D* three-dimensional, *F/U* follow-up, *fx* fraction, *IMRT* intensity-modulated radiation therapy reported on 14 patients with JA managed with radiation therapy [5]. Eleven of 14 were managed with radiation for a local recurrence after surgery and the remaining patients were treated with primary radiation therapy. Radiation therapy doses ranged from 32 to 46 Gy at 2 Gy per fraction. Four of 14 (29 %) patients experienced a local failure. All four patients who were treated to 32 Gy or less failed locally, while each patient treated to 36–46 Gy achieved local control with follow-up ranging from 1.5 to 13 years [5]. No late complications were reported at any dose level.

A study by Lee et al. [3] recently demonstrated excellent local control rates after radiation therapy for locally advanced JA. The authors reported the results of 27 patients treated with fractionated radiation therapy at University of California, Los Angeles, between 1960 and 2000. Twenty-three of 27 patients had intracranial extension of JA at the time of diagnosis. Surgical resection was not attempted before radiation therapy. The mean follow-up was 6 years. Radiation therapy was delivered either with 3D conformal radiation therapy or conventional therapy using a cobalt-60 unit. Radiation doses ranged between 30 and 50 Gy delivered at 1.8–2 Gy per fraction. Four of the 27 patients developed a local recurrence and the time to recurrence ranged between 2 and 5 years. All four patients were treated with salvage therapy. Two patients were managed with surgical resection. One patient with negative margins was noted to be tumor-free 12 months after salvage surgery. The second patient recurred after surgery and received re-irradiation to 45 Gy, which provided local control during the 7 years of follow-up. The other two local recurrences were managed with re-irradiation to 20 Gy and 36 Gy, and both patients achieved local control with 2 and 7 years of follow-up, respectively. A few serious complications occurred after treatment in this series and they included panhypopituitarism, growth retardation, and cataract formation. The most serious complication occurred after re-irradiation for locally recurrent tumor. The patient developed symptomatic brain necrosis, seizure, and keratopathy that led to orbital exenteration. Although re-irradiation appears to provide local control, it should be delivered cautiously and only when surgical resection is not feasible.

Malignant transformation after fractionated radiation therapy has been reported although it appears to be a rare outcome and potentially associated with high cumulative doses of radiation therapy. Makek et al. [31] reported on a 15-year-old male treated for JA. The patient had a transpalatal resection at the time of diagnosis, but he developed locally recurrent disease 17 years later. He underwent a second resection and the tumor was confirmed to be nasopharyngeal angiofibroma once again. He recurred again 3 months later and then underwent radiation therapy to 45 Gy delivered with conventional fractionation. Over the next 5 years, he underwent two more salvage surgeries and each histologic evaluation confirmed recurrent JA. After the fourth surgical procedure, he underwent re-irradiation to 40.5 Gy. Two years later, the tumor recurred in his nasal vestibule and this was confirmed to be fibrosarcoma. Chen et al. [32] reported on a 48-year-old man with JA involving the left nasal cavity who was treated with 66 Gy using conventionally fractionated radiation therapy. The patient showed no signs of recurrence until 12 years later when he developed a tumor in the left maxillary sinus that was confirmed to be a fibrosarcoma at the time of surgical resection. A similar case published by Batsakis et al.

[33] reported on a 48-year-old man treated with 90 Gy of radiation therapy for a JA of the nasal cavity; after 5 years of follow-up, a locally recurrent tumor was found and confirmed to be fibrosarcoma at the time of surgical salvage. Although these cases demonstrate that radiation therapy can potentially lead to malignant degeneration of JA, in each case the prescribed dose was much higher than currently recommended doses [31–33]. Furthermore, there have been cases of JA transforming to fibrosarcoma in patients without a history of radiation therapy, which suggests that malignant transformation may be a characteristic of recurrent JA as opposed to a complication following moderate-dose radiation therapy [34, 35].

Stereotactic Radiosurgery

The reported experience with SRS in the management of JA is limited and summarized in Table 18.4. Dare et al. [27] reported the outcomes of two patients with JA treated with single-fraction SRS. The first patient was an 18-year-old male initially treated with a craniofacial resection for JA that involved the left nasal cavity, nasopharynx, orbit, and cavernous sinus. Postoperatively, he had residual disease in the left cavernous sinus that measured approximately 3.0 cm^3. The residual tumor was treated to 20 Gy in a single fraction using Gamma Knife SRS. After 2 years of follow-up, the patient had no evidence of recurrent tumor or of a serious complication. The second patient was initially treated with a lateral rhinotomy and resection for JA involving the right nasal cavity, nasopharynx, and infratemporal fossa. Residual tumor was present after surgery in the infratemporal fossa and it was treated with 20 Gy using single-fraction SRS. After 2 years of follow-up, no signs of tumor recurrence or complication were found [27]. Park et al. [28] reported results of SRS in a 48-year-old patient treated for JA. The patient was initially treated with surgical resection for JA involving the right orbit. Four years after surgical resection, he recurred locally within the same orbit. He was treated with single-fraction SRS to 17 Gy using Gamma Knife SRS. After 4 years of follow-up, no signs of recurrent disease or serious complication were noted [28]. These cases and the extensive use of SRS for other skull base tumors suggest that further study is warranted regarding SRS for locally advanced or recurrent JA [25].

Posttreatment Surveillance

We recommend close clinical follow-up and serial imaging after completion of therapy. A follow-up clinical examination including nasopharyngoscopy and MRI should be performed at 3 months after completing radiation therapy and every 6 months thereafter for 5 years. MRI should be performed in follow-up in lieu of CT to reduce the patient's cumulative radiation exposure [1]. After definitive radiation

Table 18.4 Stereotactic radiation surgery results for juvenile angiofibroma

Study	No. of pts	Therapy	Tumor location	RT dose	Median follow-up	Local recurrences	Late complications
Dare et al. 2002 (University of Buffalo) [27]	2	SRS using Gamma Knife	Right nasal cavity; right cavernous sinus	20 Gy in 1 fraction	2 years	0/2	None
Park et al. 2000 (Seoul National University) [28]	1	SRS using Gamma Knife	Right orbit	17 Gy in 1 fraction	4 years	No local recurrence	None
Min at al. 2014 (Severance Hospital, Seoul Korea) [29]	1	SRS using Gamma Knife	Right nasal cavity	40 Gy maximum dose in 1 fraction	4 years	No local recurrence	CSF leak 4 years after treatment
Deguchi et al. 2002 (Kagoshima University, Japan) [30]	1	SRS using Cyberknife	Nasal cavity and nasopharynx	45 Gy maximum dose in 3 fractions	2 years	No local recurrence	None

Abbreviations: *RT* radiation therapy, *SRS* stereotactic radiosurgery, *CSF* cerebrospinal fluid leak

therapy, residual masses seen on physical examination or MRI may remain visible for several years [1, 10, 36]. Biopsy is not recommended unless tumor growth is noted or if clinical symptoms reappear. The remnants of JA following radiation therapy may remain stable in size and morphology, but they typically decrease in volume by 50 % or more [10, 36]. Spontaneous resolution of these masses is possible after puberty [7]. An example of the tumor response seen after fractionated radiation is provided in Fig. 18.5.

Increased signal intensity on T2-weighted images at the initial site of disease tends to occur over time, suggesting that part of the response to radiation therapy is fibrotic [36]. A complete radiographic response is not necessarily predictive for ultimate local control. Patients with a complete response to radiation therapy can subsequently recur locally [1].

If the patient shows no signs of tumor regrowth into his or her second or third decade of life, recurrence is very unlikely. Nevertheless, the goal should be to strive for long-term clinical follow-up since the risk for late complications after radiation therapy increases with time. In general, we recommend continuing follow-up indefinitely with scheduled visits every 5 years and with a focus on monitoring for second tumor development [1, 37, 38].

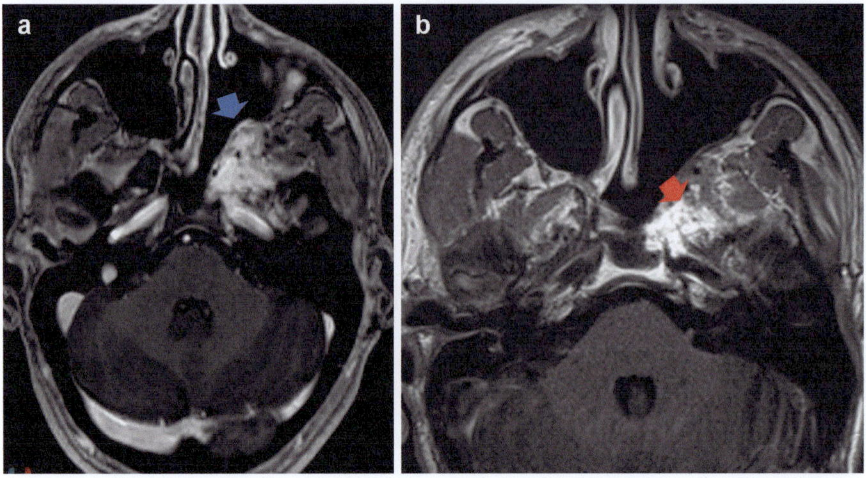

Fig. 18.5 Pre- and postradiation therapy imaging. Young male treated with radiation therapy for locally recurrent JA after surgical resection. (**a**) The pre-radiation therapy T1 contrast-enhanced MRI shows an enhancing mass involving the left nasopharynx and extending into the left pterygopalatine fossa (*blue arrow*). (**b**) Two years later, the postradiation therapy contrast-enhanced T1-weighted MRI showed a significant reduction in the size of the mass but with a small remnant of residual enhancing tissue (*red arrow*) involving the left nasopharynx. The patient was asymptomatic at this time and observation was recommended. The patient remains disease-free 4 years after radiation therapy

References

1. Amdur RJ, Yeung AR, Fitzgerald BM, Mancuso AA, Werning JW, Mendenhall WM. Radiotherapy for juvenile nasopharyngeal angiofibroma. Pract Radiat Oncol. 2011;1:271–8.
2. Kuppersmith RB, Teh BS, Donovan DT, Mai WY, Chiu JK, Woo SY, et al. The use of intensity modulated radiotherapy for the treatment of extensive and recurrent juvenile angiofibroma. Int J Pediatr Otorhinolaryngol. 2000;52:261–8.
3. Lee JT, Chen P, Safa A, Juillard G, Calcaterra TC. The role of radiation in the treatment of advanced juvenile angiofibroma. Laryngoscope. 2002;112(7 Pt 1):1213–20.
4. Mallick S, Benson R, Bhasker S, Mohanti BK. Long-term treatment outcomes of juvenile nasopharyngeal angiofibroma treated with radiotherapy. Acta Otorhinolaryngol Ital. 2015;35:75–9.
5. McGahan RA, Durrance FY, Parke Jr RB, Easley JD, Chou JL. The treatment of advanced juvenile nasopharyngeal angiofibroma. Int J Radiat Oncol Biol Phys. 1989;17:1067–72.
6. Schiff M. Juvenile nasopharyngeal angiofibroma. A theory of pathogenesis. Trans Am Laryngol Rhinol Otol Soc. 1959;1959:791–826.
7. Million RR, Cassisi NJ. Management of head and neck cancer: a multidisciplinary approach. 2nd ed. 1994. Lippincott Williams and Wilkins. Philadelphia, PA p. 627–41.
8. Neel 3rd HB, Whicker JH, Devine KD, Weiland LH. Juvenile angiofibroma. Review of 120 cases. Am J Surg. 1973;126:547–56.
9. Snyderman CH, Pant H, Carrau RL, Gardner P. A new endoscopic staging system for angiofibromas. Arch Otolaryngol Head Neck Surg. 2010;136:588–94.

10. Cummings BJ, Blend R, Keane T, Fitzpatrick P, Beale F, Clark R, et al. Primary radiation therapy for juvenile nasopharyngeal angiofibroma. Laryngoscope. 1984;94(12 Pt 1):1599–605.
11. Tyagi I, Syal R, Goyal A. Staging and surgical approaches in large juvenile angiofibroma – study of 95 cases. Int J Pediatr Otorhinolaryngol. 2006;70:1619–27.
12. Wiatrak BJ, Koopmann CF, Turrisi AT. Radiation therapy as an alternative to surgery in the management of intracranial juvenile nasopharyngeal angiofibroma. Int J Pediatr Otorhinolaryngol. 1993;28:51–61.
13. Andrews JC, Fisch U, Valavanis A, Aeppli U, Makek MS. The surgical management of extensive nasopharyngeal angiofibromas with the infratemporal fossa approach. Laryngoscope. 1989;99:429–37.
14. Radkowski D, McGill T, Healy GB, Ohlms L, Jones DT. Angiofibroma. Changes in staging and treatment. Arch Otolaryngol Head Neck Surg. 1996;122:122–9.
15. Chandler JR, Goulding R, Moskowitz L, Quencer RM. Nasopharyngeal angiofibromas: staging and management. Ann Otol Rhinol Laryngol. 1984;93(4 Pt 1):322–9.
16. Sessions RB, Bryan RN, Naclerio RM, Alford BR. Radiographic staging of juvenile angiofibroma. Head Neck Surg. 1981;3:279–83.
17. 4. Definition of volumes. J ICRU. 2010;10:41–53.
18. Mendenhall WM, Amdur RJ, Palta JR. Intensity-modulated radiotherapy in the standard management of head and neck cancer: promises and pitfalls. J Clin Oncol. 2006;24:2618–23.
19. Fung-Kee-Fung SD, Hackett R, Hales L, Warren G, Singh AK. A prospective trial of volumetric intensity-modulated arc therapy vs conventional intensity modulated radiation therapy in advanced head and neck cancer. World J Clin Oncol. 2012;3:57–62.
20. Ladra MM, Edgington SK, Mahajan A, Grosshans D, Szymonifka J, Khan F, et al. A dosimetric comparison of proton and intensity modulated radiation therapy in pediatric rhabdomyosarcoma patients enrolled on a prospective phase II proton study. Radiother Oncol. 2014;113:77–83.
21. Chung CS, Yock TI, Nelson K, Xu Y, Keating NL, Tarbell NJ. Incidence of second malignancies among patients treated with proton versus photon radiation. Int J Radiat Oncol Biol Phys. 2013;87:46–52.
22. Romesser PB, Cahlon O, Scher E, Zhou Y, Berry SL, Rybkin A, et al. Proton beam radiation therapy results in significantly reduced toxicity compared with intensity-modulated radiation therapy for head and neck tumors that require ipsilateral radiation. Radiother Oncol. 2016;118:286–92.
23. Mendenhall WM, Friedman WA, Amdur RJ, Antonelli PJ. Management of acoustic schwannoma. Am J Otolaryngol. 2004;25:38–47.
24. Ulm AJ, Friedman WA, Bova FJ, Bradshaw P, Amdur RJ, Mendenhall WM. Linear accelerator radiosurgery in the treatment of brain metastases. Neurosurgery. 2004;55:1076–85.
25. Scheick SM, Morris CG, Amdur RJ, Bova FJ, Friedman WA, Mendenhall WM. Long-term outcomes after radiosurgery for temporal bone paragangliomas. Am J Clin Oncol. 2015. http://www.ncbi.nlm.nih.gov/pubmed/26650779
26. Showalter TN, Werner-Wasik M, Curran Jr WJ, Friedman DP, Xu X, Andrews DW. Stereotactic radiosurgery and fractionated stereotactic radiotherapy for the treatment of nonacoustic cranial nerve schwannomas. Neurosurgery. 2008;63:734–40; discussion 40.
27. Dare AO, Gibbons KJ, Proulx GM, Fenstermaker RA. Resection followed by radiosurgery for advanced juvenile nasopharyngeal angiofibroma: report of two cases. Neurosurgery. 2003;52:1207–11; discussion 11.
28. Park CK, Kim DG, Paek SH, Chung HT, Jung HW. Recurrent juvenile nasopharyngeal angiofibroma treated with gamma knife surgery. J Korean Med Sci. 2006;21:773–7.
29. Min HJ, Chung HJ, Kim CH. Delayed cerebrospinal fluid rhinorrhea four years after gamma knife surgery for juvenile angiofibroma. J Craniofac Surg. 2014;25:e565–7.
30. Deguchi K, Fukuiwa T, Saito K, Kurono Y. Application of cyberknife for the treatment of juvenile nasopharyngeal angiofibroma: a case report. Auris Nasus Larynx. 2002;29:395–400.

31. Makek MS, Andrews JC, Fisch U. Malignant transformation of a nasopharyngeal angiofibroma. Laryngoscope. 1989;99(10 Pt 1):1088–92.
32. Chen KT, Bauer FW. Sarcomatous transformation of nasopharyngeal angiofibroma. Cancer. 1982;49:369–71.
33. Batsakis JG, Klopp CT, Newman W. Fibrosarcoma arising in a juvenile nasopharyngeal angiofibroma following extensive radiation therapy. Am Surg. 1955;21:786–93.
34. Donald PJ. Sarcomatous degeneration in a nasopharyngeal angiofibroma. Otolaryngol Head Neck Surg. 1979;87:42–6.
35. Allensworth JJ, Troob SH, Lanciault C, Andersen PE. High-grade malignant transformation of a radiation-naive nasopharyngeal angiofibroma. Head Neck. 2016;38:E2425–7.
36. Mancuso AA, Mendenhall WM, Vaysberg M. Nasopharynx: Juvenile Angiofibroma. In: Mancuso AA, Hanafee WN, editors. Philadelphia, PA. Head and Neck Radiology; 2010.
37. Chakraborty D, Bhattacharya A, Kamaleshwaran KK, Agrawal K, Gupta AK, Mittal BR. Single photon emission computed tomography/computed tomography of the skull in malignant otitis externa. Am J Otolaryngol. 2012;33:128–9.
38. Fields JN, Halverson KJ, Devineni VR, Simpson JR, Perez CA. Juvenile nasopharyngeal angiofibroma: efficacy of radiation therapy. Radiology. 1990;176:263–5.

Chapter 19
Adjuvant Chemotherapy and Hormonal Therapy

Alok Thakar

Abstract The near exclusivity of juvenile angiofibroma to adolescent and young adult males points to an obvious hormonal influence. Immunohistochemical evaluations on tumor specimens have demonstrated receptors to testosterone and other sex hormones. Treatment with the anti-testosterone agent flutamide is currently the most accepted and efficacious modality to bring about presurgical tumor reduction. Six-week treatment with oral flutamide has been documented to be effective in bringing about tumor volume shrinkage in the postpubertal population (mean 16 %, maximum 40 %), but is expectedly ineffective in the prepubertal population who have negligible circulating testosterone levels. Presurgical tumor volume reduction has the potential to enable tumor excision by a less invasive approach, to facilitate tumor dissection from vital nerves and vessels, and to limit surgical complications and blood loss.

Keywords Juvenile angiofibroma • Testosterone • Flutamide • Antiandrogen • Adjuvant treatment

Though we remain uncertain with regard to the exact tissue of origin of juvenile angiofibroma (JA), the near exclusivity of the tumor to males and its predominance in the adolescent years has pointed toward an obvious hormonal influence. It has been over 50 years since clinical reports demonstrated an increased tumor growth with testosterone and a regression with estrogens [1–3]. Diethylstilbestrol, an estrogen analogue, was therefore used to bring about tumor regression [2, 3], but did not find wide acceptance because of its feminizing effects on the young male patients. Further, it is not quite clear as to whether the effect of estrogen was by a direct action on the tumor or secondary to feedback inhibition on the pituitary and a consequent decrease in gonadotropin and testosterone levels.

Subsequent to this initial experience, multiple laboratory studies have since demonstrated receptors for androgen, estrogen, and progestogen on surgical specimens

A. Thakar, MS, FRCSEd
Department of Otolaryngology and Head-Neck Surgery, All India Institute of Medical Sciences, New Delhi 110029, India
e-mail: drathakar@gmail.com; drathakar.orlhns@aiims.edu

S.P. Dubey, B. Schick (eds.), *Juvenile Angiofibroma*,
DOI 10.1007/978-3-319-45343-9_19

of juvenile angiofibroma [4–10]. A clear picture of the hormonal receptors on the tumor has however not yet emerged as a wide variation is noted with regard to the detection of these receptors in different reported studies. Initial studies looking at hormonal receptors on the tumor may have suffered from technological limitations because of cross-reactivity between the different sex hormone receptors. Current investigations using monoclonal antibody-based techniques have demonstrated to the predominant presence of androgen receptors on JA [5–8]. These receptors are thermostable and can bind both dihydrotestosterone (DHT) and testosterone with a higher affinity toward DHT. In patients with familial adenomatous polyposis wherein an association has been noted with juvenile angiofibroma, it is proposed that an alteration of the adenomatous polyposis coli/β-catenin gene pathway may increase tumor androgen sensitivity [11]. Recently, the ER-b estrogen receptor has also been demonstrated in stromal pericytic and endothelial cells [9].

No alterations in the serum hormonal levels of any of the sex hormones have however been noted [12, 13].

Therapeutic Interventions Based on Hormone Manipulation

Surgical excision remains the primary treatment for juvenile angiofibroma. The demonstrated responsiveness of the tumor to hormonal manipulation and the understanding of various receptors on tumor tissue however open the door to using hormones and antihormone agents in an adjuvant setting with the intent to modify tumor growth.

Presurgical Hormone Therapy

Laboratory experiments have demonstrated that the growth rate of juvenile angiofibroma tumor fibroblasts in culture media increases with the addition of testosterone and is inhibited by the antiandrogens cyproterone acetate and flutamide [7]. Flutamide (2-methyl-n-[4-nitro-3{trifluoromethyl}phenyl] propanamide) is an orally active nonsteroidal androgen antagonist (NSAA). Unlike the previously used diethyl stilbestrol, flutamide is a pure antiandrogen compound and therefore causes no suppression of gonadotropin or testosterone levels [14]. Testosterone levels are rather increased with therapy [12, 14, 15]. The loss of libido and sexual potency noted with the previous therapies and any temporary feminizing effects are therefore very significantly decreased [14].

Flutamide is used mainly in the treatment of prostate cancer and benign prostatic hypertrophy (BPH). It is also recommended for use in adolescents and children for conditions such as congenital adrenal hyperplasia, hirsutism, and acne [16–19]. Common reported side effects include nausea and hepatotoxicity [14, 19]. The increased levels of gonadotropin lead to increased testicular production of testosterone and estrogen, and the increased estrogen levels may lead to mild breast tenderness and gynaecomastia with prolonged use [14, 19].

Clinical literature regarding the use of flutamide in juvenile angiofibroma is sparse and limited to 3 studies and 31 cases. Conflicting results were reported in the initial literature. Gates et al. [13] in 1992 observed an average tumor reduction of 44 % (maximum 62 %) in four of five cases receiving a 6-week treatment course. The remaining one of the five cases demonstrated tumor progression on the same treatment. All tumors were relatively small and pre- and posttreatment volume assessments were undertaken by CT scanning. Labra et al. [20] used flutamide for 3 weeks in six cases with advanced intracranially extending juvenile angiofibroma and noted much more modest responses with an average tumor reduction of only 7.2 % (maximum 11.1 %). Pre- and posttreatment volume assessments were again undertaken by CT scanning.

Thakar et al. [12] conducted a phase II, single-arm, before-after evaluation on 20 consecutive patients with advanced juvenile angiofibroma (Radkowski stages IIC and III) receiving a 6-week treatment course of flutamide (10 mg/kg in three divided doses, oral). Precise measurements of pre- and post-therapy tumor volumes were undertaken by MR imaging, with the reporting radiologist blinded to the pre-flutamide/post-flutamide status of the patient.

A significant variation in response was noted in the prepubertal and postpubertal groups. Prepubertal cases (with minimal testosterone levels) had inconsistent and minimal responses and 2/5 prepubertal patients demonstrated mild tumor progression while on treatment. No postpubertal patient demonstrated tumor progression, and 13/15 postpubertal cases demonstrated significant tumor volume reduction (mean volume reduction 16.5 %, maximum 40.1 %) (Fig. 19.1). Ten out of 15 patients had greater than 10 % reduction in tumor volume, and 5/15 patients had greater than 25 % reduction in tumor volume. Additionally, symptomatic improvements in nasal obstruction were also noted, and two cases with recent visual impairment secondary to optic nerve compression had documented improvements in visual acuity and visual fields (Fig. 19.2). In five cases, the reduction in tumor size led to the adoption of a more conservative surgical approach leading to the avoidance of a formal craniotomy in one and the avoidance of a facial incision in three.

The degree of tumor volume reduction was noted to correlate with serum androgen levels (Pearson's correlation coefficient $r=0.53$). A trend was noted for testosterone serum levels to rise with flutamide treatment, indicating to successful receptor blockade and consequent rise in serum levels brought about by the pituitary gonadotropin feedback loop. Testosterone levels returned to normal after cessation of treatment [12].

Transient breast tenderness was the only adverse event noted in five cases. No patient developed gynaecomastia with 6-week treatment. No alterations in liver or kidney functions were noted [12].

On the basis of the above reports, it is reasonable to use 6 weeks of flutamide for pretreatment volume reduction for all postpubertal patients with juvenile angiofibroma. Clinical response can be anticipated in both early and advanced tumors [12, 13]. Significant responses (>25 %) can be anticipated in about one-third of patients with obvious benefits in limiting surgical morbidity and probably blood

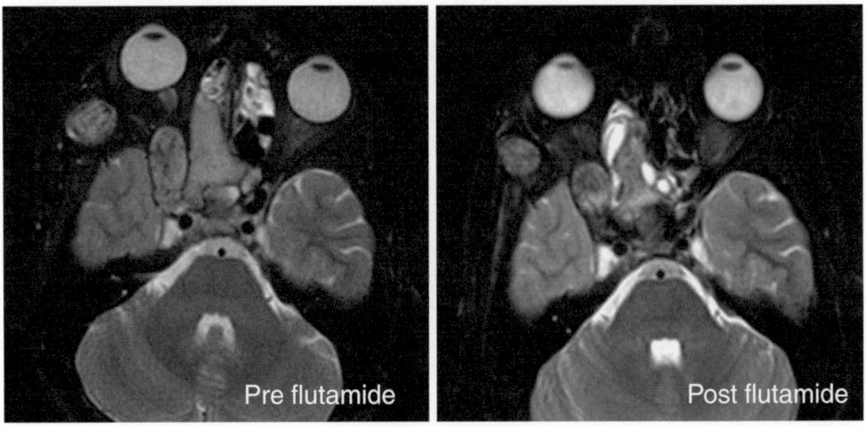

Fig. 19.1 Pre- and post-flutamide axial MR scans (stage IIIB disease, scans at level of the internal carotid artery, C3 lacerum segment). Post-flutamide tumor regression is noted in the temporal fossa, ethmoid-sphenoid, superior orbital fissure, and cavernous sinus areas. Post-flutamide the tumor is noted to regress away from the ICA and so enable surgical dissection at this area

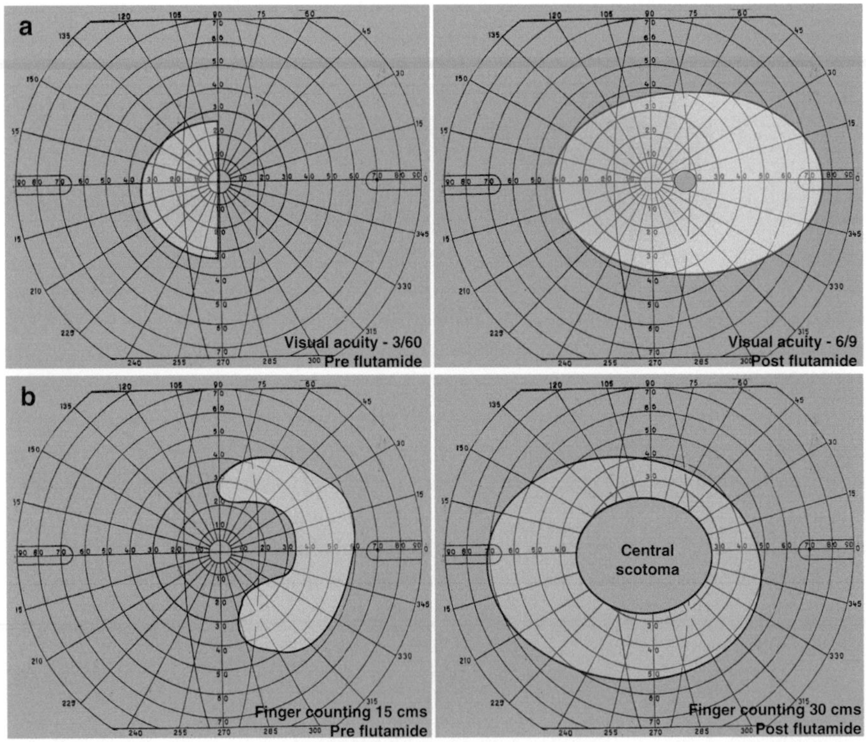

Fig. 19.2 (**a**, **b**) Demonstrating improvements in visual acuity and visual fields following flutamide therapy in two separate patients with visual loss

loss. Other patients who have milder degrees of response are also benefitted as even mild tumor regression can aid surgery by enhancing the surgical plane between the tumor and the surrounding tissues and so easing surgical dissection and facilitating tumor dissection from vital structures such as the dura and optic nerve.

The optimal duration of treatment remains not precisely defined. A treatment course of 3 weeks [20] seems less effective than treatment for 6 weeks [12, 13]. Treatment with 6 weeks at 10 mg/kg/day has been noted to be both efficacious [12, 13] and well tolerated. A further prolonged course of flutamide beyond 6 weeks has the potential to deliver even greater volume regression, but this is likely to be at the cost of increased feminizing side effects.

Postsurgical Hormone Therapy for Recurrent/Residual Juvenile Angiofibroma

High rates of recurrence have been noted with juvenile angiofibroma. The lack of a clear understanding of the tumor's tissue of origin, the unencapsulated nature of the tumor on histology, and also its propensity to invade the cancellous bone and the vidian canal are all attributed as reasons for microscopic tumor residue following surgery [21, 22]. Improvements in imaging techniques have further enhanced the detection of small and asymptomatic residual tumors in the skull base. The natural history of such small residual tumors remains unclear, and there is debate as to whether a repeat surgical excision with its potential morbidity is appropriate in such situations with radiologically demonstrable but clinically asymptomatic and possibly nonprogressive tumor recurrences [23]. Surveillance with serial MR scans is recommended as one of the treatment options in this situation, with surgical excision recommended only in cases with documented progression. An uncertain tendency for decrease in tumor growth and tumor regression is speculated with patients advancing onto the third decade, and the occasional tumor regression and also complete spontaneous involution has been previously documented [24–27]. Such a tendency for regression and involution is however not constant and many tumors may show progression over follow-up.

One of the possibilities for therapeutic intervention in this scenario is to use antiandrogen treatment to inhibit growth of the residual tumor. Flutamide has been used similarly in patients with metastatic prostatic cancer with the intent of blocking the androgenic growth stimulus to the tumor. This experience with prolonged androgen receptor blockade by flutamide has however been noted to lead to gynaecomastia and some regression of secondary sexual characteristics [14, 19]. Such an effect is often acceptable in the elderly cohort with metastatic prostatic cancer, but would not be acceptable in the young males with juvenile angiofibroma.

Nonhormonal Systemic Interventions

Systemic chemotherapy has been used previously and has been noted to bring about volume reduction in juvenile angiofibroma. The agents used include doxorubicin, vincristine, dactinomycin, cyclophosphamide, adriamycin, and dacarbazine [28, 29]. Such treatments with their attendant toxicity and risks are however not likely to find a place in contemporary practice, wherein they would generally be deemed as unsafe to use for a benign tumor with an uncertain growth potential such as JA.

An improving understanding of the hormonal receptors on the tumor opens up further possibilities of tumor growth modification in this above scenario. Other than receptors for androgen, estrogen, and progesterone, current literature also notes of the role of vascular endothelial growth factor (VEGF), transforming growth factor (TGF β1), basic fibroblast growth factor, platelet-derived growth factor (PDGF), and insulin-like growth factors (IGFs) in the growth of these tumors. It has been proposed that inhibition of these factors may find a therapeutic role in the near future [30].

VEGF expression on JA has recently been noted to be near-universal [31, 32] and offers a potential target for tumor growth inhibition by the well-established anti-VEGF monoclonal antibody – bevacuzimab. Glucocorticoids have demonstrated in vitro activity on JA tissue culture toward reducing microvascular density, reducing tumor volume, and downregulating VEGF expression [33]. Tissue culture experiments have also demonstrated an antiproliferative effect of tamoxifen [10]. Other targets which are speculated to have potential include the mTOR inhibitors (sirolimus/rapamycin) and perhaps beta-blockers which may exert an anti-vasoproliferative effect similar to the effect noted in proliferative haemangiomas [34]. None of these agents have however yet made the transition from "bench to bedside," and none has been tested for clinical efficacy. It is possible that, similar to the situation with flutamide, long-term use of many of these agents could well be restricted by toxicity considerations and cost considerations.

Conclusions

On current evidence, the authors advocate a 6-week course of flutamide as adjuvant therapy in the postpubertal patient, so as to bring about presurgical volume shrinkage. A further prolongation of treatment would be expected to be additionally effective but may run the risk of leading to gynaecomastia. Prepubertal patients are not expected to benefit from this therapy.

References

1. Johnson S, Kloster J, Schiff M. The action of hormones on juvenile nasopharyngeal angiofibroma. A case report. Acta Otolaryngol (Stockh). 1966;61:153–60.
2. Martin H, Ehrlich H, Ables J. Juvenile nasopharyngeal angiofibroma. Ann Surg. 1948;127:513–36.
3. Schiff M. Juvenile nasopharyngeal angiofibroma- a theory of pathogenesis. Laryngoscope. 1959;69:981–1016.
4. Brentani MM, Butugan O, Oshima CT, et al. Multiple steroid receptors in nasopharyngeal angiofibromas. Laryngoscope. 1989;99:398–401.
5. Hwang HC, Mills SE, Patterson K, Sown AM. Expression of androgen receptors in nasopharyngeal angiofibroma; an immunohistochemical study of 24 cases. Mod Pathol. 1998;11: 1122–6.
6. Farag MM, Ghanimah SE, Ragaie A, Saleem TH. Hormonal receptors in juvenile nasopharyngeal angiofibroma. Laryngoscope. 1987;97:208–11.
7. Hagen R, Romalo G, Sehwab B, Hoppe F, Schweikert H. Juvenile nasopharyngeal fibroma: androgen receptors and their significance for tumor growth. Laryngoscope. 1994;104: 1125–9.
8. Gatalica Z. Immunohistochemical analysis of steroid hormone receptors in nasopharyngeal angiofibromas. Cancer Lett. 1998;127:89–93.
9. Montag AG, Tretiakova M, Richardson M. Steroid hormone receptor expression in nasopharyngeal angiofibromas. Consistent expression of estrogen receptor beta. Am J Clin Pathol. 2006;125:832–7.
10. Schick B, Dlugaiczyk J, Wendler O. Expression of sex hormone receptors in juvenile angiofibromas and antiproliferative effects of receptor modulators. Head Neck. 2014;36:1596–603.
11. Valanzano R, Curia MC, Aceto G, et al. Genetic evidence that juvenile nasopharyngeal angiofibroma is an integral FAP tumor. Gut. 2005;54:1046–7.
12. Thakar A, Gupta G, Bhalla AS, Jain V, Sharma SC, Sharma R, Bahadur S, Deka RC. Adjuvant therapy with flutamide for presurgical volume reduction in juvenile nasopharyngeal angiofibroma. Head Neck. 2011;33:1747–53.
13. Gates GA, Rice DH, Koopmann CF, Schuller DE. Flutamide-induced regression of angiofibroma. Laryngoscope. 1992;102:641–4.
14. Chabner BA, Ryan DP, Paz-Ares L, et al. Antineoplastic agents. In: Hardman JG, Limbird LE, editors. Goodman and Gilman's the pharmacological basis of therapeutics. 10th ed. New York: McGraw-Hill publishers; 2001. p. 1389–459.
15. Kerrigan JR, Veldhuis JD, Rogol AD. Androgen-receptor blockade enhances pulsatile luteinizing hormone production in late pubertal males: evidence for a hypothalamic site of physiologic androgen feedback action. Pediatr Res. 1994;35:102–6.
16. Muderris BF, Guven M. A prospective, randomized trial comparing flutamide (250 mg/d) and finasteride (5 mg/d) in the treatment of hirsutism. Fertil Steril. 2000;73:984–7.
17. Thiboutot D, Chen W. Update and future of hormonal therapy in acne. Dermatology. 2003;206:57–67.
18. Merke DP, Keil MF, Jones JV, Fields J, Hill S, Cutler Jr GB. Flutamide, testolactone, and reduced hydrocortisone dose maintain normal growth velocity and bone maturation despite elevated androgen levels in children with congenital adrenal hyperplasia. J Clin Endocrinol Metab. 2000;85:1114–20.
19. Chu E, Sartorelli AC. Cancer chemotherapy. In: Katzung BG, editor. Basic and clinical pharmacology. 10th ed. New York: McGraw- Hill publishers; 2006. p. 878–907.
20. Labra A, Chavolla-Magaña R, Lopez-Ugalde A, Alanis-Calderon J, Huerta-Delgado A. Flutamide as a preoperative treatment in juvenile angiofibroma with intracranial invasion. Otolaryngol Head Neck Surg. 2004;130:466–9.
21. Howard DJ, Lloyd G, Lund V. Recurrence and its avoidance in juvenile angiofibroma. Laryngoscope. 2001;111:1509–11.

22. Thakar A, Hota A, Bhalla AS, Gupta SD, Sarkar C, Kumar R. Overt and occult Vidian canal involvement in juvenile angiofibroma and its possible impact on recurrence. Head Neck. 2016;38:E421–5.
23. Marshall AH, Bradley PJ. Management dilemmas in the treatment and follow-up of advanced JNA (review). ORL. 2006;68:273–8.
24. Spielmann PM, Adamson R, Cheng K, Sanderson RJ. Juvenile nasopharyngeal angiofibroma: spontaneous resolution. Ear Nose Throat J. 2008;87:521–3.
25. Weprin LS, Siemers PT. Spontaneous regression of juvenile nasopharyngeal angiofibroma. Arch Otolaryngol Head Neck Surg. 1991;117:796–9.
26. Dohar JE, Duvall AJ. Spontaneous regression of juvenile nasopharyngeal angiofibroma. Ann Otol Rhinol Laryngol. 1992;101:469–71.
27. Gullane PJ, Dacidson J, O'Dwyer T, Forte V. Juvenile angiofibroma: a review of the literature and a case series report. Laryngoscope. 1992;102:928–33.
28. Goepfert H, Cangir A, Lee YY. Chemotherapy for aggressive juvenile nasopharyngeal angiofibroma. Arch Otolaryngol. 1985;111:285–9.
29. Schick B, Kahle G, Hassler R, et al. Chemotherapy of juvenile angiofibroma—an alternative? HNO. 1996;44:148–52.
30. Daniel W, Scholfield DW, Brundler M, McDermott A, Mussai F, Kearns P. Adjunctive treatment in juvenile nasopharyngeal angiofibroma: how should we approach recurrence? J Pediatr Hematol Oncol. 2016;38:235–9.
31. Saylam G, Yu¨cel OT, Sungur A, et al. Proliferation, angiogenesis and hormonal markers in juvenile nasopharyngeal angiofibroma. Int J Pediatr Otorhinolaryngol. 2006;70:227–34.
32. Hota A, Sarkar C, Gupta SD, Kumar R, Bhalla AS, Thakar A. Expression of vascular endothelial growth factor in juvenile angiofibroma. Int J Pediatr Otorhinolaryngol. 2015;79:900–2.
33. Wendler O, Dlugaiczyk J, Birk S, et al. Anti-proliferative effect of glucocorticoids on mesenchymal cells in juvenile angiofibromas. Head Neck. 2012;34:1615–21.
34. Margolin JF, Soni HM, Pimpalwar S. Medical therapy for pediatric vascular anomalies. Semin Plast Surg. 2014;28:79–86.

Part IV
Other Issues

Chapter 20
Recurrence of Juvenile Angiofibroma and its Prevention

José F. Carrillo, Liliana C. Carrillo, and Margarita C. Ramirez-Ortega

Abstract At present, the treatment of choice for juvenile angiofibroma (JA) is surgery, which has evolved to endoscopic approaches, performed at referral centers.

The epicenter of JA is located in the sphenopalatine foramen, and its patterns of extension are medial and lateral, complicated due to the deep location of the structures involved and close proximity to critical vascular and neural elements.

These facts frequently predispose to incomplete tumor resection and disease recurrence, especially in advanced stages and extensive lateral invasion patterns (INCan stage IIB and more advanced). The majority of series report a mean recurrence rate of 35 %, mostly in advanced stages.

Several prognostic factors have been described that predispose to recurrence, in addition to advanced stages and extensive lateral dissemination in the central skull base. These additional factors include blood loss, tumor size, surgical margins, the expertise of the surgical team – the latter closely related with a rational application of endoscopic approaches for resection – and nonsurgical treatment.

Consequently, a rational design of the treatment strategy should be performed from the first surgical attempt, based on surgical expertise, comprising the use of endoscopy in medial and minor lateral extensions, and the utilization of open surgical approaches such as osteoplastic maxillotomy (medial and anterolateral), according to the major invasion of tumors. In very advanced cases, a maxillotomy or neuro-otological procedure (Fisch C), combined with an anterolateral and/or transtemporal neurosurgical approach, should be carried out. Radiotherapy is used for multiple recurrences and in major medial encasement of the cavernous sinus and carotid artery (INCan stage IVb).

J.F. Carrillo, MD (✉)
Departamento de Tumores de Cabeza y Cuello, Mexico, Mexico

Head and Neck Department, Instituto Nacional de Cancerología, Av. San Fernando 22, Deleg. Tlalpan, 14080 México, DF, Mexico
e-mail: josecarr@prodigy.net.mx

L.C. Carrillo, MD
Subdirección de Investigación Clínica, Mexico, Mexico

M.C. Ramirez-Ortega, PhD
Departamento de Farmacología, Instituto Nacional de Cardiología Ignacio Chávez, Mexico, Mexico

S.P. Dubey, B. Schick (eds.), *Juvenile Angiofibroma*,
DOI 10.1007/978-3-319-45343-9_20

Keywords Nasopharyngeal tumors • Nasopharyngeal angiofibroma • Angiofibroma surgery • Angiofibroma staging

Introduction

Juvenile angiofibroma (JA) is a rare vascular lesion that presents in young males aged within the range of 12–35 years, and whose incidence is 0.05–0.5 % of all head and neck neoplasms [1, 2].

These tumors originate from the posterolateral wall of the roof of the nose, where the pterygoid process of the sphenoid bone and the sphenoid process of the palatine bone constitute the sphenopalatine foramen [2]. From there, several patterns of extension occur, mainly toward the nasopharynx, and give rise to signs and symptoms that frequently produce confusion for the non-aware clinician [2, 3]. The most frequent presentation of these patients is with a nasal mass and bleeding, which can be misdiagnosed as a nasal polyp, a hypertrophic turbinate, or as maxillary and nasopharyngeal neoplasms. The low frequency of presentation of this entity, its deep epicenter location and origin, and its patterns of anatomic extension into the skull base and ethmoidomaxillary structures compel the treating physician to acquire an integrated understanding of these concepts in order to offer the best treatment strategy and surgical approach, with the latter providing the best outcome and long-term quality of life (QOL) in this young population [4].

Unfortunately, experience and efficiency with the management of these benign lesions are limited in the majority of centers throughout the world, although multiple case reports and small cohort series exist in the literature [3, 5]. Adding to these hindrances with regard to JA treatment, several staging systems have been published, which reflect the progressive and evolving understanding on real patterns of extension, its significance, and real outcomes to be expected [6, 7]. The acquisition of novel, conservative surgical approaches, and the impressive results obtained by several groups of exceptionally skilled surgeons in selected cases contribute some confusion concerning the surgical approach to be applied in each particular case.

This latter issue is especially important, due to the recurrence rate reported to date for these tumors, which ranges from 3 to 35 % in some series [8]. In addition to this, some authors report case series in which the residual tumor is left in place to preserve vascular and neural structures, and the regression of lesions is described in an anecdotal manner [8, 9].

Thus, it is imperative for surgeons involved in the treatment of these neoplasms, in addition to a deep understanding of skull base anatomy, staging systems in evolution, and new open and endoscopic surgical techniques, to develop an adequate clinical and imaging method to detect tumor persistence in the postoperative short-term (or posttreatment) period and tumor recurrences.

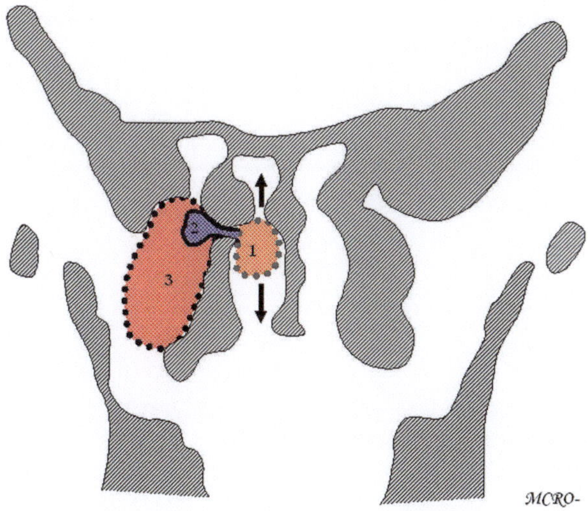

Fig. 20.1 Computed tomography (CT) coronal view diagram showing extension patterns of juvenile angiofibroma. Number *1* and *arrows* correspond to medial and anterior skull base invasion, number *2* to pterygomaxillary fissure extension, and number *3* to infratemporal fossa extensions and skull base invasion (Reprinted with permission from Copyright Elsevier. *Eur J of Surg Oncol.* Carrillo et al. [4])

Definition and Location of Recurrences

Residual disease is defined as disease detected clinically endoscopically in the immediate postoperative period or with imaging studies. Recurrence is defined as tumor lesion detected after negative, postoperative clinical and imaging evaluation and at a 6-month follow-up [7, 10].

Because no single individual author or institution has reported a sufficiently large cohort series [5], the majority of reports focuses on surgical approaches and frequencies and do not specifically address the epicenter of recurrences. However, reports from our institution and others [11, 12], which treat a fair amount of patients referred from other surgical centers, have observed that the majority of frequencies occur in the basisphenoid and sphenoid sinus (medial and lateral extension of primary lesion), root of pterygoids (lateral extension of primary tumors), roof of infratemporal fossa (major lateral extension of primary neoplasm, with invasion of vidian canal, foramen ovale, and lacerum), and cavernous sinus (especially in patients with medial cavernous carotid artery encasement). This is correlated with the patterns of extension already described by our group (Fig. 20.1) and has also been analyzed according to tumor size in our staging system, on which we will elaborate later (Tables 20.1 and 20.2).

Table 20.1 Multivariate analysis of factors associated to disease-free survival using the Cox Proportional Hazards Model ($p = 0.002$)

Prognostic factor	RR	*p*	95 % CI
INCan stages	–	0.078	–
INCan stages I–IIA	0.000	0.960	0.0–7.92
INCan stage IIB	0.185	0.033	0.039–0.870
INCan stage III	0.289	0.039	0.089–0.941
INCan stage IV[a]	1	–	–
Surgical margins	–	0.029	–
Negative surgical margins[a]	1	–	–
Positive surgical margins	2.962	0.194	0.576–15.234
No surgical resection	7.275	0.013	1.523–34.737

Reprinted with permission from John Wiley & Sons, Carrillo et al. [7]
RR risk ratios, *p* probability value, *CI* confidence intervals
[a]Reference category

Table 20.2 Proposed staging system definitions and stage-specific recurrence frequencies

Stage	Extension and size	Recurrence frequency (%)
I	Location in the nasopharynx, nasal fossae, maxillary antrum, anterior ethmoid cells, and sphenoid sinus	0/2 (0 %)
IIa	Invasion to pterygomaxillary fossae or infratemporal fossae anterior to pterygoid plates, with major diameter <6 cm	0/8 (0 %)
IIb	Invasion to pterygomaxillary fossae or infratemporal fossae anterior to pterygoid plates, with major diameter ≥6 cm	2/14 (14.3 %)
III	Invasion to infratemporal fossae posterior to pterygoid plates or posterior ethmoid cells	5/12 (41.7 %)
IV	Extensive skull base invasion >2 cm or intracranial invasion	11/18 (61.1 %)

Reprinted with permission from John Wiley & Sons. Carrillo et al. [7]

Prognostic Factors Related with Recurrence

Several prognostic factors have been related with recurrences, which include age, residual vascularity after carotid artery embolization, extension patterns, tumor size, blood loss, stage, surgical margins, endoscopic and open approaches, and surgical and nonsurgical therapy, specifically radiation therapy [8, 13].

Age has been described in very few reports [3, 10], indicating that younger ages (mean age, 14 years) present higher recurrence frequency. This, to our knowledge, has not been reproduced in other groups of patients.

Residual vascularity after preoperative embolization as well has been described by some authors [10]. However, this has not been validated or supported by multivariate analyses and has been explored only in more advanced-stage cases, and their performance is feasible in patients subjected to preoperative angiography embolization [14]. Despite these facts, it has been repeatedly reported that preoperative embolization decreases blood loss, and probably, in an indirect manner, better exposure and a clear surgical field result in improved rates of clear resection and recurrences, on which we will also elaborate later.

Extension patterns comprise one of the most significant factors that exert an influence on recurrence, and their understanding is basic in defining strategy and undertaking minimally invasive [15], conservative, or open major surgical procedures [16]. This has been proven in bivariate and multivariate analyses [4]. Specifically, lateral extensions that have been divided into minor invasion toward the pterygomaxillary fissure, and those that invade the infratemporal fossa up to its roof or posterior to pterygoid plates have been found highly significant. Invasion to the orbit, as well as to skull base and its extension, and distinction of extradural extensive and intradural invasion [7] and to cavernous sinus should be considered for the design of the therapeutic strategy.

JA, as demonstrated in Fig. 20.1, also follows a longitudinal, vertical pattern of extension, with minimal lateral invasion in some cases, or lateral invasion to maxillary antrum, as has been defined previously [7, 17, 18]. These cases have been considered as the most adequate for tumor resection with endoscopic approaches, on which we will elaborate later.

Tumor size had not been described, to our knowledge, as being of major importance for recurrence until the analyses of our work group [4, 7], in which we demonstrated that a tumor size of ≥6 cm was determinant for recurrence, and on incorporating this factor into a novel staging system, recurrence reached statistical significance in multivariate analyses (Tables 20.1 and 20.2). Subsequently, reports appeared [19] to have explored the impact of tumor size in relation to recurrence and the selection of the surgical approach, finding significance only in bivariate analyses. Other authors, such as Carrau and Snyderman [10], point out the lack of tumor size significance in their study, but, to our knowledge, no real analyses or elaboration exist regarding this issue, although their study attempts to establish a new staging system and the endoscopic approach as the first choice for surgery in these neoplasms. It is clear, however, in very recent reports, that with the adoption of endoscopic procedures, tumor size is considered as increasingly important in the selection of a therapeutic strategy, especially by groups who intend to establish the endoscopic approach as first-choice surgical modality [19].

Blood loss is another factor that is recently being increasingly studied [20]. Because the mainstay of treatment is surgery in this neoplasm, a clear surgical field that encompasses all lesion extensions and reduced the chance of leaving tumor remnants is imperative. Within this context, in recent reports, the majority of authors note the need for performing preoperative embolization in order to obtain tumor shrinkage and a bloodless field [14]. These facts, although of utmost importance in all surgical approaches, have acquired special importance since the advent of endoscopic and conservative procedures, in which major bleeding and a consequently obscure surgical field with risk for morbidity, and even mortality, could indicate conversion to an open or more extensive procedure in an emergency situation, with a possible increase in recurrence rates.

Staging has been defined in several ancillary systems [17, 18, 21] according to known extension patterns at the time of the proposal of a specific classification, and

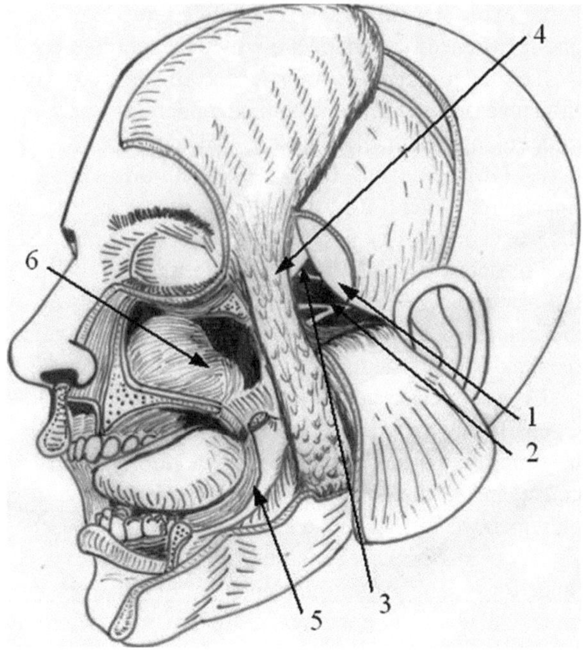

Fig. 20.2 Final development of anterolateral osteoplastic maxillotomy with drilling and dissection of roof of infratemporal fossa (minimal craniotomy has been performed). *1* Temporal lobe dura; *2* mandibular division of trigeminal nerve; *3* maxillary division of trigeminal nerve; *4* frontalis-cervico-parotid tissue, which envelops the frontalis branch of the facial nerve; *5* orbital floor; and *6* nasal septum (Reprinted with permission from Sage Publications. Carrillo et al. [16])

logically, the majority of these were incomplete. With knowledge of the real extension patterns, recurrence factors, and reports on recurrence epicenters, and with the need to define accurately the anatomic dissemination of these tumors due to the advent of novel endoscopic approaches, new classifications have been described [7, 10, 12], which attempt to aid in the design of therapy and, if indicated, in the selection of the most suitable surgical approach for a given tumor, according to the expertise of the surgical team. A balance between recurrence rates and QOL should be obtained with the help of future staging systems.

We think, based on our published work [4, 7, 11], that, at present, other factors, such as tumor size, should be considered in staging systems. We concur with other authors [10, 14] that vascularity and preoperative embolization could be included in staging systems in the future, specifically at more advanced stages. The National Institute of Cancerology Mexico (INCan) staging system proposed by our group [7] was compared with the Radkowski, Chandler, and Fisch systems [17, 18, 21]; our INCan system was found to define and predict better for recurrence rate. However, the evolution of surgical endoscopy and the increasing expertise and rational use of open procedures such as osteoplastic maxillotomy with low morbidity and good QOL (Fig. 20.2) [16], combined with neurosurgical approaches, when indicated, will decrease the recurrence rate and increase the QOL of patients with advanced tumors, which are those most frequently reported in the majority of series to date [5].

Another aim and virtue of any proposed classification – aside from better definition of therapeutic strategies, definition of surgical approaches, and aiding in results and peer communication – should be simplicity and logical grading of prognostic factors, especially in areas where therapy is found in a developmental state. We believe that the INCan classification [7] accomplishes this objective.

Our group has also demonstrated the significance of obtaining negative surgical margins in multivariate analyses [4, 7], an aspect that, although previously mentioned, has not been adequately analyzed in previous series.

A proposal has been made by Our group has defined a negative margin as no macroscopic residual tumor remaining after resection, confirmed with surgical bed histology, as well as when in follow-up and after complying the previous requirements, a suspicious residual tumor was observed in the CT scan or in magnetic resonance imaging (MRI) <0.5 cm in diameter, with no clinical translation or evidence of growth in subsequent imaging studies [7].

Recurrence is defined as a clinical or imaging study that demonstrated tumor presence in nasopharynx, nasal fossa, or neighboring structures, with confirmed growth accompanied by major symptoms including epistaxis, or nasal obstruction, or facial deformity after 6 months of follow-up of the initial treatment [4, 22, 23].

In spite of the previous considerations, there are reports and reviews that attempt to compare the recurrence rate according to the surgical technique employed, specifically endoscopic vs. open approaches [5]. The majority of these analyses consequently focus on early, medial extension tumors without adequate dissection or precise assessment of lateral extensions.

Moreover, some reports analyze another subset of surgical procedures: **endoscopic-assisted open approaches** [5], which some authors have considered an important addition to the surgical armamentarium for extensive lesions [24]. Given the previously described extension patterns and other prognostic factors such as tumor size, performance of preoperative embolization, as well as lesion stage, we think that these comparisons have added confusion to the already existent controversy on surgical approach and choice of therapeutic strategy. Logically, studies that aim for this comparison are biased, and endoscopic-assisted approaches are utilized most frequently in advanced stages, with no analyses of the expertise of surgical team members or the patient's recurrence history.

Additionally, the use of radiation therapy has also been compared with surgical endoscopic and open approaches. In a previous study conducted by our group [4], on multivariate analyses of prognostic factors, lack of surgery (treatment with radiation therapy alone) was found associated with a higher recurrence rate. Given the retrospective nature of our study, a selection bias existed for treating patients with less advanced tumors exclusively with surgery. Despite this, patients with extensive recurrence had post-radiation surgery with a 90 % salvage rate [4], which underscores the possible role of radiotherapy in very advanced cases.

Selection of Treatment Strategy to Prevent Recurrence

There is general consensus [8] that recurrence is principally associated with residual disease after surgical treatment. Consequently, prevention of residual disease is a major objective when designing the surgical approach.

Previous reports [7, 18] have found that tumor stage is the most important factor for recurrence, and, in recent reports, the feasibility of and the low morbidity existing for endoscopic approaches have been established [5]. These results have been achieved with a combination of expertise in endoscopic techniques, as well as adequate selection of the approach in tumors with predominant medial extension, medium-to-small size, few prior surgical procedures, and the employment of preoperative embolization.

However, in cases with medium-to-major lateral extensions, prior treatment (either surgical or with radiation therapy), tumor size ≥6 cm, and no preoperative embolization, the surgical approach of choice should consider an open procedure, especially at centers where endoscopic expertise is median to low.

In a recent paper by Huang [3] that evaluated 162 patients with JA, a comparison between endoscopic procedures and open surgical approaches was carried out for recurrences, and no difference in recurrence rate was found for patients in Radkowski stage IIB and higher. It is noteworthy that the open procedures described were transpalatal and medial maxillectomy by means of the degloving approach. Interestingly, and despite their results, the authors recommended endoscopic approaches for Radkowski stages I–IIB and only for select cases – which are equivalent to stages I and IIA in our system [7] – in more advanced stages. In extensive lesions (stages IIB and more advanced according to our system), our open methods differ from those described in this series, in that we use osteoplastic maxillotomy, either medial or anterolateral [16, 25], as modified by our group, combined as necessary with lateral and anterolateral skull base approaches (orbitozygomatic or transtemporal), with no recurrences reported in our last 20 cases [7].

Regarding major extensions (IVa and IVB in the INCan system) [7], alternative, open approaches that could be successful in obtaining negative surgical margins are those described by Fisch (infratemporal fossa approach type C) [26], especially regarding stage IVa, which refers to extensive skull base invasion with no intradural or cavernous sinus invasion. Patients with these latter structures affected (stage IVB), especially those with lateral invasion to cavernous sinus structures, are candidates for the same approach where extensive experience exists for neuro-otological procedures. Medial cavernous sinus invasion under these circumstances should be attempted by surgical teams with extensive expertise in neuro-otological approaches and endoscopic surgery.

Some patients in stages IIB and III (INCan system) at centers where endoscopic surgery expertise is high are candidates for a conservative, non-open approach. If doubt exists in the transoperative period on leaving residual tumor or if significant bleeding ensues, osteoplastic maxillotomy, either medial or lateral [16] according to preoperative extension, could be used, transforming the procedure into a combined endoscopic approach.

Surgery alone in advanced stages, as has been mentioned previously, has been reported with high recurrence rates, specifically due to residual tumor left in critical neural and vascular areas. Fagan et al. [27] reported a very high recurrence rate (37.5 %) in cases with extensive skull base and dural invasion. Tyagi et al. [28] reported a residual tumor rate of 84.6 % for patients with tumors with major invasion to the clivus, medial cavernous sinus extensions, and in patients with widened pterygoid fissure (Fisch stages III, IVA, and B). In INCan stages III and IV, radiation therapy has been employed as an alternative treatment, either to decrease the recurrence rate or the progression of the residual lesion when an R1 resection has been performed or even as primary treatment under special circumstances [29, 30]. Major criticisms to radiation include immediate morbidity, late sequelae for facial bones in a state of development, and the possibility of second malignancies. With the introduction of conformal radiotherapy techniques and intensity-modulated radiation (IMR) [30] and the consequent decrease in morbidity rates, radiation therapy has appeared again as a feasible treatment, usually administered in dosages 35–50 Gy.

For INCan stage IVB recurrent/persistent cases [30], conformal radiation is indicated, especially in rapidly growing lesions. In advanced stages IVA and IVB, when surgery is not feasible or when the possibility of residual lesion is not accepted by the patient, administration of up-front radiotherapy could be considered.

Recurrence Treatment and Prevention

An aphorism exists in tumor surgery, noting that the best way to prevent recurrences is the design of an adequate strategy and, consequently, efficient resection of the lesion from the very first procedure.

One issue of utmost importance and one not very often addressed is the expertise of the surgical team. As stated previously, juvenile angiofibroma is an infrequent lesion whose patterns of extension are complicated, which is consequently not easily understood by all head and neck surgeons. All reported series are plagued by recurrent lesions that have been already resected, which pose a formidable task for which surgery is not always feasible.

We think that endoscopy and open procedures, as described previously, are not easily mastered by surgical teams for these lesions and should be attempted at referral centers. Briefly, endoscopy should be consigned to lesions with minor lateral extensions (INCan stages I–IIA). Open procedures (such as medial osteoplastic maxillotomy and medial maxillectomy) should be reserved for INCan stages IIB and III. Skull base surgical neuro-otological procedures, osteoplastic maxillotomy, and neurosurgical approaches could be assigned to INCan stages III and IV. Stage IVB should be resected by highly expert surgical teams, especially when medial invasion to the cavernous sinus exists (probably combined with endoscopy). Otherwise, treatment of these lesions could be attempted with conformal radiotherapy up front.

On evaluating a recurrent tumor and the design of the surgical approach, we restage the lesion according to the INCan system [7] and follow same indications and approaches as stated in the previous paragraph for non-treated lesions. However, indications for endoscopic procedures are more stringent, and patients are counseled on the high probability of procedure conversion or a combination of endoscopic and open surgery. In cases with lateral invasion to the cavernous sinus, a cranio-orbitozygomatic approach combined with anterolateral osteoplastic maxillotomy is a must. We do not recommend resection of recurrences of medial cavernous sinus invasion due to the dense, fibrous adhesions produced by prior treatments, including radiotherapy. In asymptomatic patients with medium-to-small-sized tumors, we could adopt a conservative follow-up for 3–6 months. If tumor volume is small (<3 cm), Gamma Knife could be used. In cases of medial cavernous sinus invasion where no previous radiotherapy has been administered, conformal or intensity-modulated radiation therapy (IMRT) is indicated.

Aside from recurrence prevention with efficient surgery, follow-up is undertaken carefully to detect persistent lesions and recurrences in the following manner:

I. Clinical and endoscopic examination is performed at 3-month intervals during the first year after surgery, with the first imaging study performed at 10 weeks posttreatment. If minor suspicious lesions ≤2 cm in diameter are detected, follow-up continues unless tumor growth occurs at 6 months.
II. If involution or no growth occurs of the suspicious lesion detected, negative margins are considered.
III. If lesion growth occurs, surgical resection is attempted if feasible, according to the schema described previously. If lesions abut the medial cavernous sinus, or if the patient refuses surgery, radiotherapy could be attempted.

Conclusion

Juvenile angiofibroma is a vascular lesion that has a very high recurrence rate despite the establishment of new endoscopic techniques, which have provided a better QOL to patients afflicted by these tumors, especially in early stages. Unfortunately, unclear understanding of the extension of JA to skull base and inadequate selection of surgical strategies to treat these tumors constitute the main explanation for high recurrence frequency. Surgical procedures for the treatment of JA should be attempted by expert surgical teams, at referral centers, and especially endoscopy, because of the low frequency of the disease. Recurrent disease due to a poorly designed treatment strategy produces a significant decrease in the QOL of these young individuals.

References

1. Lund VJ, Stammberger H, Nicolai P, et al. European position paper on endoscopic management of tumours of the nose, paranasal sinuses and skull base. Rhinol Suppl. 2010;22:1–143.
2. Nicolai P, Schreiber A, Bolzoni Villaret A. Juvenile angiofibroma: evolution of management. Int J Pediatr. 2012;2012:412545.
3. Huang Y, Liu Z, Wang J, Sun X, Yang L, Wang D. Surgical management of juvenile nasopharyngeal angiofibroma: analysis of 162 cases from 1995 to 2012. Laryngoscope. 2014;124:1942–6.
4. Carrillo JF, Albores O, Ramírez-Ortega MC, Aiello-Crocifoglio V, Oñate-Ocaña LF. An audit of nasopharyngeal fibromas. Eur J Surg Oncol. 2007;33:655–61.

5. Boghani Z, Husain Q, Kanumuri VV, Khan MN, Sangvhi S, Liu JK, Eloy JA. Juvenile nasopharyngeal angiofibroma: a systematic review and comparison of endoscopic, endoscopic-assisted, and open resection in 1047 cases. Laryngoscope. 2013;123:859–69.
6. Alshaikh NA, Eleftheriadou A. Juvenile nasopharyngeal angiofibroma staging: an overview. Ear Nose Throat J. 2015;94:E12–22.
7. Carrillo JF, Maldonado F, Albores O, Ramírez-Ortega MC, Oñate-Ocaña LF. Juvenile nasopharyngeal angiofibroma: clinical factors associated with recurrence, and proposal of a staging system. J Surg Oncol. 2008;98:75–80.
8. Marshall AH, Bradley PJ. Management dilemmas in the treatment and follow-up of advanced juvenile nasopharyngeal angiofibroma. ORL J Otorhinolaryngol Relat Spec. 2006;68:273–8.
9. Önerci TM, Yücel ÖT, Ögretmenoglu O. Endoscopic surgery in treatment of juvenile nasopharyngeal angiofibroma. Int J Pediatr Otorhinolaryngol. 2003;67:1219–25.
10. Snyderman CH, Pant H, Carrau RL, Gardner P. A new endoscopic staging system for angiofibromas. Arch Otolaryngol Head Neck Surg. 2010;136:588–94.
11. Ochoa-Carrillo FJ, Carrillo JF, Frías M. Staging and treatment of nasopharyngeal angiofibroma. Eur Arch Otorhinolaryngol. 1997;254:200–4.
12. Onerci M, Oğretmenoğlu O, Yücel T. Juvenile nasopharyngeal angiofibroma: a revised staging system. Rhinology. 2006;44:39–45.
13. Leong SC. A systematic review of surgical outcomes for advanced juvenile nasopharyngeal angiofibroma with intracranial involvement. Laryngoscope. 2013;123:1125–31.
14. Lutz J, Holtmannspötter M, Flatz W, Meier-Bender A, Berghaus A, Brückmann H, Zengel P. Preoperative embolization to improve the surgical management and outcome of Juvenile Nasopharyngeal Angiofibroma (JNA) in a single center: 10-year experience. Clin Neuroradiol. 2015;29:1–9.
15. Nicolai P, Villaret AB, Farina D, Nadeau S, Yakirevitch A, Berlucchi M, Galtelli C. Endoscopic surgery for juvenile angiofibroma: a critical review of indications after 46 cases. Am J Rhinol Allergy. 2010;24:e67–72.
16. Carrillo JF, Celis MA, Ramírez-Ortega M, Rivas B, Ochoa FJ. Osteoplastic maxillotomy for treatment of neoplasms of the nasopharynx and infratemporal fossa. Ann Otol Rhinol Laryngol. 2005;114(1 Pt 1):58–64.
17. Chandler JR, Goulding R, Moskowitz L, Quencer RM. Nasopharyngeal angiofibromas: staging and management. Ann Otol Rhinol Laryngol. 1984;93:322–9.
18. Radkowski D, McGill T, Healy GB, Ohlms L, Jones DT. Angiofibroma. Changes in staging and treatment. Arch Otolaryngol Head Neck Surg. 1996;122:122–9.
19. Sun XC, Wang DH, Yu HP, Wang F, Wang W, Jiang JJ. Analysis of risk factors associated with recurrence of nasopharyngeal angiofibroma. J Otolaryngol Head Neck Surg. 2010;39:56–61.
20. Ye D, Shen Z, Wang G, Deng H, Qiu S, Zhang. Analysis of factors in successful nasal endoscopic resection of nasopharyngeal angiofibroma. Acta Otolaryngol. 2016;136:205–13.
21. Andrews JC, Fisch U, Valavanis A, Aeppli U, Makek MS. The surgical management of extensive nasopharyngeal angiofibromas with the infratemporal fossa approach. Laryngoscope. 1989;99:429–37.
22. Herman P, Lot G, Chapot R, Salvan D, Huy PT. Long-term follow-up of juvenile nasopharyngeal angiofibromas: analysis of recurrences. Laryngoscope. 1999;109:140–7.
23. Kasper ME, Parsons JT, Mancuso AA, et al. Radiation therapy for juvenile angiofibroma: evaluation by CT and MRI, analysis of tumor regression and selection of patients. Int J Radiat Oncol Biol Phys. 1993;25:689–94.
24. Sun XC, Li H, Liu ZF, Hu L, Yu HP, Wang JJ, Liu Q, Liu J, Wang DH. Endoscopic assisted sublabial and buccolabial incision approach for juvenile nasopharyngeal angiofibroma with extensive infratemporal fossa extension. Int J Pediatr Otorhinolaryngol. 2012;76:1501–6.
25. Catalano PJ, Biller HF. Extended osteoplastic maxillotomy. A versatile new procedure for wide access to the central skull base and infratemporal fossa. Arch Otolaryngol Head Neck Surg. 1993;119:394–400.

26. Fisch U. The infratemporal fossa approach for nasopharyngeal tumors. Laryngoscope. 1983;93:36–44.
27. Fagan JJ, Snyderman CH, Carrau RL, Janecka IP. Nasopharyngeal angiofibromas: selecting a surgical approach. Head Neck. 1997;19:391–9.
28. Tyagi I, Syal R, Goyal A. Recurrent and residual juvenile angiofibromas. J Laryngol Otol. 2007;121:460–7.
29. Reddy KA, Mendenhall WM, Amdur RJ, Stringer SP, Cassisi NJ. Long-term results of radiation therapy for juvenile nasopharyngeal angiofibroma. Am J Otolaryngol. 2001;22:172–5.
30. Mallick S, Benson R, Bhasker S, Mohanti BK. Long-term treatment outcomes of juvenile nasopharyngeal angiofibroma treated with radiotherapy. Acta Otorhinolaryngol Ital. 2015;35:75–9.

Chapter 21
Extranasopharyngeal Angiofibroma

Jochen P. Windfuhr

Abstract Angiofibromas in the head and neck area are acknowledged to originate from the superior aspect of the sphenopalatine foramen, typically presenting in male adolescents, and to grow with a highly predictable spreading pattern. They may also originate from or localized elsewhere than the nasopharynx, commonly labeled *extranasopharyngeal angiofibroma* (ENA). A review of the current literature indicates that the nasal septum is most commonly involved in the disease besides the maxillary sinus, inferior tubinate, ethmoid sinus, nasal cavity, and various other sites. ENA presents late ata median age of 23 years with a more balanced sex ratio compared to juvenile angiofibromas. Symptoms develop shortly in a median time of 4 months, most commonly as nasal obstruction, either in combination with epistaxis (25.8 %) or other symptoms (12.6 %). Surgery is rarely complicated by bleeding requiring major surgical approaches or preoperative embolization. Transnasal or transmaxillary resection is feasible in most cases and multidisciplinary approaches rarely indicated. Tumor recurrence is extremely rare and usually occurs within the first postoperative year. Although extremely rare, ENAs have to be encountered in the differential diagnosis, particularly if adult patients present with a rapidly developing nasal obstruction resulting from a nasal septum tumor. Female gender or normal vascularity does not exclude diagnosis. Further research is indicated to clarify the origin of this rare entity.

Keywords Extranasopharyngeal angiofibroma • Atypical angiofibroma • Maxillary tumor • Nasal septum • Arteriography • Carotid ligation • Embolization • Immunohistochemistry • Biopsy

---

J.P. Windfuhr, MD
Department of Otorhinolaryngology, Plastic Head and Neck Surgery, Kliniken Maria Hilf, Sandradstraße43, 41061 Mönchengladbach, Germany
e-mail: jochen.windfuhr@mariahilf.de

S.P. Dubey, B. Schick (eds.), *Juvenile Angiofibroma*,
DOI 10.1007/978-3-319-45343-9_21

Introduction

Angiofibromas in the head and neck region are nonencapsulated, highly vascular tumors which usually present in the nasopharynx and affect male patients at an average age of 14–17 years, correctly labeled as *juvenile angiofibroma* (JA) [1–3]. They account for 0.05–0.5 % of all head and neck tumors [4, 5] and grow locally aggressive, although histologically benign. Microscopical examination of angiofibroma tissue reveals thin-walled, angulated vessels lined by plump endothelium contained within a dense stroma of abundant, plump, stellate-shaped fibroblasts. This is the most important criterion to distinguish angiofibromas from other tumors. The relative absence of the smooth muscle cells in the walls of the vessels precludes vasoconstriction and contributes to brisk episodes of uncontrollable bleeding, the commonest clinical feature [6]. JA can readily be identified with transnasal endoscopy as a lobulated pinkish or bluish mass, occasionally ulcerated with superficial slough in situations with epistaxis and nasal packing [5]. The tumor is considered to arise from the superior margin of the sphenopalatine foramen [2, 4, 7, 8] and to expand in highly predictable patterns resulting in nasal obstruction, epistaxis, skeletal deformities, anosmia, and rhinolalia [9, 10]. In contrast to atypical appearances of JAs in very young [11–20], very old [21–23], female [22, 24–27], or pregnant [28] patients, angiofibromas may also originate from or localized elsewhere than the nasopharynx, commonly labeled as *extranasopharyngeal angiofibromas* (ENAs). This chapter aims to summarize the current knowledge about this rare entity.

Sites

Angiofibromas may present as a swelling of the cheek [29–32] or as a mass in the oral [33, 34] or nasal cavity [35]. However, findings in computed tomography (CT) or magnetic resonance imaging (MRI) will clarify the origin of these lesions in the proximity of the sphenopalatine foramen and frequently disclose a large tumor volume. The first case of a true ENA, i.e., involvement of the sphenopalatine foramen, can be excluded and was reported by de Kleyn and Van Ryssel in 1918 [36]. Since then, approximately 174 cases were published [37], allowing a more precise differentiation between JA and ENA (Table 21.1). In contrast to earlier publications [15, 38–44], it can now be stated that most cases of ENA affected the nasal septum [15, 37, 42, 45–74]. Other sites were less frequently involved (Table 21.2) and encompassed the maxillary sinus [12, 16, 39, 41, 43, 75–91], inferior turbinate [46, 92–109], ethmoid [12, 13, 36, 71, 110–117], nasal cavity [118–128], oral cavity [129–137], oropharynx [14, 44, 46, 97, 138–142], larynx [46, 143–148], sphenoid sinus [41, 149–154], cheek [155–159], infratemporal fossa [46, 160–163], neck [164–167], hypopharynx [52, 168, 169], middle turbinate [40, 170, 171], eye [172, 173],external ear [174], esophagus [175], facial

Table 21.1 Juvenile angiofibroma vs. extranasopharyngeal angiofibroma

	JA	ENA
Median age	15–17 y	23 y
Female patients	Uncommon	31 %
Origin	Sphenopalatine foramen	Variable
Symptoms	Epistaxis, nasal obstruction	Variable
Spreading pattern	Yes	No
Median symptom duration	>6 months	4 months
First line treatment	Surgery	Surgery
Radiotherapy	Unresectable cases, recurrences	Uncommon
Chemotherapy	Anecdotal	Not reported
Hormonal therapy	Anecdotal	Anecdotal
Arteriography, MR angiography	Common	Uncommon
Preoperative embolization	Common	Uncommon
Staging system	Radkowski	None
Recurrence rate	25 %	<5 %
Intracranial extension	20 %	<2 %
Differential diagnoses	Pyogenic granulomas, nasal polyps, hemangiopericytomas Skull base tumors (craniopharyngioma, chordoma, chondrosarcoma, nasopharyngeal carcinoma, olfactory neuroblastoma, rhabdomyosarcoma)	Intraoral: primary bone lesions, odontogenic neoplasms or gingival hyperplastic processes Intranasal: lobular capillary hemangioma, pyogenic granuloma, angiomatous polyps, neurofibromas, and hemangiopericytomas for intranasal lesions CD34 staining: low-grade vascular lesions, spindle cell neoplasms, comprising of a large range of benign and low-grade malignant soft tissue lesions, including cellular angiofibroma, solitary fibrous tumor, fibromyxoid sarcoma, myxofibrosarcoma, myxoid liposarcoma, giant cell angiofibroma, angiomyolipoma, and angiomyofibroblastoma

JA juvenile angiofibroma, *ENA* extranasopharyngeal angiofibroma, *y* years

nerve [176], trachea [177], lacrimal sac [178], middle cranial fossa [179], external nose [180], and parotid [181]. One report did not specify the exact site of the lesion within the nasal cavity [182]. There was a slight preponderance of the right side (87 vs. 73 left side; one bilateral case; side not specified for 6 patients or not applicable in 7 cases).

Table 21.2 Extranasopharyngeal angiofibromas – sites

Site	*n*	%
Septum	39	22.4
Maxilla	23	13.2
Inferior turbinate	20	11.5
Ethmoid	14	8.1
Nasal cavity	11	6.3
Oral cavity	9	5.2
Oropharynx	9	5.2
Larynx	7	4.0
Sphenoid	7	4.0
Cheek	5	2.9
Infratemporal fossa	5	2.9
Not specified	5	2.9
Neck	4	2.3
Hypopharynx	3	1.7
Middle turbinate	3	1.7
Eye	2	1.1
External ear	1	0.6
Esophagus	1	0.6
Facial nerve	1	0.6
Trachea	1	0.6
Lacrimal sac	1	0.6
Middle cranial fossa	1	0.6
Nasal dorsum	1	0.6
Lesions may encounter more than one site		

Demographics

In contrast to JA with an almost exclusive presentation in male adolescents, 31.6% of all patients with an ENA were female. The lesion may be present at birth or at an age of 87 years (Table 21.3).

Most commonly, young adults were affected with a mean age of 28.7 and a median age of 23 years [37].

Presentation

One to two years elapse, when diagnosis of JA is established in contrast to only several months in case of ENA [38]. Unilateral nasal obstruction with rhinorrhea and recurrent unilateral epistaxis in a male adolescent is highly suspicious for JA, variably accompanied by headache, facial pain, and Eustachian tube dysfunction with secondary otitis media. Other symptoms include swelling of the

Table 21.3 Extranasopharyngeal angiofibroma – age distribution

Age (years)	*n*
≤10	21
≤20	52
≤30	37
≤40	17
≤50	10
≤60	19
≤70	8
≤80	3
≤90	1

Age range, 0–87 y; mean, 28.7 y; median, 23 y
Age not specified for six patients

cheek, neurological deficits, alteration in olfaction, rhinolalia clausa, and otalgia, respectively [183]. Signs of chronic rhinosinusitis may result from tumor growth into the paranasal sinuses with proptosis and/or vision impairment indicating involvement of the orbit in 10–20 % of all JA cases [1–4, 184, 185] which in contrast to 6.9 % advanced stages of ENA require surgical approaches like craniotomy, maxillectomy, transmandibular, or transzygomatic resection, respectively [37].

The majority of patients with an ENA presented with nasal obstruction, either in combination with epistaxis (25.8 %) or variable symptoms (12.6 %). Other symptoms were less frequently reported like nasal obstruction (9.8 %) or epistaxis without any other symptoms (6.9 %), painless facial swelling with (3.4 %) or without any other symptoms (4.6 %), dysphagia (3.4 %), and miscellaneous (32.4 %). Diagnosis by chance was reported for two patients, including one case with correct diagnosis after adenoidectomy [41, 131]. Six patients presented as emergency cases [51, 84, 96, 98, 107, 177], four with a congenital lesion [13, 16, 111, 173]. Symptom duration was not stated/available for 19 cases (10.9 %) or labeled as "weeks"[36], "long history"[55], "recurrent episodes"[70], "several months"[60, 139], "several weeks"[174], or "slowly progressing"[106], respectively. The remainder developed symptoms within 13.1 months on average (range, 2 days–360 months; median, 4 months) [37].

Histology and Biopsy

The pinkish/bluish surface of ENAs compares to JAs, sometimes with a visible tumor pedicle to the septum or ethmoid suggesting surgical removal without preoperative radiological examination.

While biopsy in patients suspicious for JA should be avoided due to the inherent risk of excessive bleeding [183], excisional biopsies were not followed by bleeding complications in patients with a finally diagnosed ENA [119, 129, 173, 174].

Moreover, repeated serious bleeding events stopped after autoamputation of an ENA from the nasal septum [60].

Correct diagnosis after biopsy prior to therapy was established in 35 patients, and the clinical course was either uneventful [12, 14, 41, 49, 58, 89, 97, 99, 121–123, 126, 134, 136, 137, 143, 147, 149, 161] or complicated by bleeding [12, 42, 76, 79, 80, 82, 88, 94, 114, 124, 151, 171, 179] with two authors reporting more than one case [12, 41].

As reported for JA, surface biopsy can be misleading since typical histologic appearance is only seen internally. Dogan et al. stated that ENAs have interstitial stromal predominance with less vascular elements on histopathologic examination, like that of long-standing JA [67]. The diameter of the vessels decreases from the center to the surface of the tumor. Bigger vessels may have irregular or incomplete muscular layers but do not contain elastic fibers like hemangiomas. Immunohistochemistry for diagnosis of an ENA with a positive reaction to vimentin and CD34 and a negative reaction to actin and desmin has been identified [186] with CD34 detecting endothelial cell proliferation. Garcia-Rodriguez et al., however, denied the necessity of immunohistochemical analysis [63]. Until today, immunohistochemistry was performed in only 13.8 % of all 174 reported patients with an ENA, including CD34, vimentin, actin, β-catenin, CD31, S-100, glial fibrillary acidic protein, factor VIII, desmin, CD117, anti-smooth muscle antibodies, Ki-67, D2-40, and NSE, respectively [37, 187].

In a recent review, a variety of initial diagnoses after biopsy, different from the final report, was made such as *granulation tissue* [87, 115], *inflammatory tissue* [77], *unspecific inflammation* [91], *benign tumor* [148], *capillary hemangioma* [64, 156], *hemangioma* [46], *pyogenic granuloma* [93], *solitary fibrous tumor* [128], *unspecific* [16], *vascular tumor* [127], and *PNET* [83], respectively. In one case, diagnosis was established fortuitously after adenoidectomy, and a biopsy 6 months after surgery revealed normal tissue in this case [41]. Only 4 of this group of 13 patients had experienced bleeding complications after biopsy [16, 91, 93, 115].

Differential Diagnosis

A wide array of other neoplasms can masquerade as JA or ENA, such as inflammatory polyps, angiomatous polyps, nasopharyngeal cysts/malignancies/benign tumors, upper maxillary malignancies, esthesioneuroblastoma, chordomas, neurofibromas, hemangiomas, and retropharyngeal tuberculosis [137, 188]. Hemangiomas generally consist of small amount of fibrous tissue, show lobulation in different degrees, and are most commonly seen on the skin of pregnant females but can occur also on nasal mucosa [97, 137]. A positive staining for CD34 expands the number of differential diagnosis including low-grade vascular lesions and spindle cell neoplasms, comprising of a large range of benign and low-grade malignant soft tissue lesions, including cellular angiofibroma, solitary fibrous tumor, fibromyxoid sarcoma, myxofibrosarcoma, myxoid liposarcoma, giant cell angiofibroma, angiomyolipoma, and angiomyofibroblastoma [181]. A positive staining for vimentin and negative staining for CD34 and actin is acknowledged as a typical finding in a hemangiopericytoma [187]. Hemangiopericytomas originate from extravascular cells and may grow in the nasal cavity. Pathologically these tumors have only a small amount of interstitial stroma with many spindle-shaped cells and dilated vascular spaces [60]. Expression of vascular endothelial growth factor (VEGF) is elevated in the tissue of human hemangiomas but not in vascular malformations [187]. Intraoral lesions may result from primary bone lesions, odontogenic neoplasms, or gingival hyperplastic processes in the differential diagnosis [137].

Hypervascularity

Hypervascularity is without doubt the most common clinical feature of JAs, emphasized by the commonly reported history of epistaxis. In addition, a strong enhancement of contrast in arteriography, CT or MRI is a typical finding. Moreover, intraoperative bleedingof 300–3500 ml despite "temporary occlusion of the external carotid artery" has been reported [189]. Today, intraoperative bleeding is prevented with preoperative embolization as a routine and managed with a readily available cell saver system and preoperative autologous blood donation [190]. According to Gleeson, the role of preoperative embolization is prudent only in JA patients with an extensive tumor size but doubtful in medium-sized tumors. He noted that the recurrence risk is associated with embolization, and, alternatively, larger vessels can easily be ligated in open approaches [191]. However, his statement is contradicted by the report of Liu et al. who could not identify a significant difference concerning blood loss after ligation of the external carotid artery compared to preoperative embolization in advanced stage JAs. In this study, embolization was advantageous only in early stages of JA [6].

Concerning patients with an ENA, hypervascularity was identified in only 19 cases patients by radiological means. Moreover, it has been stated that significant bleeding had complicated only few surgical procedures [46, 48, 77, 88, 96, 104, 117, 124, 153, 155, 192] and was associated to biopsy taking in only one third of all patients [37].

Staging and Radiology

Various systems of classification systems for JA have been suggested in the past [3, 193–195]. One of the most commonly adopted systems was proposed by Radkowski in 1996 [196]. However, some newer staging systems are based on advances in technology and surgical approaches [197–199] and have shown promising utility [200]. Since ENAs develop at different sites and are apparently extremely rare, a comparable classification is virtually impossible.

A high index of suspicion is warranted when patients – preferably male adolescents – present with epistaxis and a mass in the nasal cavity/nasopharynx. CT and/or MRI with contrast will readily establish the correct diagnosis of a JA dispensing any biopsy, sometimes confirmed by angio-MRI and/or arteriography. JA will demonstrate an intense homogenous contrast enhancement on CT with an anterior bowing of the posterior maxillary wall (Holman-Miller sign) and a widening of the sphenopalatine foramen. A homogenous and intense contrast enhancement is also noted on T1-/T2-weighted MRI [183].

While JA is associated with a strong and homogeneous enhancement on CT or MRI, contrast enhancement is less and inhomogeneous in patients with an ENA. Normal findings in arteriography do not exclude an ENA [8, 93]. This statement is supported by a review of 23 arteriographies in 174 patients with a verified ENA [37]. Hypervascularity was identified in only 19 cases in patients and followed by simultaneous embolization in 13 patients (Table 21.4). While Schick and Kahle identified multiple arteries as blood supply of JA [190], only few feeding arteries in patients with an ENA were identified, most commonly branches of the internal maxillary artery. Moreover, there were only two cases with a bilateral blood supply (Table 21.4; [37]). Ligation of the external carotid artery was performed in six patients [112, 122, 134, 163], including one case with a bilateral ligation of the external carotid artery prior to radiotherapy followed by surgery with a unilateral ligation of the common carotid artery [76] and one case with a simultaneous ligation of the anterior ethmoid artery [88]. Other authors reported ligation of the facial and lingual artery [130] and ligation of the maxillary artery [161], and there was also one report of a resection of the external carotid artery [167]. Angiographic findings of tumor blood supply are described in Table 21.4.

Surgery

Management of JA has become more refined by high-resolution CT/MRI, angio-MRI, preoperative embolization, improved anesthesia, and an increased familiarity with skull base surgical approaches including endoscopic surgical techniques [201]. Preoperative tumor embolization, cell saver systems, and preoperative autologous blood donation have contributed to secure hemostatic control and to prevent complications associated with significant intraoperative bleeding [190, 201].

Size, location, stage of surgery (primary/revision), surgical experience, and blood supply of the tumor are significant factors when the best surgical approach is considered. This can be either a transpalatal (with or without sublabial extension), transmaxillary (lateral rhinotomy, medial maxillectomy, midfacial degloving, Le Fort I osteotomy), or lateral skull base approach (subtemporal-infratemporal, infratemporal), alone or in combination [5, 20, 191]. Endoscopic techniques were introduced in the 1990s and are associated with a reduced postoperative morbidity and maximum preservation of the anatomy responsible for facial growth [187, 202–208]. ENA presenting within the nasal cavity including nasal septum and turbinates,

Table 21.4 Angiographic findings of tumor blood supply (alphabetical order)

Author	Gender, age	Site	Involved arteries
Antoniades	m, 14	Hard palate, molar region	Maxillary artery (superior maxillary/pterygopalatine branches)[a]
Beeden	m, 13	Posterior wall of oropharynx and hypopharynx	Hypervascularity excluded
Cho	m, 72	Ethmoid	Hypervascularity excluded
Chung YS	m, 21	Soft palate	Maxillary/facial artery[a]
Crespo-Hiero	m, 17	Lateral nasal cavity	Maxillary artery (pterygopalatine branches; bilateral)[a]
DeBlanc	m, 52	Carotid bifurcation	Hypervascularity excluded, displacement of the internal and external carotid artery
Isherwood	m, 13	Infratemporal fossa, pterygomaxillary fissure	Maxillary artery
Johnson	m, 25	Parapharyngeal space	Maxillary artery[a]
Karthikeyan	m, 13	Sphenoid sinus	Maxillary artery[a]
Keskin	m, 21	Sphenoid sinus	Maxillary artery[a]
Lim	f, 41	Middle turbinate	Maxillary artery[a]
Marcos-Garcia	f, 60	Inferior turbinate	Maxillary artery[a]
Nomura	m, 62	Inferior turbinate	Maxillary artery (sphenopalatine branch)
Rho	m, 23	Oropharynx	Maxillary artery[a]
Somdas	m, 27	Nasal septum (BCJ)	Maxillary artery (sphenopalatine branch)[a]
Steele	f, 64	Pyriform sinus/aryepiglottic fold	Left superior laryngeal artery
Supiyaphun	m, 14	Oral cavity (mandible)	Maxillary/facial/lingual artery
Szymanska	m, 24	Infratemporal fossa	Maxillary artery[a]
Szymanska	m, 23	Infratemporal/pterygopalatine fossa/cheek	Maxillary artery (presumably)
Taggarshe	m, 30	Inferior turbinate	Maxillary artery[a]
Tsunoda	m, 12	Sphenoid sinus	Maxillary artery (sphenopalatine branch)[a]
Ulubil	f, 35	Retropharyngeal mass	Lingual branch (right) + lingual/maxillary branch (left)
Windfuhr	f, 13	Maxilla	Hypervascularity excluded

[a] = arteriography was followed by simultaneous embolization; gray shaded: hypervascularity excluded

endonasal surgery was sufficient, and only few cases were accompanied by selective arteriography and embolization (Table 21.4). Lesions involving the paranasal sinuses frequently demanded transmaxillary approaches, sometimes combined with endonasal techniques and rarely requiring a multidisciplinary approach due to intracranial extension [118, 163]. There was one anecdotal case of “successful” autoamputation emphasizing that the tumor cells were located within or distal to the tumor pedicle, not at the basis of the tumor originating from the nasal septum [60].

Radiotherapy

Radiotherapy has been recommended for unresectable tumors, failure of complete tumor removal, or for extensive intracranial extension [4, 209–211]. According to a most recent publication, the potential of a malignant transformation of a JA has to be included in the informed consent [212]. A local control rate of 80–85 % in terms of symptom regression after radiotherapy has been reported which is comparable to surgical procedures [123, 213, 214]. A dose of 30–35 Gy is recommended but may be increased to 40–45 Gy for extensive lesions [123, 211, 215]. Radiotherapy was rarely indicated for ENA and first results published between 1961 and 1979 for six patients [12, 14, 78, 149]: Alajmo and Storchii used “3 tubi da 10 mgdi radium” for 72 h after partial resection of an ethmoid lesion. Another patient was treated with 10 mg radium for 36 h after lateral rhinotomy. A third case with previous ineffective radiotherapy 3 years before the patient underwent surgical removal of an ethmoid ENA. Finally, one 14-year-old boy received “Roentgenterapia (1.500 r)” since the family refused surgery but this could not prevent recurrence after 2 years mandating surgery [12]. Reddy treated a patient with an intracranial extension of an ENA with “6100 r of cobalt radiation” after a biopsy, but 18 months later the patient died [149]. Perko did not specify a 2-month and effective radiotherapy in a patient who had undergone revision surgery “because invasion of the tumor into soft tissues and the remaining part of the left maxilla made further surgery impossible”[78]. Beeden and Alexander used “a dose of 1.029 r in eight treatments over 4 weeks” 1 month before transoral resection of the ENA. Biopsies were positive only 1 month after surgery but the pharynx unsuspicious after 18 months [14]. Reddy mentioned that he used “a small dose of 600 r” to reduce the bleeding of an oral ENA which finally was ineffective during surgery [130]. Later, there were only three other cases published between 1986 and 1992, with a various outcome [82, 123, 134]. Gudea irradiated a large maxillary lesion successfully (40 Gy) with curative intention [123]. Kitano reported of a maxillary angiofibroma which was treated with 20 Gy after biopsy was taken to shrink the tumor and manage profuse bleeding [82]. Supiyaphun tried to shrink a huge ENA in the oral cavity “with radiation of 3.000 rad over 3-week period” but therapy was ineffective and repeated surgery required in the following course [134]. It can be concluded from the case collection that radiotherapy was before (four patients) and after (five patients) surgery/biopsy [37].

Alternative Therapy

Other treatment modalities and instruments were implemented for JA and include cryotherapy [209, 216], KTP laser [217], brachytherapy [218–221], harmonic scalpel [222], coblation [223–226], Gamma Knife [227–230], hormone therapy [216, 231–236], arterial ligation, sclerotherapy [209, 237], and observation with hope of spontaneous regression of JA [184, 238–242]. Chemotherapy with doxorubicin and dacarbazine has been suggested for recurrences or locally aggressive JA [243–245]. Only one author reported of an attempt to stop rapid tumor growth with the application of diethylstilbestrol for one week, which was ineffective [124]. There was only one case of a misdiagnosed ENA with presurgical chemotherapy which turned out to be ineffective [83].

Recurrences and Death

Diagnosis of recurrent or residual JA remains challenging, especially in cases with a negative finding in an asymptomatic patient with an enhanced mass on the first CT done several months after surgery. Repeated CT examination is mandatory in these cases to assess whether or not a tumor progression exists to indicate revision surgery [246]. Recurrence is reported for approximately 25 % of JA cases regardless the method of treatment [190, 246]. Further recurrences may develop in roughly 40 % of these patients and are more likely in patients with advanced stage disease and in those treated by inexperienced surgeons. The recurrence risk decreases with age, and most recurrences develop as a consequence of invasion of the basisphenoid. Therefore, drilling out the basisphenoid at the time of primary surgery has been highly recommended. In view of the very high incidence of recurrent disease, prolonged clinical and radiological monitoring is necessary for all these patients. Disease-free status 5 years after primary surgery probably represents cure which is not valid for those who have experienced recurrent disease [191].

In contrast to the aforementioned data, recurrence of an ENA was reported for only 2.3 % in a series of 174 patients with an ENA, all within 12 months after diagnosis [39, 43, 78, 102]. The remainder was followed for 3 weeks to 8 years and presented without recurrence (mean: 20.7 months; median: 12 months; follow-up unspecified/not stated for 41.4 %). A progressive disease was reported for one single case after 24 months [174]. One patient died within 1 h after initial presentation as a result of acute respiratory compromise [177]. Two other patients died due to endocranial extension of the ENA within 5 [179] and 18 months [149] after initial diagnosis. In one single patient a malignant course of an initially confirmed ENA was identified 9 years after therapy, maybe as a consequence of implantation of radium seeds at the age of 6 years. However, no evidence of disease was found two years later [12].

Open Questions

Concerning the origin and histogenesis of JA, developmental, hormonal imbalance, and genetic causes are still under discussion [137, 186, 187, 247, 248]. JA are considered by some authors as a true neoplasm exposing androgen receptors or activated transforming growth factor beta-1 within the neoplasm [1–4, 249]. Others suggested a vascular origin [250], specific variant of angioma [251], reactive over growth of connective tissue [209], irregular vessels set in fibrous stroma typical for vascular malformation [252], result of pituitary-dependent sex hormone dysfunction [27], or hamartoma [26, 253]. Finally, angiofibromas are acknowledged as a vascular malformation that derives from an incomplete regression of the first branchial arch artery. This hypothesis is supported by the finding of a discontinuous vascular basal lamina, focal lack of pericytes, and pronounced irregularity of the smooth muscle layers. However, the predilection for adolescent males with JA suggests a relationship with sex hormones for JA and a protective value of high estrogen levels in females [4]. The influence of sexual hormones has repeatedly been described [254, 255], and Schiff speculated that angiofibroma is a testosterone-dependent tumor that arises from a fibrovascular nidus in the nasopharynx that is inactive until the onset of puberty [9]. Another hypothesis suggests that JA originates in the tissue of the anterior margin of the atlas at the lower surface of the sphenoid bone (fascia basalis). During its development, this tissue extends up to the posterior part of the vomer and the ethmoid bone and the middle concha.

Many of these considerations may sufficiently explain the etiology of JA, but the clinical data of ENAs favor the possibility of other etiological factors; as there is a much more balanced sex ratio, tumors occur in female and very young/old patients and may present far away from an assumed nidus and the sphenoid bone. It was suggested that embryonic ectopic tissue remnants during the development of the nasal septum were the origin of septal ENAs [52, 67]. Probably, the periosteum of the perpendicular plate of the ethmoid bone is an abnormal presentation of the fascia basalis [15, 42]. While the theory may explain a presentation at the bony cartilaginous junction [15, 47–51] and bony part of the septum [52–58], it is insufficient for lesions at the cartilaginous part [42, 52, 59–74]. Unfortunately, the subsite was not specified for 12 patients [45, 46, 182]. Moreover, further research is desirable to explain presentation of an ENA at the inferior turbinate, facial nerve, larynx, palatine tonsil, trachea, external nose, external ear, oropharynx, hypopharynx, and esophagus. Finally, all considerations are challenged by reports of spontaneous involution of JA [184, 238–242].

References

1. Lloyd G, Howard D, Phelps P, Cheesman A. Juvenile angiofibroma: the lessons of 20 years of modern imaging. J Laryngol Otol. 1999;113:127–34.
2. Economou TS, Abemayor E, Ward PH. Juvenile nasopharyngeal angiofibroma: an update of the UCLA experience,1960–1985. Laryngoscope. 1988;98:170–5.

3. Andrews JC, Fisch U, Valavanis A, Aeppli U, Makek MS. The surgical management of extensive nasopharyngeal angiofibromas with the infratemporal fossa approach. Laryngoscope. 1989;99:429–37.
4. Gullane PJ, Davidson J, O'Dwyer T, Forte V. Juvenile angiofibroma: a review of the literature and a case series report. Laryngoscope. 1992;102:928–33.
5. Thakar A, Hota A, Pookamala S. Nasopharyngeal Angiofibroma. Otorhinolaryngol. 2013;6:25–34.
6. Liu L, Wang R, Huang D, Han D, Ferguson EJ, Shi H, et al. Analysis of intra-operative bleeding and recurrence of juvenile nasopharyngeal angiofibromas. Clin Otolaryngol. 2002;27: 536–40.
7. Sessions RB, Zarin DP, Bryan RN. Juvenile nasopharyngeal angiofibroma. Am J Dis Child. 1981;135:535–7.
8. Harrison DF. The natural history, pathogenesis, and treatment of juvenile angiofibroma. Personal experience with 44patients. Arch Otolaryngol Head Neck Surg. 1987;113: 936–42.
9. Schiff M. Juvenile nasopharyngeal angiofibroma. a theory of pathogenesis. Laryngoscope. 1959;69:981–1016.
10. Szymanska A, Szymanski M, Czekajska-Chehab E, Szczerbo-Trojanowska M. Invasive growth patterns of juvenile nasopharyngeal angiofibroma: radiological imaging and clinical implications. Acta Radiol. 2014;55:725–31.
11. Shaheen HB. Nasopharyngeal fibroma. J Laryngol Otol. 1930;45:259–64.
12. Alajmo E, Fini-Storchi O. Ilfibro angioma primitivodellefossenasaliedeiseniparanasali. Bollettinodelle Malattiedell Orecchiodella Goladel Naso. 1961;79:217–40.
13. Furstenberg AC, Boles R. Nasopharyngeal angiofibroma. Trans Am Acad Ophthalmol Otolaryngol. 1963;67:518–23.
14. Beeden AG, Alexander FW. An unusual pharyngeal tumour. J Laryngol Otol. 1971;85:733–5.
15. Sarpa JR, Novelly NJ. Extra nasopharyngeal angiofibroma. Otolaryngol Head Neck Surg. 1989;101:693–7.
16. Manjalay G, Hoare TJ, Pearman K, Green NJ. A case of congenital angiofibroma. Int J Pediatr Otorhinolaryngol. 1992;24:275–8.
17. Stern RM, Beauchamp GR, Berlin AJ. Ocular findings in juvenile nasopharyngeal angiofibroma. Ophthalmic Surg. 1986;17:560–4.
18. Gruber B, Kron TK, Goldman ME, Matz GJ. Nasopharyngeal angiofibroma in two young children. Otolaryngol Head Neck Surg. 1985;93:803–6.
19. De Vincentiis G, Pinelli V. Rhinopharyngeal angiofibroma in the pediatric age group. Clinical-statistical contribution. Int J Pediatr Otorhinolaryngol. 1980;2:99–122.
20. Huang Y, Liu Z, Wang J, Sun X, Yang L, Wang D. Surgical management of juvenile nasopharyngeal angiofibroma: analysis of 162 cases from 1995 to 2012. Laryngoscope. 2014;124:1942–6.
21. Pradillo JA, Rodriguez HA, Arroyo JF. Nasopharyngeal angiofibroma in the elderly: report of a case. Laryngoscope. 1975;85:1063–5.
22. Ewing JA, Shively EH. Angiofibroma: a rare case in an elderly female. Otolaryngol Head Neck Surg. 1981;89:602–3.
23. Zhang HK, Wang JJ, Liu ZF, Wang DH. Management of nasopharyngeal angiofibroma in a 72-year-old male through a sublabial and buccolabial incision approach: A case report and literature review. Oncol Lett. 2015;10:1267–70.
24. Rominger CJ, Santore FJ. Juvenile nasopharyngeal fibroma in female adult. Rep Case Arch Otolaryngol. 1968;88:85–7.
25. Barrios JM, Garcia J, Moreno E. Nasal angiofibroma in a 60 year-old female patient. An Otorrinolaringol Ibero Am. 1983;10:327–31.
26. Osborn DA, Sokolovski A. Juvenile angiofibroma in a female. Arch Otolaryngol. 1965;82:629–932.
27. Hicks JL, Nelson JF. Juvenile nasopharyngeal angiofibroma. Oral Surg Oral Med Oral Pathol. 1973;35:807–17.

28. Peloquin L, Klossek JM, Basso-Brusa F, Gougeon JM, Toffel PH, Fontanel JP. A rare case of nasopharyngeal angiofibroma in a pregnant woman. Otolaryngol Head Neck Surg. 1997;117:S111–4.
29. Patil RN, Agarwal AK, Prakash B, Ghosh P. Extra-nasopharyngeal extensions of angiofibroma. J Laryngol Otol. 1982;96:1053–64.
30. Yi Z, Li ZC, Lin C, Ye S. Huge lobulated juvenile angiofibroma: sites of extension and selection of procedures for management. J Otolaryngol. 2003;32:211–6.
31. Mannai C, Schwartz HC. Juvenile nasopharyngeal angiofibroma presenting as a facial swelling. A case report. J Maxillofac Surg. 1986;14:329–31.
32. Hazarika P, Nayak RG, Chandran M. Extra-nasopharyngeal extension of juvenile angiofibroma. J Laryngol Otol. 1985;99:813–7.
33. Kabot TE, Goldman ME, Bergman S, Schwartz RD. Juvenile nasopharyngeal angiofibroma: an unusual presentation in the oral cavity. Oral Surg Oral Med Oral Pathol. 1985;59: 453–7.
34. Pardhe N, Chhibber N, Agarwal D, Jain M, Vijay P. Juvenile nasopharyngeal angiofibroma extending into the oral cavity: a rare entity. J Clin Diagn Res. 2015;9:ZD31–3.
35. Stokes SM, Castle JT. Nasopharyngeal angiofibroma of the nasal cavity. Head Neck Pathol. 2010;4:210–3.
36. DeKleyn A, Van Ryssel EC. ÜberzweimerkwürdigeTumorenderEthmoidalgegend.II EinFibroangiomderEthmoidalgegend. Acta Otolaryngol. 1918;1:197–200.
37. Windfuhr JP. Extra nasopharyngeal Angiofibroma revisited. [submitted]. 2016.
38. Windfuhr JP, Remmert S. Extra nasopharyngeal angiofibroma: etiology, incidence and management. Acta Otolaryngol. 2004;124:880–9.
39. Panesar J, Vadgama B, Rogers G, Ramsay AD. HartleyBJ. Juvenile angiofibroma of the maxillary sinus. Rhinology. 2004;42:171–4.
40. Huang RY, Damrose EJ, Blackwell KE, Cohen AN, Calcaterra TC. Extra nasopharyngeal angiofibroma. Int J Pediatr Otorhinolaryngol. 2000;56:59–64.
41. Schick B, Kind M, Schwarzkopf G, Weber R, Draf W. Angiofibroma with atypical localizations in early childhood. HNO. 1997;45:1022–8.
42. Hiraide F, Matsubara H. Juvenile nasal angiofibroma: a case report. Arch Otorhinolaryngol. 1984;239:235–41.
43. Juul A, Larsen K, Illum P. Angiofibroma of the maxillary antrum. Arch Otorhinolaryngol. 1982;236:135–8.
44. Ali S, Jones WI. Extranasopharyngeal angiofibromas. (Sex incidence and age distribution). J Laryngol Otol. 1982;96:559–65.
45. Silveira MAA, Nunes AAA, Paiva FCG, Feijão MRMJ, Azevedo MA, Lima VB. Extranasopharyngeal angiofibroma: case report. Int Arch Otorhinolaryngol. 2013; 17(Suppl1):61.
46. Szymanska A, Szymanski M, Morshed K, Czekajska-Chehab E, Szczerbo-Trojanowska M. Extranasopharyngeal angiofibroma: clinical and radiological presentation. Eur Arch Otorhinolaryngol. 2013;270:655–60.
47. Shah N, Hathiram BT, Dwivedi A, Sheth K, Grewal DS, Behl NK. Nasopharyngeal angiofibroma-an unusual origin & presentation. Indian J Otolaryngol Head Neck Surg. 2000;52:179–81.
48. Handa KK, Kumar A, Singh MK, Chhabra AH. Extranasopharyngeal angiofibroma a rising from the nasal septum. Int J Pediatr Otorhinolaryngol. 2001;58:163–6.
49. Somdas MA, KetenciI, Unlu Y, Canoz O, Guney E. Extranasopharyngeal angiofibroma originating from the nasal septum. Otolaryngol Head Neck Surg. 2005;133:647.
50. Uyar M, Turanli M, Pak I, Bakir S, Osma U. Extranasopharyngeal angiofibroma originating from the nasal septum: a case report. Kulak Burun Bogaz Ihtis Derg. 2009;19:41–4.
51. Hamdan AL, Moukarbel RV, Kattan M, Natout M. Angiofibroma of the nasal septum. Middle East J Anaesthesiol. 2012;21:653–5.
52. Akbas Y, Anadolu Y. Extranasopharyngeal angiofibroma of the head and neck in women. Am J Otolaryngol. 2003;24:413–6.

53. Mahafza T. Nasal septal angiofibroma in a 20 years old female. J Bahrain Med Soc. 2007;19:84–7.
54. Tasca I, Compadretti GC. Extranasopharyngeal angiofibroma of nasal septum. A controversial entity. Acta Otorhinolaryngol Ital. 2008;28:312–4.
55. Martinez F, Argüello D, Alvarez M, Calzada. Angiofibroma of the nasal septum: An extremely unusual presentation. Rev Port Otorrinolaringol Cir Cerv Fac. 2011;49:177–9.
56. Atmaca S, Bayraktar C, Yildiz L. Extranasopharyngeal angiofibroma of the posterior nasal septum: a rare clinical entity. Kulak Burun Bogaz Ihtis Derg. 2013;23:295–8.
57. Correia FG, Simoes JC, Mendes-Neto JA, Seixas-Alves MT, Gregorio LC, Kosugi EM. Extranasopharyngeal angiofibroma of the nasal septum--uncommon presentation of a rare disease. Braz J Otorhinolaryngol. 2013;79:646.
58. Ewe S, Dayana F, Fadzilah FM, Gendeh BS. Nasal septal angiofibroma in a post-menopausal woman: a rare entity. J Clin Diagn Res. 2015;9:MD03–5.
59. Bhargava SK, Phatak S, Phatak S. Angiofibroma arising from nasal septum in adult male—a rare occurence. Indian J Otolaryngol Head Neck Surg. 1995;47:39–41.
60. Castillo MP, Timmons CF, McClay JE. Auto amputation of an extranasopharyngeal angiofibroma of the nasal septum. Int J Pediatr Otorhinolaryngol Extra. 2006;1:267–70.
61. Mohindra S, Grover G, Bal AK. Extranasopharyngeal angiofibroma of the nasal septum: a case report. Ear Nose Throat J. 2009;88:E17–9.
62. Gupta N, Vaid L, Churg N, Singh PP. Extranasopharyngeal angiofibroma from the nasal septum: a case report and a mini review. Clin Rhinol. 2010;3:169–71.
63. Garcia-Rodriguez L, Rudman K, Cogbill CH, Loehrl T, Poetker DM. Nasal septal angiofibroma, a subclass of extranasopharyngeal angiofibroma. Am J Otolaryngol. 2012;33:473–6.
64. Berkiten G, Topaloğlu I, Kamli G. Nasal Septal Angiofibroma in Pregnancy. Eur J Gen Med. 2012;9:280–2.
65. Chavan SS, Deshmukh S, Pawar V, Sarvade K, Kirpan V, Kumbhakarna NR, et al. Case Study of Clinicopathological Correlation of Benign Sinonasal Masses. 2012. http://www.waent.org/archives/2012/Vol5–1/20120115-Benign-Sinonasal-Masses/Case-3_Extra-nasopharyngeal_Angiofibroma.htm. Accessed 1 Dec 2015.
66. Madana J, Yolmo D, Gopalakrishnan S, Saxena S. Extranasopharyngeal angiofibroma of the cartilaginous nasal septum: possible origin from ectopic tissue trapped during septal development. Int J Otorhinolaryngol. 2012;14:1–5.
67. Dogan S, Yazici H, Baygit Y, Metin M, Soy FK. Extranasopharyngeal angiofibroma of the nasal septum: a rare clinical entity. J Craniofac Surg. 2013;24:e390–3.
68. Mahajan G, Ghate G, Thomas J, Shah P. Nasal angiofibroma-a rare presentation. Webmed Central Otorhinolaryngology. 2013;4:1–6.
69. Narve VP, Vyas M, Sachan MK, Kadam HS, Basu R. Extranasopharyngeal angiofibroma originating from nasal septum in a female-a rare case report. J Evol Med Dent Sci. 2013;2:6635–9.
70. Shanmugam VU, Krishnaswamy B, Shanmugam R, Mariappan RG, Swaminathan B, Srikanth N. etal. Angiofibroma of nasal septum: a case report. J Evol Med Dent Sci. 2014;3:12032–5.
71. Singhal SK, Gupta N, Verma H, Dass A, Kaur A. Extranasopharyngeal angiofibroma: report of two cases. Egypt J Ear Nose Throat. 2014;15:73–6.
72. AlOsaimi SM. Extra-nasopharyngeal angiofibroma of nasal septum: a case report. Int J Adv Case Rep. 2015;2:468–70.
73. Niedzielski AB, Horoch T, Mielnik-Niedzielska G, Brodzisz A, Zdunek M. Juvenile angiofibroma occurring in an unusual site: report of a case. Pediatr Ther. 2015;5:1–4.
74. Anand TS, Singh GB, Garg S, Yadav G, Yadav M. Extranasopharyngeal angiofibroma of nasal septum. Nat J Otorhinolaryngol Head Neck Surg. 2013;1:24–5.
75. Tsuru Y. ÜberdieBlutgeschwulstinderNasenhöhleundNebenhöhlen. Zbl Hals Nasen Ohren Hk. 1937;27:24–5.
76. Munson FT. Angiofibroma of the left maxillary sinus. Ann Otol Rhinol Laryngol. 1941;50:561–9.

77. Ogura Y, Fushimi N, Ohue H, Saito R. A very rare case of juvenile angiofibroma in the right maxillary sinus. Nippon Jibiinkoka Gakkai Kaiho. 1965;68:1234–40.
78. Perko M, Uehlinger E, Hjorting-Hansen E. Nasopharyngeal angiofibroma of the maxilla: report of case. J Oral Surg. 1969;27:645–8.
79. Maniglia AJ, Mazzarella LA, Minkowitz S, Moskowitz H. Maxillary sinus angiofibroma treated with cryosurgery. Arch Otolaryngol. 1969;89:527–32.
80. Ryc K, Malicka K, Ksiazek J. [Juvenile angiofibroma of maxillary sinus]. Otolaryngol Pol. 1973;27:543–5.
81. Krutchkoff DJ, Matteson SR, Mark H, Hasson J. Juvenile nasopharyngeal angiofibroma. An unusual presentation as an oral mass. Arch Otolaryngol. 1977;103:553–6.
82. Kitano M, Landini G, Mimura T. Juvenile angiofibroma of the maxillary sinus. A case report. Int J Oral Maxillofac Surg. 1992;21:230–2.
83. Windfuhr JP, Remmert S. Extranasopharyngeal angiofibroma of the nasal cavity and paranasal sinuses. Laryngorhinootologie. 2004;83:308–16.
84. IsmiO,ArpaciRB,YesilowaM,VayisogluV,ÖzcanC. www.entcase.org/manuscript/41/makale/rinoloji/extranasopharyngeal-angiofibroma-of-maxillary-sinus-seen- during-surgery-for-epistaxis.htm. Accessed 1 Dec 2015.
85. Malvic G, Manestar D, Krstulja M, Corak D, Candrlic B, Kujundzic M, et al. Juvenile angiofibroma of the maxillary sinus. Coll Antropol. 2012;36 Suppl 2:197–9.
86. Chakrabarti RN, Venkataramaiah NR, Ravikala P, Rao V, Ramanjaneyulu P. Extranasopharyngeal juvenile angiofibroma--a case report. Indian J Cancer. 1973;10:471–4.
87. Ramanjaneyulu P. Juvenile fibroma of antral origin. Int Surg. 1974;59:423–4.
88. Pathak PN. Extranasopharyngeal juvenile angiofibroma--a case report. J Laryngol Otol. 1970;84:449–51.
89. Veeranjaneyulu P, Yadlapalli AK, Chintapalli A. Extranasopharyngeal angiofibroma of maxillary sinus: a rare entity. J Pharm Biomed Sci. 2015;5:713–8.
90. Hora JF, Brown Jr AK. Paranasal juvenile angiofibroma. Arch Otolaryngol. 1962;76:457–9.
91. Bhagat S, Verma RK, Panda NK. Extranasopharyngeal angiofibroma in an adult: a rare presentation. Indian J Otolaryngol Head Neck Surg 2011;63(Suppl1):25–6.
92. Kim JJ, Lee KS, Kim KS. A case of angiofibroma in the nasal cavity of a pregnant woman. Korean J Otolaryngol. 1982;25:209–12.
93. Alvi A, Myssiorek D, Fuchs A. Extranasopharyngeal angiofibroma. J Otolaryngol. 1996;25:346–8.
94. Gaffney R, Hui Y, Vojvodich S, Forte V. Extranasopharyngeal angiofibroma of the inferior turbinate. Int J Pediatr Otorhinolaryngol. 1997;40:177–80.
95. MarcosGarcia M, Pino Rivero V, Pardo Romero G, Trinidad Ruiz G, Pando Pinto JM, Blasco HA. Nasal angiofibroma in a 60 year-old female. A clinical case and literature review. Acta Otorrinolaringol Esp. 2004;55:195–7.
96. Taggarshe D, Quraishi MS, Dugar JM. Inferior turbinate angiofibroma: an atypical presentation [correction of preservation]. Rhinology. 2004;42:45–7.
97. Celik B, Erisen L, Saraydaroglu O, Coskun H. Atypical angiofibromas: a report of four cases. Int J Pediatr Otorhinolaryngol. 2005;69:415–21.
98. Park YJ, Hwang SJ, Hong JH, Lee BH. A case of extranasopharyngeal angiofibroma of the inferior Turbinate. Korean J Otolaryngol. 2005;48:523–5.
99. Nomura K, Shimomura A, Awataguchi T, Murakami K, Kobayashi T. A case of angiofibroma originating from the inferior nasal turbinate. Auris Nasus Larynx. 2006;33:191–3.
100. Zhou SH, Wang SQ, Wang QY. [Atypical angiofibroma in inferior nasal turbinate: report of a case]. Zhonghua Er Bi Yan Hou Tou Jing Wai Ke Za Zhi. 2008;43:68.
101. Lee DK, Bae WY, JoK S, Rha SH. Atypical angiofibroma originating from the inferior turbinate. Korean J Otorhinolaryngol Head Neck Surg. 2012;55:382–5.
102. Kang JW, Kim YH, Kim JH. Angiofibroma of inferior turbinate as an unusual complication of CO2 laser turbinoplasty. J Craniofac Surg. 2013;24:e513–4.
103. Lee JH, Jeong HM. Extranasopharyngeal angiofibroma originating in the inferior turbinate. Ear Nose Throat J. 2013;92:E31–2.

104. Baptista MA, Pinna Fde R, Voegels RL. Extranasopharyngeal angiofibroma originating in the inferior turbinate: a distinct clinical entity at an unusual site. Int Arch otorhinolaryngol. 2014;18:403–5.
105. Debbarma S, Langstang AD, Kumar SJ. Extranasopharyngeal angiofibroma of inferior turbinate in a young female: a very rare presentation. J Otol Rhinol. 2015;4:1–2.
106. Mutlu V. Angiofibroma from the tail of the inferior turbinate. Eur J Med. 2015;47:66–8.
107. Nazar R, Naser A, Rubio F, Ortega G. Extranasopharyngeal angiofibroma of the left lower turbinate: a case report. Acta Otorrinolaringol Esp. 2015;66:56–8.
108. Salimov A, Ozer S. A rare location of angiofibroma in the inferior turbinate in young woman. Int Arch otorhinolaryngol. 2015;19:187–90.
109. Hod R, Yaniv E. Angiofibroma of the nasal vestibule in a 56 year old woman. Isr Med Assoc J. 2012;14:200–1.
110. Radcliffe A. Ethmoidal fibroangioma. J Laryngol. 1951;5:786–7.
111. Chaikovskii VK. Angiofibroma of the nose in a 14-day-old infant girl. Zh Ushn Nos Gorl Bolezn. 1967;27:103–4.
112. Hiranandani LH, Melgiri RD, Juveker RV. Angiofibroma of the ethmoidal sinus in a female. J Laryngol Otol. 1967;81:935–9.
113. Szczepanski J, Perlowski H. Vascular tumors of the ethmoid sinus. Pol Tyg Lek. 1967;22:1503–4.
114. Lerra S, Nazir T, Khan N, Qadri MS, Dar NH. A case of extra nasopharyngeal angiofibroma of the ethmoid sinus: a distinct clinical entity at an unusual site. Ear Nose Throat J. 2012;91:E15–7.
115. Cho JH, Kim CS, Ihn YK, Park YJ. A case of extra nasopharyngeal angiofibroma of the ethmoid sinus in a 72-Year-oldman. Korean J Otolaryngol. 2007;50:268–71.
116. Kamal SM, Bradley ES. Angiofibroma arising from the uncinate. Otolaryngol Head Neck Surg. 2011;145(2Supp):252.
117. GordievskiiI D, Borisenko AI, ErryshevIu N. [Juvenile angiofibroma of the ethmoidal labyrinth in a young woman]. Zh Ushn Nos Gorl Bolezn. 1980;3:72–3.
118. Rao MS, Lakshmi CR, Sonylal PE, Chakravarthy VK, Murthy PS. Recurrent angiofibroma of ethmoid region-a rare variant. J Clin Diagn Res. 2014;8:KD01–2.
119. Malipatil SR. Extranasopharyngeal angiofibroma from nasal vestibule: a rare presentation. Int J Otorhinolaryngol Clin. 2013;5:169–72.
120. Maheshwarappa RP, Gupta A, Bansal J, Kattimani MV, Shabadi SS, Baser SC. An unusual location of Juvenile angiofibroma: a case report and review of the literature. Case Rep Ortsinotolaryngol. 2013;2013:175326.
121. Hersh SP, Grimes Jr CD, Harrison WG, Iwamoto T. Angiomyofibroma of the nasal cavity: a clinical and electron micrographic study. Otolaryngol Head Neck Surg. 1995;112:603–6.
122. Nasretdinov T, Moldavskii MI, Aganova KK. Angiofibroma of nasal cavity in a woman. Vestn Otorinolaringol. 1985;4:73–4.
123. Gudea F, Vega M, Canals E, Montserrat JM, Valdano J. Role of radiation therapy for 'juvenile' angiofibroma. J Laryngol Otol. 1990;104:725–6.
124. Obiako MN, Jacobs A. An isolated case of juvenile angiofibroma in the nasal cavity. Ear Nose Throat J. 1983;62:70–4.
125. Pastor Quirante FA, Perez Martinez F, Diaz Caparros F, Montalban Romero S, Perez GM. [Nasal angiofibroma in an adult]. An Otorrinolaringol Ibero Am. 1994;21:479–86.
126. Crespodel Hierro J, Gete Garcia P, Coello Casariego G, Rivas E, Monge Jodra R, Alvarez-Vicent JJ. [Extra-naso-pharyngeal angiofibroma: report of a new case and review of literature]. Acta Otorrinolaringol Esp. 2002;53:297–301.
127. Mehta AK, Bindra MS, Ravikumar R. Nasal angiofibroma: an unusual presentation. MJAFI. 2001;57:59–60.
128. Durko M, Murlewska A, Gryczynski M, Ratynska M, Pietruszewska W. Angiofibroma of the nasal cavity and anterior ethmoid cells--problems in differential diagnosis. Otolaryngol Pol. 2007;61:736–9.
129. Bakhshi M, Basir Shabestari S, Eshghyar N. Nasopharyngeal angiofibroma in the oral cavity in a 50-year-old man: a case report. Shiraz Univ Dent J. 2011;12:90–4.

130. Reddy BK, Isaac V, Nayak MN, Prabhu SR. Juvenile oral angiofibroma in a female. J Oral Surg. 1979;37:338–41.
131. Chung YS, Kim JK, Kweon HW, Lee WS, Lee HH. Angiofibroma: an unusual presentation in soft palate. Korean J Otolaryngol. 1995;38:779–85.
132. Thakur RK, Madan E, Tomar A, Arora M. Angiofibroma on cheek mucosa: a rare entity and its management with laser. J Cutan Aesthet Surg. 2014;7:227–8.
133. Andreadis DA, Rizos CB, Belazi M, Peneva M, Antoniades DZ. Encephalocraniocutaneous lipomatosis accompanied by maxillary compound odontoma and juvenile angiofibroma: report of a case. Birth Defects Res A Clin Mol Teratol. 2004;70:889–91.
134. Supiyaphun P, Sastarasadhit V, Chochaipanichnon L, Tonsakulrungruang K. Intraoral angiofibroma: a case report. J Med Assoc Thai. 1986;69:382–5.
135. Stewart DJ, O'Brien FV. Juvenile angiofibroma. Report of a case occurring within the mouth. J Dent. 1973;1:150–2.
136. Antoniades K, Antoniades DZ, Antoniades V. Juvenile angiofibroma: report of a case with intraoral presentation. Oral Surg Oral Med Oral Pathol Oral Radiol Endod. 2002;94:228–32.
137. Capodiferro S, Faviaa G, Lacaitaa MG, LoMuziob L, Maioranoc E. Juvenile angiofibroma: report of a case with primary intra-oral presentation. Oral Oncol Extra. 2005;41:1–6.
138. Rho YS, Park IS, Kim JH, Kim SD. A case of angiofibroma arising in parapharyngeal space. Korean J Otolaryngol. 2002;45:1105–9.
139. Cejas Mendez L, Espejo Castro E, Artazkozdel Toro JJ, Gil Curbelo JA, Saavedradela Torre JA, de Miguel Hernandez B. Tonsil larangiofibroma. An Otorrinolaringol Ibero Am. 2000;27:605–11.
140. Mendoza-Ramíreza S, Martínez-Hernándeze J, Vicuna-Honoratob I, Mendoza-Ramírezd M, Murguía-Péreza M. Angiofibroma atípicodela amígdalapalatina. Rev Esp Patol. 2012;45:125–7.
141. Kim JK. A case of angiofibroma in the oropharynx. Korean J Otolaryngol. 1972;15:69–72.
142. Eftekharian A, Samiei F, Rakhshan M. Angiofibroma with oropharyngeal origin. Pak J Med Sci. 2008;24:319–20.
143. Renukananda GS, Basavaraja PK, Naik AS, Maheshwari M, Balaji NK, Thangavelu G. Atypical angiofibroma of larynx-a case report. Indian J Otolaryngol Head Neck Surg 2008;60:51–2.
144. Canciullo R. On angiomas of the larynx. Etiopathogenetic considerations on a case fibroangioma of the larynx. Arch Ital Otol Rinol Laringol Patol Cervicofacc. 1969;80:562–76.
145. Trinidad CAJ, David MJCD, Chua AH. Extranasopharyngeal angiofibroma of the larynx. Philipp J Otolaryngol Head Neck Surg. 2010;25:23–5.
146. Morita T. [A laryngeal angiofibroma]. Jibiinkoka. 1965;37:875–8.
147. Meva'a Bioué1é RC, Djomou F, Sando Z, Andjock Nkouo YC, Ndjolo A, Bengono G. Angiofibrome laryngé: À Proposd'unCasàYaoundé. Health Sci Dis. 2014;15:1–2.
148. Grishchenkov VK, Lopatin AS. Giant laryngopharyngeal angiofibroma and an organ-sparing method for its removal. Vestn Otorinolaringol. 1985;6:87–8.
149. Reddy JB, Farb S. Angiofibroma of the sphenoid sinus. A case report. Laryngoscope. 1963;73:108–19.
150. Yamagiwa M, Sakakura Y, Majima Y, Yoshii S. Angiofibroma of sphenoid sinus. A case report. Practica Otologica Kyoto. 1974;67:1103–7.
151. Tsunoda A, Kohda H, Ishikawa N, Komatsuzaki A. Juvenile angiofibroma limited to the sphenoid sinus. J Otolaryngol. 1998;27:37–9.
152. San T, Tekin M, Cam OH, Kilicaslan A, Zemheri E. Extranasopharyngeal angiofibroma originating from sphenoid sinus: a case report. J Med Updat. 2012;2:120–3.
153. Keskin IG, Ila K. Juvenile angiofibroma originating from the sphenoid sinus: a case report. Kulak Burun Bogaz Ihtis Derg. 2013;23:235–8.
154. Karthikeya P, Mahima VG, Bagewadi SB. Juvenile nasopharyngeal angiofibroma. Indian J Dent Res 2005;16:22–6.
155. Whitlock RI. Angiofibroma of cheek. Br J Dent. 1961;111:372–4.

156. Dere H, Ozcan KM, Ergul G, Bahar S, Ozcan I, Kulacoglu S. Extranasopharyngeal angiofibroma of the cheek. J Laryngol Otol. 2006;120:141–4.
157. Singh V, Ramesh V, Rohilla K, Sriram K. Angiofibroma masquerading as a cheek swelling-a diagnostic dilemma. JIMSA. 2013;26:111–2.
158. Hora JF, Weller WA. Extranasopharyngeal juvenile angiofibroma. Ann Otol Rhinol Laryngol. 1961;70:164–70.
159. Irby WB. Angiofibroma of cheek and infratemporal fossa. J Oral Surg. 1961;19:296–301.
160. Szymanska A, Szymanski M, Skomra D, Szczerbo-Trojanowska M. Extranasopharyngeal angiofibroma of the infratemporal fossa. Otolaryngol Head Neck Surg. 2009;140:433–4.
161. Isherwood I, Dogra TS, Farrington WT. Extranasopharyngeal juvenile angiofibroma. J Laryngol Otol. 1975;89:535–44.
162. Motlagh MF, Hasaniafshar A, Milani M. Extranasopharyngeal angiofibroma with lateral extension to the Buccal Region. Asian J Oral Maxillofac Surg. 2007;19:105–6.
163. Gupta M, Motwani G, Gupta P. Extranasopharyngeal angiofibroma arising from the infratemporal region. Indian J Otolaryngol Head Neck Surg 2006;58:312–5.
164. Johnson JE, Yang PJ, Koopmann Jr CF, Heffner DK. Parapharyngeal angiofibroma. AJNR Am J Neuroradiol. 1987;8:1152–3.
165. Lee BH. Parapharyngeal angiofibroma: a case report. Iran J Radiol 2015;12, e17353.
166. Ulubil SA, Ucar S, Iseri M, Ustundag E, Sari F. Retropharyngeal angiofibroma. J Otolaryngol Head Neck Surg. 2012;41:E31–4.
167. DeBlanc Jr HJ, Chretien P. Angiofibroma clinically indistinguishable from carotid body tumor. A possible embryologic relationship. Am J Surg. 1970;119:743–5.
168. Hsieh ST, Guo YC, Tsai TL, Chen WY, Huang JL. Angiofibroma of the hypopharynx. J Chin Med Assoc. 2004;67:373–5.
169. Steele MH, Nuss DW, Faust BF. Angiofibroma of the larynx: report of a case with clinical and pathologic literature review. Head Neck. 2002;24:805–9.
170. Lim DJ, Kang SH, Jung MS, Kim HG. A case of angiofibroma arising from the middle turbinate of an adult woman. Korean J Otolaryngol. 2005;46:543–6.
171. Peric A, Baletic N, Cerovic S, Vukomanovic-Durdevic B. Middle turbinate angiofibroma in an elderly woman. Vojnosanit Pregl. 2009;66:583–6.
172. Mincione G. On the subject of rare conjunctival pathology. Arch De Vecchi Anat Patol. 1964;44:1023–48.
173. Baldanzini M. Angiofibroma of the conjunctiva. Ann Ottalmol Clin Ocul. 1967;93:953–8.
174. Marill FG, Boutovsky S. Angiofibroma in a cluster on the external ear. Bull Soc Fr Dermatol Syphiligr. 1968;75:566.
175. Borisov BF. Angiofibroma of the esophagus. Klin Khir. 1968;1.
176. El-Barbary AS. Fibroangioma of the facial nerve. J Laryngol Otol. 1966;180:1265–7.
177. Voisin C, Wattel F, Cosselin B, Caron JC, Tonnel A. Tracheal haemangiofibroma. Lille Med. 1968;13:215–6.
178. Schick B, Kind M, Draf W, Weber R, Lackmann GM. Extranasopharyngeal angiofibroma in a 15- month-old child. Int J Pediatr Otorhinolaryngol. 1997;42:135–40.
179. Iyer GV, Vaishya ND, Bhaktaviziam A, Taori GM, Abraham J. Angiofibroma of the middle cranial fossa. Case report. J Neurosurg. 1971;35:90–4.
180. Bhutia TY, Singh P, Kumar R. A rare case report a typical angiofibroma-dorsum of nose. J Dent Med Sci. 2015;14(5Ver.VI):93–4.
181. Hallur NH, Zainab H, Shah A, Siddiqua A. Parotid angiofibroma. J Oral Maxillo Facial Pathol. 2014;18:295–8.
182. Mohamed AA. Angiofibroma of the nasal fossae: apropos of 12 cases observed in Mali. Med Trop(Mars). 1994;54:247–8.
183. Nicolai P, Schreiber A, BolzoniVillaret A. Juvenile angiofibroma: evolution of management. Int J Pediatr. 2012;2012:412545.
184. Jacobsson M, Petruson B, Ruth M, Svendsen P. Involution of juvenile nasopharyngeal angiofibroma with intracranial extension. A case report with computed tomographic assessment. Arch Otolaryngol Head Neck Surg. 1989;115:238–9.

185. Bathia ML. Intracranial extension of juvenile angiofibroma of the nasopharynx. J Laryngol Otol. 1967;81:1395–403.
186. Perić A, Baletić N, Cerović S, Vukomanović-Đurđević B. Middle turbinate angiofibroma in an elderly woman. Vojnosanit Pregl. 2009;66:583–6.
187. Peric A, Sotirovic J, Cerovic S, Zivic L. Immunohistochemistry in diagnosis of extranasopharyngeal angiofibroma originating from nasal cavity: case presentation and review of the literature. Acta Med. 2013;56:133–41.
188. Alves FRA, Granato L, Maia MS, Lambert E. Surgical approaches to juvenile nasopharyngeal angiofibroma-case report and literature review. Int Arch Otorhinolaryngol. 2006;10:162–6.
189. English GM, Hemenway WG, Cundy RL. Surgical treatment of invasive angiofibroma. Arch Otolaryngol. 1972;96:312–8.
190. Schick B, Kahle G. Radiological findings in angiofibroma. Acta Radiol. 2000;41:585–93.
191. Gleeson M. Juvenile Angiofibroma. In: Gleeson M, editor. Scott-brown´s otorhinolaryngology, head and neck surgery. 7th ed. London: Hodder Arnold; 2008. p. 2437–44.
192. Irby WB. Angiofibroma of cheek and infratemporal fossa. J Oral Surg Anesth Hosp Dent Serv. 1961;19:296–301.
193. Sessions RB, Bryan RN, Naclerio RM, Alford BR. Radiographic staging of juvenile angiofibroma. Head Neck Surg. 1981;3:279–83.
194. Fisch U. The infratemporal fossa approach for nasopharyngeal tumors. Laryngoscope. 1983;93:36–44.
195. Chandler JR, Goulding R, Moskowitz L, Quencer RM. Nasopharyngeal angiofibromas: staging and management. Ann Otol Rhinol Laryngol. 1984;93(4Pt1):322–9.
196. Radkowski D, McGill T, Healy GB, Ohlms L, Jones DT. Angiofibroma. Changes in staging and treatment. Arch Otolaryngol Head Neck Surg. 1996;122:122–9.
197. Onerci M, Ogretmenoglu O, Yucel T. Juvenile nasopharyngeal angiofibroma: a revised staging system. Rhinology. 2006;44:39–45.
198. Snyderman CH, Pant H, Carrau RL, Gardner P. A new endoscopic staging system for angiofibromas. Arch Otolaryngol Head Neck Surg. 2010;136:588–94.
199. Carrillo JF, Maldonado F, Albores O, Ramírez-Ortega MC, Oñate-Ocaña LF. Juvenile nasopharyngeal angiofibroma: clinical factors associated with recurrence, and proposal of a staging system. J Surg Oncol. 2008;98:75–80.
200. Alshaikh NA, Eleftheriadou A. Juvenile nasopharyngeal angiofibroma staging: an overview. Ear Nose Throat J. 2015;94:E12–22.
201. Hodges JM, McDevitt AS, El-SayedAli AI, Sebelik ME. Juvenile nasopharyngeal angiofibroma: current treatment modalities and future considerations. Indian J Otolaryngology Head Neck Surg 2010;62:236–47.
202. Khoueir N, Nicolas N, Rohayem Z, Haddad A, AbouHamad W. Exclusive endoscopic resection of juvenile nasopharyngeal angiofibroma: a systematic review of the literature. Otolaryngol Head Neck Surg. 2014;150:350–8.
203. Leong SC. A systematic review of surgical outcomes for advanced juvenile nasopharyngeal angiofibroma with intracranial involvement. Laryngoscope. 2013;123:1125–31.
204. Schick B, el Rahmanel TA, Brors D, Kahle G, Draf W. Experiences with endonasal surgery in angiofibroma. Rhinology. 1999;37:80–5.
205. Mitskavich MT, Carrau RL, Snyderman CH, Weissman JL, Fagan JJ. Intranasal endoscopic excision of a juvenile angiofibroma. Auris Nasus Larynx. 1998;25:39–44.
206. Lim IR, Pang YT, Soh K. Juvenile angiofibroma: case report and the role of endoscopic resection. Singapore Med J. 2002;43:208–10.
207. Ye D, Shen Z, Wang G, Deng H, Qiu S, Zhang Y. Analysis of factors in successful nasal endoscopic resection of nasopharyngeal angiofibroma. Acta Otolaryngol. 2016;136:205–13.
208. Garofalo P, Pia F, Policarpo M, Tunesi S, Valletti PA. Juvenile nasopharyngeal angiofibroma: comparison between endoscopic and open operative approaches. J Craniofac Surg. 2015;26:918–21.
209. Witt TR, Shah JP, Sternberg SS. Juvenile nasopharyngeal angiofibroma. A 30 year clinical review. Am J Surg. 1983;146:521–5.

210. Neel 3rd HB, Whicker JH, Devine KD, Weiland LH. Juvenile angiofibroma. Review of 120 cases. Am J Surg. 1973;126:547–56.
211. Reddy KA, Mendenhall WM, Amdur RJ, Stringer SP, Cassisi NJ. Long-term results of radiation therapy for juvenile nasopharyngeal angiofibroma. Am J Otolaryngol. 2001;22:172–5.
212. Makek MS, Andrews JC, Fisch U. Malignant transformation of a nasopharyngeal angiofibroma. Laryngoscope. 1989;99(10Pt1):1088–92.
213. Sinha PP, Aziz HI. Juvenile nasopharyngeal angiofibroma. A report of seven cases. Radiology. 1978;127:501–3.
214. De Blanc HJ, Chretien P. Angiofibroma clinically indistinguishable from carotid body tumor. Am J Surg. 1970;119:743–5.
215. Fitzpatrick PJ, Briant TD, Berman JM. The nasopharyngeal angiofibroma. Arch Otolaryngol. 1980;106:234–6.
216. Spector JG. Management of juvenile angiofibromata. Laryngoscope. 1988;98:1016–26.
217. Hazarika P, Nayak DR, Balakrishnan R, Raj G, Pillai S. Endoscopic and KTP laser-assisted surgery for juvenile nasopharyngeal angiofibroma. Am J Otolaryngol. 2002;23:282–6.
218. Voets AG, Knegt P, de Jong PC, van Andel JC, Vander Schans EJ. Juvenile angiofibroma of the nasopharynx; an overview of 20 years of management. Ned Tijdschr Geneeskd. 1988;132:296–300.
219. Chen HJ, Leung SW, Su CY. Linear accelerator based radiosurgery as a salvage treatment for skull base and intracranial invasion of recurrent nasopharyngeal carcinomas. Am J Clin Oncol. 2001;24:255–8.
220. Wei WI, Lam KH, Sham JS. New approach to the nasopharynx: the maxillary swing approach. Head Neck. 1991;13:200–7.
221. Tate DJ, Adler Jr JR, Chang SD, Marquez S, Eulau SM, Fee WE, et al. Stereotactic radiosurgical boost following radiotherapy in primary nasopharyngeal carcinoma: impact on local control. Int J Radiat Oncol Biol Phys. 1999;45:915–21.
222. Chen MK, Tsai YL, Lee KW, Chang CC. Strictly endoscopic and harmonic scalpel-assisted surgery of nasopharyngeal angiofibromas: eligible for advanced stage tumors. Acta Otolaryngol. 2006;126:1321–5.
223. Ruiz JW, Saint-Victor S, Tessema B, Eloy JA, Anstead A. Coblation assisted endoscopic juvenile nasopharyngeal angiofibroma resection. Int J Pediatr Otorhinolaryngol. 2012;76:439–42.
224. Ye L, Zhou X, Li J, Jin J. Coblation-assisted endonasal endoscopic resection of juvenile nasopharyngeal angiofibroma. J Laryngol Otol. 2011;125:940–4.
225. Pierson B, Powitzky R, Digoy GP. Endoscopic coblation for the treatment of advanced juvenile nasopharynge alangiofibroma. Ear Nose Throat J. 2012;91:432,434,436,438.
226. Cannon DE, Poetker DM, Loehrl TA, Chun RH. Use of coblation in resection of juvenile nasopharyngeal angiofibroma. Ann Otol Rhinol Laryngol. 2013;122:353–7.
227. Min HJ, Chung HJ, Kim CH. Delayed cerebro spinal fluid rhinorrhea four years after gamma knife surgery for juvenile angiofibroma. J Craniofac Surg. 2014;25:e565–7.
228. Park CK, Kim DG, Paek SH, Chung HT, Jung HW. Recurrent juvenile nasopharyngeal angiofibroma treated with gamma knife surgery. J Korean Med Sci. 2006;21:773–7.
229. Dare AO, Gibbons KJ, Proulx GM, Fenstermaker RA. Resection followed by radiosurgery for advanced juvenile nasopharyngeal angiofibroma: report of two cases. Neurosurgery. 2003;52:1207–11; discussion 11.
230. El Morsy SM, Khafagy YW. Transnasal endoscopic management of angiofibroma extending to pterygopalatine and infra temporal fossae. J Laryngol Otol. 2011;125:701–5.
231. Hagen R, Romalo G, Schwab B, Hoppe F, Schweikert HU. Juvenile nasopharyngeal fibroma: androgen receptors and their significance for tumor growth. Laryngoscope. 1994;104:1125–9.
232. Gates GA, Rice DH, Koopmann Jr CF, Schuller DE. Flutamide-induced regression of angiofibroma. Laryngoscope. 1992;102:641–4.
233. Kuttner K, Katenkamp D, Stiller D. Hormone therapy of the juvenile angiofibroma (author'stransl). Arch Otorhinolaryngol. 1977;214:331–8.
234. Quade R, Kuttner K. Nasopharyngeal angiofibroma. Histochemical observations and hormone therapy (author'stransl). Acta Histochem. 1977;59:201–9.

235. Correa A, LorenziI A. Radiotherapy & hormone therapy in juvenile nasopharyngeal angiofibroma. Med Cir Farm. 1957;19:389–96.
236. Labra A, Chavolla-Magana R, Lopez-Ugalde A, Alanis-Calderon J, Huerta-Delgado A. Flutamide as a preoperative treatment in juvenile angiofibroma (JA) with intracranial invasion: report of 7 cases. Otolaryngol Head Neck Surg. 2004;130:466–9.
237. Chen WL, Huang ZQ, Li JS, Chai Q, Zhang DM. Percutaneous sclerotherapy of juvenile nasopharyngeal angiofibroma using fibrin glue combined with OK-432 and bleomycin. Int J Pediatr Otorhinolaryngol. 2010;74:422–5.
238. Dohar JE, Duvall 3rd AJ. Spontaneous regression of juvenile nasopharyngeal angiofibroma. Ann Otol Rhinol Laryngol. 1992;101:469–71.
239. Weprin LS, Siemers PT. Spontaneous regression of juvenile nasopharyngeal angiofibroma. Arch Otolaryngol Head Neck Surg. 1991;117:796–9.
240. Spielmann PM, Adamson R, Cheng K, Sanderson RJ. Juvenile nasopharyngeal angiofibroma: spontaneous resolution. Ear Nose Throat J. 2008;87:521–3.
241. Tosun F, Onerci M, Durmaz A, Ugurel S. Spontaneous involution of nasopharyngeal angiofibroma. J Craniofac Surg. 2008;19:1686–9.
242. Herman P, Lot G, Chapot R, Salvan D, Huy PT. Long-term follow-up of juvenile nasopharyngeal angiofibromas: analysis of recurrences. Laryngoscope. 1999;109:140–7.
243. Goepfert H, Cangir A, Lee YY. Chemotherapy for aggressive juvenile nasopharyngeal angiofibroma. Arch Otolaryngol. 1985;111:285–9.
244. Goepfert H, Cangir A, Ayala AG, Eftekhari F. Chemotherapy of locally aggressive head and neck tumors in the pediatric age group. Desmoid fibromatosis and nasopharyngeal angiofibroma. Am J Surg. 1982;144:437–44.
245. Schick B, Kahle G, Hassler R, Draf W. Chemotherapy of juvenile angiofibroma--an alternative? HNO. 1996;44:148–52.
246. Chagnaud C, Petit P, Bartoli J, Champsaur P, Gaubert J, Dessi P, et al. Postoperative follow-up of juvenile nasopharyngeal angiofibromas: assessment by CT scan and MR imaging. Eur Radiol. 1998;8:756–64.
247. Schick B, Plinkert PK, Prescher A. Aetiology of angiofibromas: reflection on their specific vascular component. Laryngorhinootologie. 2002;81:280–4.
248. Schick B, Brunner C, Praetorius M, Plinkert PK, Urbschat S. First evidence of genetic imbalances in angiofibromas. Laryngoscope. 2002;112:397–401.
249. Farag MM, Ghanimah SE, Ragaie A, Saleem TH. Hormonal receptors in juvenile nasopharyngeal angiofibroma. Laryngoscope. 1987;97:208–11.
250. Martin HM, Ehrlich HE, Abel JC. Juvenile nasopharyngeal angiofibroma. Ann Surg. 1948;127:513–36.
251. Steinberg SS. Pathology of the juvenile nasopharnygeal angiofibroma: a lesion of adolescent males. Cancer. 1954;7:15–28.
252. Beham A, Beham-Schmid C, Regauer S, Aubock L, Stammberger H. Nasopharyngeal angiofibroma: true neoplasm or vascular malformation? Adv Anat Pathol. 2000;7:36–46.
253. Maurice M, Milad M. Pathogenesis of juvenile nasopharyngeal fibroma. (Anewconcept). J Laryngol Otol. 1981;95:1121–6.
254. Härmä RA. Nasopharyngeal angiofibroma. A clinical and histopathological study. Acta Otolaryngol. 1958;146(Suppl):1–74.
255. Waldman SR, Levine HL, Astor F, Wood BG, Weinstein M, Tucker HM. Surgical experience with nasopharyngeal angiofibroma. Arch Otolaryngol. 1981;107:677–82.

Chapter 22
Remaining Controversies

Siba P. Dubey

Abstract Juvenile angiofibroma (JA), rarely, can undergo involution and malignant transformation. Occasionally, the tumor may be encountered in female. Literature showed seven cases of involution of angiofibroma. It was postulated that when the patient reaches the age of 20–25 years, the tumor undergo resorption and disintegration. Among these seven patients, three underwent surgical excision (one with bilateral external carotid artery ligation with multivessel embolization and another with ipsilateral external carotid artery ligation), two refused any treatment, and one each underwent biopsy and maxillary artery embolization. Spontaneous resolution took place in two patients who opted for no treatment; regression of the tumor started after 3 years in one patient, and complete involution took place over a 12-year period in another.

Literature showed six cases of malignant transformation in juvenile angiofibroma. In three patients, JA was diagnosed at the fifth decade and in the rest in the second decade. Five out of six patients had multiple operations. The minimum time interval between operation and malignant transformation was 1 year. Five out of six patients received external irradiation, the dose of which was between 3,000 and 12,000 cGy. Two patients also received exogenous hormone therapy. The time interval between irradiation to malignancy was 11 months to 21 years. One patient developed malignant fibrous histiocytoma and the rest of them had fibrosarcoma.

Angiofibroma in female was found in the age between second and eighth decade. The tumor in this group of patients is usually localized in the nasal cavity with extension into the nasopharynx, maxillary antrum, ethmoid sinus, and oropharynx. In one patient the condition was diagnosed during pregnancy; the tumor was removed after delivery. Intranasal, Caldwell-Luc, lateral rhinotomy, midfacial degloving, and craniofacial resection were the various approaches by which these tumors were dealt with surgically. Two patients also received irradiation.

Keywords Angiofibroma • Juvenile • Involution • Malignant transformation • Female

---

S.P. Dubey, MS
Department of Otolaryngology-Head and Neck Surgery, Port Moresby General Hospital, Boroko, NCD, Papua New Guinea
e-mail: dr_sp_dubey@yahoo.com

S.P. Dubey, B. Schick (eds.), *Juvenile Angiofibroma*,
DOI 10.1007/978-3-319-45343-9_22

Introduction

One of the highly controversial aspects in juvenile angiofibroma (JA) has been the possibility of spontaneous regression of JA [1]. But the radiologic proof was lacking until the advent of CT scan. Another rare event is malignant transformation of JA with or without irradiation. JA occurring in females, though neglected for long time, has also been observed. These three findings are described in the following sections of this chapter.

Involution of Juvenile Angiofibroma

At the beginning, it was the idea of spontaneous regression of JA that has been stated without the opinion to prove it. Ringertz [2] postulated that spontaneous regression of JA usually occurs, when the patient reaches the age of 20–25 years, by both resorption and disintegration with the breaking off of the peripheral processes of the tumor. Martin et al. [3] felt that it is probable that some cases of JA of moderate size occur and regress spontaneously. Dane [4] reported a JA in the process of regression. The spontaneous regression in this case, however, was noted with only on the basis of the patient's history. In the next step, first documentation of the fate of residual tumor was given in the literature that pointed on possible tumor regression. Stansbie and Phelps [5] documented involution of residual JA by means of serial CT scans over a period of 3 years. However, there was no histologic confirmation of the residual tumor in their case. Jacobsson et al. [6] mentioned the regression of JA which recurred following surgical resection. The recurrent tumor in this patient, showing a middle cranial fossa extension, was treated with embolization of all branches of the external carotid artery. The patient was followed up with serial CT scan over the next 6 years. For a period of 2 years following embolization, there was no change in the size of the tumor. The extracranial part of the tumor started regressing in the third year after embolization. One and a half years later, the intracranial part started regressing in this patient. Jacobsson et al. [6] felt that the embolization undertaken evidently had no effect on the tumor growth and should be regarded as an adjunct to operative procedure or to be used to reduce the risk of major hemorrhage in inoperable cases. Weprin and Siemens [7] described in detail the spontaneous tumor regression in an 11-year-old boy and followed it up over a 12-year period during which the process was complete. The boy had presented with nasal obstruction and frequent epistaxis and the diagnosis of JA had been proven on biopsy. The patient's parents refused both surgical intervention and hormonal therapy.

Dohar and Duvall [8] reported a case of JA who after surgical excisions developed recurrences. Subsequently, he was lost in follow up; but returned after 22 years with an unrelated otolaryngologic condition. A CT scan at that time showed complete resolution of the tumor.

Spielmann et al. [9] described a 17-year-old male who presented with recurrent nasal obstruction and epistaxis. The CT and MRI showed an enhancing lesion in the nasopharynx, pterygopalatine, and infratemporal fossae. The patient refused resection and/or radiotherapy. After 2 years, the mass gradually decreased in size and was confined mainly in the nasopharynx with limited extension in the infratemporal fossa. Tosun et al. [10] published a case in which a 25-year-old patient whose tumor underwent almost complete involution within 5 years. This tumor occupied the nasal cavity, pterygopalatine and infratemporal fossae, and sphenoid sinus and extended into the cavernous sinus. The said patient repeatedly refused surgery and irradiation; only maxillary artery was embolized. The data of the above patients are summarized in Table 22.1.

It has been claimed early that JA may regress spontaneously. Especially the hormonal changes have been in the focus to speculate on tumor regression after adolescence. One should be aware that spontaneous tumor regression is a rare event and no indicators are up to now available to define tumors that might decrease in size or diminish without therapy. Nevertheless, the so far available knowledge justifies to follow up the residual tumor to define the tumor growth and stabilize the disease or tumor regression before further treatment is planned.

Malignant Transformation of JA

Review of literature showed six cases of malignant transformation of a JA [11–16]. Three patients were at the fifth decade at the time of diagnosis of JA [12–14]. The other three patients were in the second decade at the time of diagnosis of JA [11, 15, 16]. It is not very clear and very difficult to understand why the malignant transformation were detected in third decade of life or beyond in all patients. The minimum interval between the diagnosis of JA and its malignant form was 1 year [13]. Five out of seven patients had multiple operations. One patient had a single procedure [13]. The dosage of irradiation varied between 3,000 cGy to as high as 12,000 cGy; no irradiation was given to one patient [13]. Two patients received exogenous hormone therapy [12, 15]. The time interval between irradiation to the diagnosis of malignancy ranged from 11 months to 21 years. One patient had malignant fibrous histiocytoma [15]; the rest developed fibrosarcomas [11–14, 16]. The findings of these patients are mentioned in Table 22.2.

Angiofibroma in Female

The clinical, radiological, and operative findings of ten cases of angiofibroma in females are summarized in Table 22.3 [17–26]. The angiofibroma in these females was localized in the nasal cavity with occasional extension into the nasopharynx, maxillary and ethmoid sinuses, and oropharynx; in one patient it was attached at the inferior turbinate. One patient presented during pregnancy and was operated upon after delivery [21]. These tumors were removed by peroral and intranasal, Caldwell-Luc with lateral rhinotomy, midfacial degloving, and lateral rhinotomy with craniofacial approaches. Two patients also received irradiation [17, 19].

Table 22.1 Involution of JA

Author (s)	Age (year) at diagnosis	Therapy (surgery, irradiation, and hormone)	Recurrence	Interval between diagnosis and onset of regression
Dane [4]	12	Biopsy	Nil	19 years
Stansbie and Phelps [5]	13	Excision by lateral rhinotomy	Recurrence	Follow-up CT scan showed progressive reduction in size over 3 years
Jacobsson et al. [6]	15	Excision of extracranial part by (i) Denker's approach (ii) Lateral rhinotomy (iii) Ligation of both external carotid arteries (iv) Multivessel embolization	Recurrence after first surgery	Regression of extracranial part after 5 years and intracranial part regressed by 8 years
Weprin and Siemens [7]	11	Patient's parents refused any therapy	Nil	Tumor bulk started regressing after 2 years; CT scan showed complete involution of both extra- and intracranial part over a 12-year period
Dohar and Duvall [8]	13	Resection by (i) Transpalatal approach (ii) Transnasal approach (iii) Intraoral tripartite approach and ligation of external carotid artery	Recurrences after first and second surgery and then lost in follow-up for 16 years	CT scan confirmed complete tumor resolution over 22 years
Spielmann et al. [9]	17	Opted for no treatment	Nil	Gradual reduction in size after 3 years
Tosun et al. [10]	21	Refused surgery or irradiation; maxillary artery embolized	Nil	Near total involution within 5 years

Table 22.2 Malignant transformation of JA

Author (s)	Age (in years) of diagnosis of JA	Therapy (surgery, irradiation, hormone)	Age (in years) of diagnosis of malignancy	Type of malignancy
Gisslesson et al. [11]	12	First excision by Denker's approach and another five excisions subsequently; 12,000 cGy irradiation	33	Fibrosarcoma
Batsakis et al. [12]	48	Surgery, 9,000 cGy irradiation, and androgen	54	Fibrosarcoma
Donald [13]	47	Removal of JA by transpalatal approach. Repeat transpalatal and external ethmoidectomy approach to remove the recurrence	48	Low-grade fibrosarcoma
Chen and Bauer [14]	48	Lateral rhinotomy for partial excision. 3,000 cGy irradiation. Re-exploration and removal and repeat lateral rhinotomy and partial maxillectomy. Excision of recurrence	66	Fibrosarcoma
Spagnolo et al. [15]	19	Surgery, 9,400–10,400 cGy irradiation, androgen, and estrogen	23	Malignant fibrous histiocytoma
Makek et al. [16]	15	Two times transpalatal approach; 4,500 cGy irradiation; excision by transethmoidal-transsphenoidal approach; 4,050 cGy irradiation; debulking performed	39	Fibrosarcoma

Table 22.3 Angiofibroma in female

Author (s)	Age (in years) at diagnosis of JA	Clinical, radiological, and operative features
Finerman [17]	13	Mass in nasal cavity and nasopharynx and hanging into oropharynx; patient treated with low-dose irradiation
Osborn and Sokolovski [18]	15	Nasal and nasopharyngeal mass; peroral and intranasal removal
Rominger and Santore [19]	60	Repeated epistaxis from choanal and nasopharyngeal mass; mass removed by Caldwell-Luc and lateral rhinotomy approach; irradiation was also given
Ewing and Shirley [20]	71	Fungating firm and rubbery nasal mass; nasal and maxillary antral mass; removed by combined Caldwell-Luc and lateral rhinotomy procedure
Peloquin et al. [21]	31	Nasal mass in pregnant patient; following delivery, MRI done and the mass removed by degloving approach; tumor pedicle attached near the sphenopalatine foramen
Garcia et al. [22]	60	CT and MRI showed enhancing mass attached to the ipsilateral inferior turbinate; turbinectomy done after clamping the external carotid artery
Madhavan et al. [23]	45	Tender, firm and 4×3 cm swelling of hemiface; CT scan showed tumor occupying maxillary antrum, nasal cavity, and inferolateral aspect of the orbit; biopsy confirmed the diagnosis of nasopharyngeal angiofibroma
Patrocinio et al. [24]	64	Mass in nasal cavity, nasopharynx, and ipsilateral maxillary and ethmoid sinus; removed by midfacial degloving
Szymanska et al. [25]	57	CT and MRI showed enhancing mass in nasal cavity and nasopharynx; preoperative embolization done and the tumor removed by sublabial degloving approach; its pedicle attached near sphenopalatine foramen
Rao et al. [26]	27	Bilateral proptosis and telecanthus; MRI showed enhancing bilateral nasal mass; previous operation by lateral rhinotomy; craniofacial resection done and mass separated from the anterior cranial fossa dura

References

1. Chandler JR, Goulding R, Moskowitz L, Quencer RM. Nasopharyngeal angiofibromas: staging and management. Ann Otol Rhinol Laryngol. 1984;93:322–9.
2. Ringertz N. Pathology of malignant tumors arising in the nasal and paranasal cavities and maxilla. Acta Otolaryngol (Stockh). 1938;27:158–61.
3. Martin H, Ehrlich HE, Abels JC. Juvenile nasopharyngeal angiofibroma. Ann Surg. 1948;127:513–36.
4. Dane WH. Juvenile angiofibroma in state of regression. Ann Otol Rhinol Laryngol. 1954;63:997–1014.
5. Stansbie JM, Phelps PD. Involution of residual juvenile nasopharyngeal angiofibroma: a case report. J Laryngol Otol. 1986;100:599–603.

6. Jacobsson M, Petruson B, Ruth B, Svendsen P. Involution of juvenile nasopharyngeal angiofibroma with intracranial extension. Arch Otolaryngol Head Neck Surg. 1989;115:238–9.
7. Weprin LS, Siemens PT. Spontaneous regression of juvenile nasopharyngeal angiofibroma. Arch Otolaryngol Head Neck Surg. 1991;117:796–9.
8. Dohar JE, Duvall III AJ. Spontaneous regression of juvenile nasopharyngeal angiofibroma. Ann Otol Rhinol Laryngol. 1992;101:469–71.
9. Spielmann PM, Adamson R, Cheng K, Sanderson RJ. Juvenile nasopharyngeal angiofibroma: spontaneous resolution. Ear Nose Throat J. 2008;87:521–3.
10. Tosun F, Onerci M, Dumaz A, Ugurel S. Spontaneous involution of nasopharyngeal angiofibroma. J Craniofac Surg. 2008;19:1686–9.
11. Gisslesson L, Lindgren M, Stenram U. Sarcomatous transformation of a juvenile nasopharyngeal angiofibroma. Acta Pathol Microbiol Scand. 1958;42:305–12.
12. Batsakis JG, Klopp CT, Newman W. Fibrosarcoma arising in a "juvenile" nasopharyngeal angiofibroma following extensive radiation therapy. Am Surg. 1976;21:786–93.
13. Donald PJ. Sarcomatous degeneration in a nasopharyngeal angiofibroma. Otolaryngol Head Neck Surg. 1979;87:42–6.
14. Chen KT, Bauer FW. Sarcomatous transformation of nasopharyngeal angiofibroma. Cancer. 1982;49:369–71.
15. Spagnolo DV, Papadimitriou JM, Archer M. Postradiation malignant fibrous histiocytoma arising in juvenile nasopharyngeal angiofibroma and producing alpha-1-antitrypsin. Histopathology. 1984;8:339–52.
16. Makek MS, Andrew JC, Fisch U. Malignant transformation of a nasopharyngeal angiofibroma. Laryngoscope. 1989;99:1088–92.
17. Finerman WB. Juvenile nasopharyngeal angiofibroma in the female. Arch Otolaryngol. 1951;54:620–3.
18. Osborn DA, Sokolovski A. Juvenile nasopharyngeal angiofibroma in a female. Arch Otolaryngol. 1965;82:629–32.
19. Rominger CJ, Santore FJ. Juvenile nasopharyngeal angiofibroma in female adult. Arch Otolaryngol. 1968;88:85–7.
20. Ewing JA, Shively EH. Angiofibroma: a rare case in an elderly female. Otolaryngol Head Neck Surg. 1981;89:602–3.
21. Peloquin L, Klossek J-M, Barsa-Brusa F, Gougeon J-M, Toffel PH, Fontanel J-P. A rare case of nasopharyngeal angiofibroma in a pregnant woman. Otolaryngol Head Neck Surg. 1997;117:S111–4.
22. Garcia MM, Rivero VP, Romero GP, Ruiz GT, Pinto JMP, Huelva AB. Nasal angiofibroma in a 60 year old female. A clinical case and literature review. Acta Otorrinolaringol Esp. 2004;55:195–7.
23. Madhavan NR, Veeravarmal V, Santha Devy A, Ramachandran CR. Unusual presentation of nasopharyngeal (juvenile) angiofibroma in a 45 year old female. Indian J Dent Res. 2004;15:145–8.
24. Patrocinio JA, Patrocinio LG, Borba BHC, Bonatti BDS, Guimaraes AHB. Nasopharyngeal angiofibroma in an elderly woman. Am J Otolaryngol Head Neck Med Surg. 2005;26:198–200.
25. Szymanska A, Korobowicz E, Golabek W. A rare case of nasopharyngeal angiofibroma in an elderly female. Eur Arch Otorhinolaryngol. 2006;263:657–60.
26. Rao MS, Laksmi CR, Sonylal PK, Chakravarthy VK, Murthy PSN. Recurrent angiofibroma of ethmoid region – a rare variant. J Clin Diagn Res. 2014;8:1–2.

Index

S.P. Dubey, B. Schick (eds.), *Juvenile Angiofibroma*,
DOI 10.1007/978-3-319-45343-9

J

K

L

M

N

MIX
Papier aus verantwortungsvollen Quellen
Paper from responsible sources
FSC® C105338

If you have any concerns about our products,
you can contact us on
ProductSafety@springernature.com

In case Publisher is established outside the EU,
the EU authorized representative is:
Springer Nature Customer Service Center GmbH
Europaplatz 3, 69115 Heidelberg, Germany

Printed by Libri Plureos GmbH
in Hamburg, Germany